A Century of Service

AND BEYOND

A History of One Hundred Years of Leadership for Independent Pharmacy

BY C. FRED WILLIAMS, PH.D.
Professor of History
University of Arkansas at Little Rock

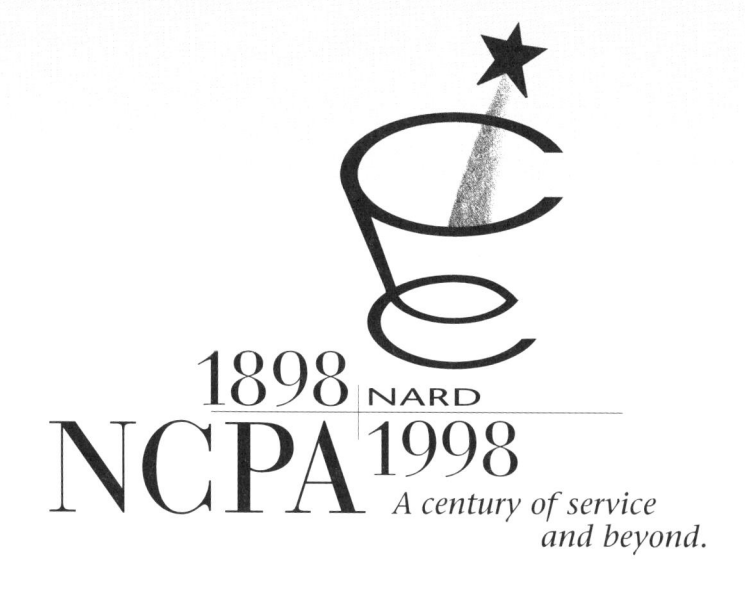

1898 | NARD
NCPA 1998
A century of service and beyond.

NARD/NCPA: A Century of Service and Beyond
ISBN 0-9668067-0-0

Copyright © 1998 National Community Pharmacists Association. ALL RIGHTS RESERVED. Printed in the U.S.A. No part of this publication may be reproduced, stored in a retrieval system, or transmitted in any form or by any means, electronic, mechanical, photocopying, recording or otherwise without the prior written permission of the publisher and the authors.

For information on purchase of this book at a cost of $25.00, which includes shipping, please contact NCPA at 1-800-544-7447 or write to NCPA, 205 Daingerfield Road, Alexandria, Virginia 22314.

TABLE OF CONTENTS

ACKNOWLEDGMENTS v

PREFACE vii

CHAPTER ONE — NARD MEETS ITS DESTINY IN ST. LOUIS: 1898
A Beginning Built on a Bedrock of Principles, Beliefs, and Action 1

CHAPTER TWO — THE FIRST DECADE: 1899 – 1908
In Search of Galvanizing Issues: Taking on the "Cutters" 17

CHAPTER THREE — THE SECOND DECADE: 1909 – 1918
Economic Forces Reshape the Marketplace 47

CHAPTER FOUR — THE THIRD DECADE: 1919 – 1928
Prohibition and Retail Pharmacy:
The "Great War" in the Marketplace 65

CHAPTER FIVE — THE FOURTH DECADE: 1929 – 1938
"Great Depression" Yields a New General
and a Great NARD Victory: The Robinson-Patman Act 83

CHAPTER SIX — THE FIFTH DECADE: 1939 – 1948
Emerging Marketplace Challenges Reshape Association Priorities 109

CHAPTER SEVEN — THE SIXTH DECADE: 1949 – 1958
More NARD Victories in Repelling Assaults on Fair Trade 127

CHAPTER EIGHT — THE SEVENTH DECADE: 1959 – 1968
NARD Grapples with Seismic Change in the Marketplace 149

CHAPTER NINE — THE EIGHTH DECADE: 1969 – 1978
NARD Meets the Storm's Center in Washington 175

CHAPTER TEN — THE NINTH DECADE: 1979 – 1988
NARD Wins Battles in the Legislative Trenches 195

CHAPTER ELEVEN — THE CENTENNIAL DECADE: 1989 – 1998
Community Pharmacists Tackle the New Marketplace 221

EPILOGUE 251

HIGHLIGHTS FROM THE 100–YEAR HISTORY
OF NARD/NCPA 253

PAST PRESIDENTS OF NARD/NCPA 275

Acknowledgments

The National Community Pharmacists Association
wishes to acknowledge the generous support of

The NCPA Foundation

in helping to make this Centennial History possible.

NCPA also wishes to extend its sincere thanks to NCPA Historian

C. Fred Williams, Ph.D.

of the University of Arkansas at Little Rock Department of History
for his tireless research and editorial contributions
as the author of this Centennial History.

MANAGING EDITOR
Todd Dankmyer
Senior Vice President, Communications, NCPA

EDITOR
Robert A. Malone

Preface

The story of independent retail pharmacy in the United States is perhaps as heroic and powerful a saga as any written in the twentieth century about American business. Independent retail pharmacists played — and continue to play — a signal role in enhancing and maintaining the health care needs of the nation, often amid extraordinary challenges that would have fazed, demoralized, and destroyed lesser industries and professions.

Independents were — and still are — bedrocks of their communities. They are as inextricably linked to the health and welfare of their patients as they are to the local community groups, civic organizations, and state legislatures they so admirably serve. It's no wonder that independent pharmacists came to be viewed by the American public as the "number one" most trusted of all professions.

With roots as deep as the nation itself, independent pharmacy would have had a difficult path toward survival in this century — given the formidable adversaries it faced over a 100-year period — had its practitioners not banded together to protect their professional practice and economic livelihood. In 1898, a small group of "true believers" in the profession issued a call to others amid an economic crisis — a stamp tax on proprietary medicines to fund the Spanish-American war. That call to arms, predictably over a legislative matter, was the genesis of the National Association of Retail Druggists (NARD). From this modest beginning effort to organize a national group representing both the professional and proprietary interests of independent retail pharmacy grew one of the most powerful national associations — pharmacy or otherwise — ever to grace the halls of Congress. In 1937, in the wake of two extraordinary congressional victories, *Business Week* labeled NARD "the nation's most powerful trade association."

Due to its tenacity, singularity of purpose (promoting the cause of the independent), and the grassroots strength of its active and vocal membership, NARD earned the respect of its adversaries as well as of its allies, including several U.S. Presidents.

The issues confronting independent pharmacists at the turn of the century have a remarkably familiar ring to today's practitioners — price-cutting, price protection, price discrimination, fair trade, mail order, physician dispensing, and an encroaching federal government. On issue after issue, NARD scratched, fought, struggled, and, as often as not, overcame those seeking to undermine the independents of America.

Ensuring the economic survival and prosperity of its members was one focus of NARD. An ever-vigilant, tenacious political agenda was generally employed to accomplish that. But another was its stewardship of the profession. Throughout its history, NARD created and promoted a host of programs to help pharmacists become better managers and marketers — something they only rarely learned about in pharmacy school. Increasingly, the association also sought to help its members discover new avenues of professional expertise — promoting a vast array of specialty niches as well as certification programs in health supports and appliances and today in disease state management.

Whether the focus was economic or political, managerial or professional, NARD, throughout the decades, brought a practical real-world perspective to all that it touched. That approach mirrors the outlook of the neighborhood pharmacists and small business men and women it represents. Similarly, a can-do attitude dominated the outlook of NARD's leaders throughout the century. Again, a reflection of the membership.

Of course, an association should mirror its members. But it should also lead. NARD has been nudging and cajoling its members to political action since its beginnings in St. Louis. In recent decades, it has also been pushing the professional horizons of the profession. Leadership of the political and professional kind are the stuff of a strong association.

To reach the first 100 years in any organization's lifespan is a considerable achievement. To have continuity of leadership throughout those years residing in the hands of only eight individuals — Thomas Wooten, Thomas Potts, Samuel Henry, John Dargavel, Willard Simmons, William Woods, Charles West, and now Calvin Anthony — is truly remarkable.

The steadfastness of its leaders and endurance of the constitution, almost without alteration since 1898, speak volumes about the correctness of the original purpose of NARD: to ensure the economic and professional survival and prosperity of the independent pharmacists of America.

The extraordinary story begins in St. Louis, Missouri, and unfolds — for the first 100 years.

CHAPTER ONE

NARD Meets Its Destiny In St. Louis: 1898

A Beginning Built on a Bedrock of Principles, Beliefs, and Action

*O*ne hundred years ago community pharmacists in Chicago, Illinois, were in an angry mood. The federal government had implemented a "stamp tax" on proprietary medications and cosmetics to help finance the Spanish-American War, and both manufacturers and wholesalers had found a way to pass the costs of the tax on to pharmacists. Although the fee was minimal, it nevertheless reduced the small margin of profit that independent druggists earned. Decades of battling department stores, large mail order houses, proprietary medicine companies, physicians who dispensed prescriptions, and aggressive price cutters had left most community pharmacists with little margin of profit. The stamp tax was the last straw, and a small group in Chicago decided to organize in protest.

Leonard Tillotson, editor of the *Western Druggist,* published in Chicago, was the catalyst for action. From his vantage point, he had watched numerous attempts to organize in the past — all ending in disappointment. Retail members of the American Pharmaceutical Association (APhA) formed an organization in 1883 in an effort to forge agreement on prices for proprietary medicines. Calling itself the National Retail Druggists Association, the new organization sought to bring some control to the ruinous atmosphere of competition. But the new organization was fraught with disagreements from the beginning and became so divided in opinion over strategy that it could never effectively achieve its mission. It died an ungrieved death in 1887.

APhA then tried to organize a commercial section within its framework. But APhA was far more interested in the academic and pharmacological aspects of the profession and its new retail division became less than a stepchild in the organization. This led to a new group of retailers forming the Interstate Druggists League in 1891, but again individual differences led the group to disband in 1894. Four years later, as aggressive price cutting from department stores and wholesalers continued, a new group organized the National Retail Druggists Congress. But, subsequent to its first meeting, the group again failed to develop into an organization.

This was the backdrop for Tillotson's call in 1898 for yet another effort at organization. Not surprising, many pharmacists greeted his editorial with skepticism, but this time circumstances were different. An issue affecting the economic livelihood — and possibly the survival of independent retail pharmacy — was thrust upon the profession and required a coordinated response from pharmacist practitioners. The issue — the new stamp tax — was an inflammatory and seminal event that served as a catalyst for organizational action among all pharmacists.

Tillotson also moved beyond the editorial voice of his magazine and engaged in discussions with Thomas V. Wooten, who owned a pharmacy near Tillotson's offices. Wooten was president of the Chicago Retail Drug Association, a group that had been in existence since 1886 and that had earned a reputation as a respected voice in the health delivery system in Chicago. One of the strengths of the organization was its emphasis on cooperation and on teamwork among its members.

Wooten embraced the concept of concerted action based on commonly pooled interests among its members and asked the association for approval to appoint a committee to plan the procedures and format for developing a national community of pharmacists. Although many pharmacists, if not most, were pessimistic about the potential of yet another attempt to organize na-

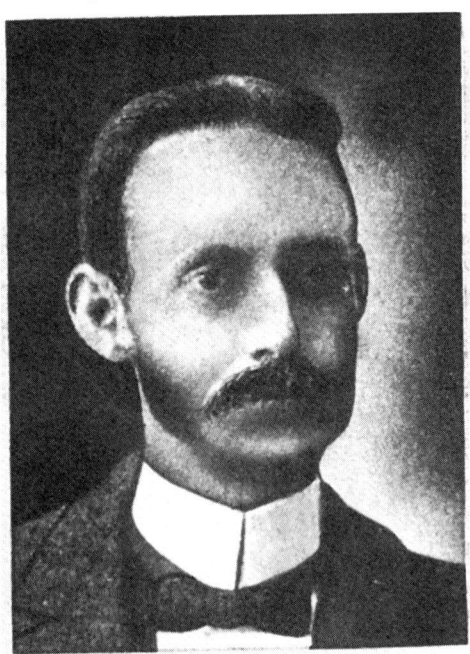

Leonard Tillotson, the founder of the National Association of Retail Druggists

tionally, all agreed that action had to be taken to counter the greatly despised stamp tax. Thus, the members gave support to their president. Wooten appointed a committee of fifteen colleagues and, along with Tillotson, this ad hoc group met in the basement of the local Masonic Temple on the evening of August 11, 1898. The group included George P. Engelhard, publisher of the *Western Druggist,* who was also Tillotson's boss, and Thomas N. Jamieson, a friend of Englehard with connections to the Illinois Central Railroad.

The group wasted little time debating "if" there was a need for a national meeting and instead focused its energy on how to make a prospective organization work. Everyone agreed that the time for talking about "insidious trade evils" and the arrogance of the manufacturers and wholesalers was over. Something of significance had to be done.

Tillotson offered his magazine as a vehicle for nationwide communication calling for a national meeting of pharmacists — an organized call to arms. He believed the invitation should be made to existing organizations rather than individuals in an effort to enlist those who had already shown a predilection for organized action. The group from Chicago agreed to invite every druggists' association to elect delegates, a maximum of five, for the organizational meeting.

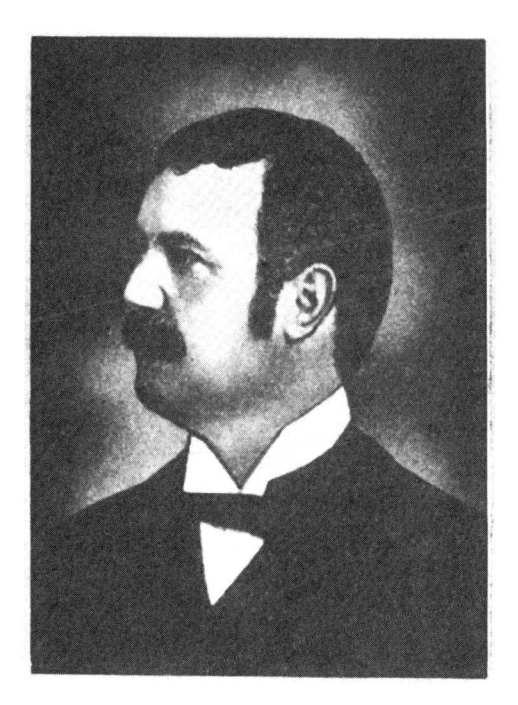

Thomas V. Wooten, the first NARD Executive Secretary, 1898 – 1908

As a final action, the group set the date for the meeting for the third week in October in St. Louis, Missouri. That date gave Tillotson time to contact other editors of drug trade publications to elicit their help in promoting the meeting. He also knew that the National Wholesale Druggists' Association (NWDA) and the Proprietary Association of America (PA) were having their annual meetings in St. Louis in October and had no doubt many retail druggists would already be there to attend one or both of those meetings.

Englehard agreed to underwrite the printing and mailing costs for the announcement. Tillotson subsequently elicited cooperation from his fellow editors to print an announcement calling for this national meeting and asking other locally organized associations of retail druggists to indicate their support by completing a prospective registration form and returning it to him.

In the nine weeks that followed the Chicago meeting, Tillotson and Wooten anxiously watched the mail to see how their fellow retailers were responding. They also contacted colleagues in other cities and encouraged them to promote the meeting. Wooten was particularly interested in having in attendance members of APhA, and he contacted J.M. Good, president of that organization and a St. Louis resident as well, inviting him to attend and address the meeting. When it became apparent that there was sufficient interest to hold a meeting, Wooten and his colleagues drafted a tentative agenda to facilitate the organization. Wooten also contacted John H. Allen, president of the St. Louis Apothecaries Association, and asked him to make local arrangements for the meeting.

Prior to his travel by train to St. Louis, Tillotson had received responses from pharmacists in twenty-one states, representing more than sixty associations. Based on those returns, he estimated that approximately 200 delegates would attend. Jamieson, although not actively involved in the organizing strategy, agreed to cover the transportation costs of the Chicago delegation attending the meeting.

Arriving in St. Louis on Sunday, October 16, 1898, Tillotson, Wooten, and other pharmacists checked in at the St. Nicholas Hotel located at the northwest corner of Locust and 8th streets. The banquet hall of the hotel had been reserved for the meeting, and there at 11:00 a.m. Monday morning, October 17, this ad hoc group that was to become the National Association of Retail Druggists (NARD) held its first meeting. In later years, those present remembered the somber, serious mood of the participants. Most had been demoralized by the past failures at organizing members of their profession to respond to serious issues challenging the economic viability of their business. Accordingly, they were less than confident about the success of this meeting.

Wooten was prepared for this mood of pessimism. As chairman of the founding group in Chicago, he took the prerogative to address the delegates first and remind them why they had assembled. In a brief ten-minute speech, one that he stayed up all night rehearsing, he told the delegates, "The great problem to be solved (is) how to make such a beginning in the work of organizing the retail trade of the country as (will) command universal respect, universal support." The greatest barrier to improving conditions "has been the unorganized state of the retail drug trade." He said it was also imperative that pharmacists "overcome indifference born of years of disheartening experience."

The imposition of the special war tax on medicines was sufficient grounds to spur pharmacists to action. Wooten further challenged the delegates by saying, "We come to you today with the firm conviction forced upon us by years of thought, discussion, and observation, that the first work and the great work of the men here assembled is to perfect an organization which shall be strong in plan and liberal in character. Everything depends on organization."

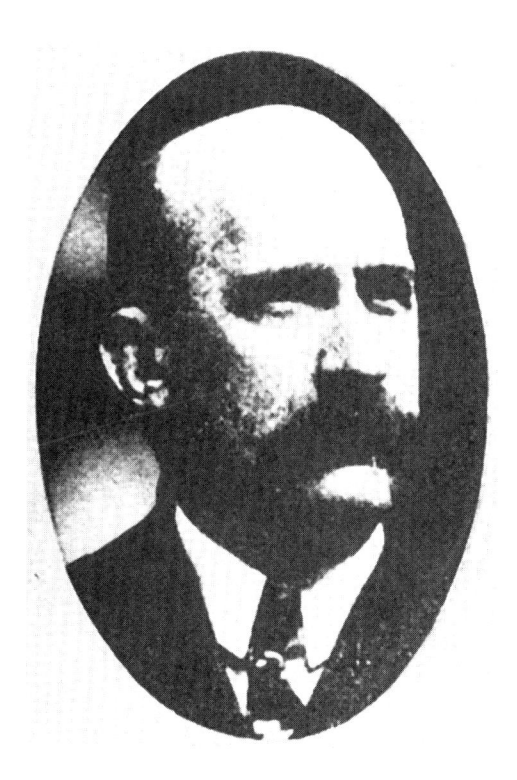

Henry P. Hynson, first president of the National Association of Retail Druggists

J.M. Good was then invited to address the delegates as part of his official functions with APhA. But he had also been chosen as a delegate by the St. Louis Apothecaries Association and it was from that position that he addressed the delegates. He pledged APhA's support, but he also reminded the group that "whatever has been done for the retailer has been done through the American Pharmaceutical Association...." Before closing his speech, he admitted that "the retail druggists (have) been repeatedly ignored by other bodies, including our government."

After the opening addresses, temporary chairman Wooten declared the first order of business to be an election of a permanent chairman for the new (but not yet formalized) organization. He opened the floor for nominations. William Bodemann, a member of the Chicago Apothecaries Society, nominated J.M. Good. This was an interesting move on Bodemann's part. While a member of the original Chicago planning committee, he had never been one of the inner circle. An independent-minded, hard-driving personality, Bodemann did not always see eye to eye with his fellow druggists and may have harbored some hard feelings toward Wooten's strong leadership. Over the next two decades he frequently disputed official policy and was often at odds with the association's leadership.

Good declined and nominated Thomas Wooten for the position. Wooten was elected by acclamation. William Muir, representing the Kings County (Brooklyn) New York Pharmaceutical Association, then nominated John H. Allen of the St. Louis Apothecaries Association for vice chairman, and Allen was elected by acclamation. E.B. Heimstreet of the Wisconsin Pharmaceutical Association nominated John W. Lowe of the Connecticut State Pharmaceutical Association for secretary. With that nomination and election, the officers' slate was complete.

Delegates then selected a committee to prepare a constitution and adjourned until 5:30 p.m. that afternoon to give the committee time to draft a document. Beyond name and purpose, a nettlesome point for this group centered on representation in the new organization. Henry P. Hynson, representing the Baltimore Druggists Association, noted that most of the major cities had strong druggist associations for many years and represented the greatest concentration of pharmacists who met on a regular basis. He believed that was a critical factor in sustaining an organization. His "Baltimore Plan" called for proportional representation that would be weighed in favor of the cities. By contrast, N.A. Kuhn of Omaha, Nebraska, proposed a "Nebraska Plan," which favored equal representation by state population.

After debating these and a number of other variations, the committee finally agreed on a compromise known as the "Chicago Plan." Under this proposal every organized pharmacy group received at least one representative, but larger associations were also accommodated by allowing incremental representation based on membership.

Commencing a second session, Chairman Wooten called the delegates together and recognized A. Timberlake of the Will County (Indiana) Pharmaceutical Association and chairperson of the committee to present the report. The preamble called for "united action" of all retail druggists in the nation: Article I identified the new organization as the "National Association of Retail Druggists," and Article II stated that the group planned to "unite...in a central body for the improvement of the business conditions of the retail drug trade." Membership was based on a delegate system and vested in "regularly organized associations of retail druggists." Each association was entitled to one delegate for each 100 active members, provided they were "actively engaged in the retail drug business." APhA was allotted "five delegates to all the meetings of the association."

The new association was to be administered by a president, three vice presidents, a secretary, a treasurer, and an executive committee of five members. These officers were to be elected annually to a one-year term and were eligible for re-election. Seven standing committees were also proposed to assist the officers with policy issues. The executive committee was authorized to assess "the different associations on the basis of their membership" in or-

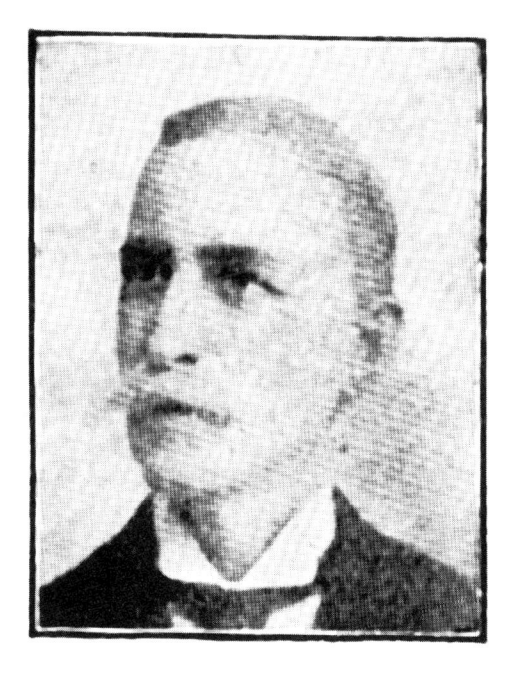

Simon N. Jones, another NARD pioneer, second vice president in the original slate of officers

der to generate funds to operate the organization. When Timberlake finished presenting the committee's report, N.A. Kuhn (Omaha, Nebraska) moved to table the document until 8:00 p.m. to give the delegates time for informal discussion.

Wooten called the group back into session promptly at the appointed time and the proposed constitution was debated paragraph by paragraph. Only two sections presented any real division of thought. Henry P. Hynson (Baltimore Druggists Association) moved to change the name to the "National Retail Druggists Congress," but his motion was defeated. A.A. Pardee (Madison, Wisconsin Pharmaceutical Association) moved to delete the section giving membership to APhA, but after extensive discussion his motion was also defeated. The remaining document was adopted virtually as submitted by the committee and as of Monday evening, October 17, NARD was born.

One item of business remained — appointing a nominating committee to recommend officers for the new organization. As prescribed in the newly adopted constitution, each state was allowed one member, chosen by the respective intrastate associations. After each state selected its delegate, the meeting adjourned for the evening.

The nominating committee elected F.H. Burton (Evansville [Will County] Indiana Pharmaceutical Association) chairperson and worked late into the night to select officers for the new association. At 10:00 a.m. on Tuesday, October 18, the slate was ready. Henry P. Hynson (Baltimore Druggists Association) for president; George L. Hechler (Ohio Pharmaceutical Association), first vice president; Simon N. Jones (Louisville [Kentucky] Botanical Club), second vice president; Norman A. Kuhn (Omaha, Nebraska — registered without identifying an association), third vice president; Thomas V. Wooten (Chicago Retail Druggists Association), secretary; and John W. Lowe (Connecticut Pharmaceutical Association), treasurer.

Names submitted for the executive committee included F.E. Holliday (Kansas City [Missouri] Pharmaceutical Association); John H. Allen (St. Louis Apothecaries Association); D.E. Prall, (Saginaw [Michigan] Pharmaceutical Society); and A. Timberlake (Will County [Indianapolis, Indiana] Pharmaceutical Association).

On a motion from J.M. Good, the nominations were accepted, and Wooten turned the meeting over to the new leaders. As his first action, President Hynson recognized Leonard Tillotson for a motion to appoint a committee on resolutions. The motion carried without dissent; Hynson appointed the committee, then adjourned the meeting until 2:00 p.m.

Reconvening, a committee on constitution and bylaws reported that it had now completed its work on the organization's bylaws, and President

Hynson recognized E.B. Heimstreet (Wisconsin Pharmaceutical Association) to present the report. There were no objections to the seven "laws" presented, but W.C. Anderson (Kings County [Brooklyn, New York] Pharmaceutical Association) used the occasion to propose an amendment to Article VII of the constitution to clarify the language and ensure that state associations would only be assessed fees for members not affiliated with a local pharmacy association. Anderson's amendment passed unanimously, but such could not be said for the committee on resolutions' report.

The committee had carefully sorted its work into resolutions that should be referred to one of the standing committees and those items on which the committee as a whole could respond. But feelings ran high on the seven statements that the committee brought to the floor and after "extended discussions" and motions to "amend," "strike out," and "substitute," the entire report was referred back to the committee with instructions for the group to be prepared to report again the next day at 9:30 a.m.

In an effort to be more responsive to the membership committee, Chairman Heimstreet announced that his group would hold an open meeting during the evening to hear anyone wishing to make a statement. Before adjournment, Thomas Stoddard (Erie County [N.Y.] Pharmaceutical Association) noted that the new organization had no money to fund its operations and suggested that a "collection" be taken to help defray expenses. The suggestion was met favorably and while the amount of money collected was not reported, the secretary did note it was "sufficient to defray the immediate expenses of the secretary's office." Hynson then reminded the membership about the committee on resolutions' plan to conduct hearings and adjourned the delegates until the following morning.

The third full day of deliberations found the committee on resolutions (after an all-night session) still not ready to report, and President Hynson turned to Delegate Heimstreet to introduce a plan for organizing the new group. Heimstreet recommended that each state association be organized into county societies and that NARD, in turn, be a composite of the state societies. After extended debate, the item was referred to the executive committee for further discussion. By this time, the resolutions were ready, and the president called on Chairman Tillotson for the recommendations.

The committee had prepared seven resolutions. The first addressed the burdensome war-time stamp tax by making a request to Congress that it find a substitute mechanism for financing the war. A follow-up resolution suggested that the tax be shifted to the manufacturers, and still another identified a formula for pricing retail goods. A fourth recommended that the various state boards of pharmacy be urged to promote a uniformity of standards among the states and that higher qualifications be established for newcomers wishing to become members of NARD. The remaining resolutions were essentially concerned with public relations or routine business of the convention.

In the midst of the floor debate on the various resolutions, there was another event that presaged relationships between the new organization of retail druggists (NARD) and their counterparts in the wholesale druggists and proprietary manufacturer arenas (NWDA and PA, respectively). Delegates from the regional Western Wholesale Druggist Association (WWDA), who were attending the convention of the NWDA nearby, arrived on the NARD convention floor. President Hynson interrupted the proceedings to introduce the representatives, welcomed them on behalf of NARD, and invited representatives of the group to speak. F.A. Faxon, a Missouri wholesaler and chairman of the delegation, spoke first and emphasized the wholesalers' interest in promoting harmony among each segment of the drug trade. He invited the NARD delegates to attend the WWDA's meeting still in progress at the nearby Charles Hotel.

Another spokesman, W.H. Torbert also of Missouri, said that "the interests of (his) association and that of the retail druggist were identical" and noted that NARD members might well wish to hear a report prepared by Faxon's committee on proprietary goods, which was to be presented to the WWDA convention within the hour. But the NARD delegates were not so easily swayed. Although cordial to their guests, the retailers had been caught on the wrong side of this triangle before and viewed the kudos with a degree of skepticism. President Hynson did accept Chairman Faxon's invitation for representatives of NARD to make an appearance at the WWDA and hear the report. At 11:30 a.m., NARD adjourned its meeting for an hour to allow a delegation from its group to return the visit to WWDA.

At the wholesalers' meeting, President Hynson was invited to speak on behalf of NARD. In a hastily organized speech, he said, "You will note the wholesaler and retailer with clasped hands, which is typical of the future...there is a place for all classes of the drug trade." He then with other members of the delegation listened as Faxon presented the committee on proprietary goods' report. The most salient point of that presentation was "the insistence that proprietors refuse to sell to any retailer direct, no matter how large his order might be, at the lowest quantity prices."

The report touched off considerable discussion among WWDA members and with that discussion, Hynson noted that NARD was "actively engaged in a most important session" and asked "that you allow us to retire." Returning to the Nicholas Hotel, Hynson had scarcely called the afternoon session to order before hearing that a committee from PA, the proprietary manufacturers' association, was in the building and wished to be recognized.

Hynson had little choice but to invite those representatives to address the convention as well. Two committeemen spoke with high praise for NARD's efforts to organize retail pharmacists, and one noted that the PA was reserving time at 4:30 that afternoon to take up any questions that NARD "desired to consider."

Hynson called upon Delegate Stoddard to respond to the PA remarks. Stoddard, while cordial to the guests, nevertheless noted "the great advantage to the manufacturer of proprietary goods in having those goods distributed to the public over the counters of the pharmacists," and he hoped the manufacturers realized "that such advantage did not attend their distribution through other channels."

Stoddard had hardly finished his remarks before Tillotson was on his feet to present a motion. In a carefully worded statement, he moved that "the formal response (from NARD)...to the committee of the Proprietary Association of America be that the question upon which united action was desired now lay on President McKinley's desk" — a clear reference to the odious stamp tax, the burden of which retail pharmacists, not wholesalers or manufacturers, would have to bear. The motion passed. Lest they be misunderstood, NARD delegates were clearly telling the PA that their timing was a bit

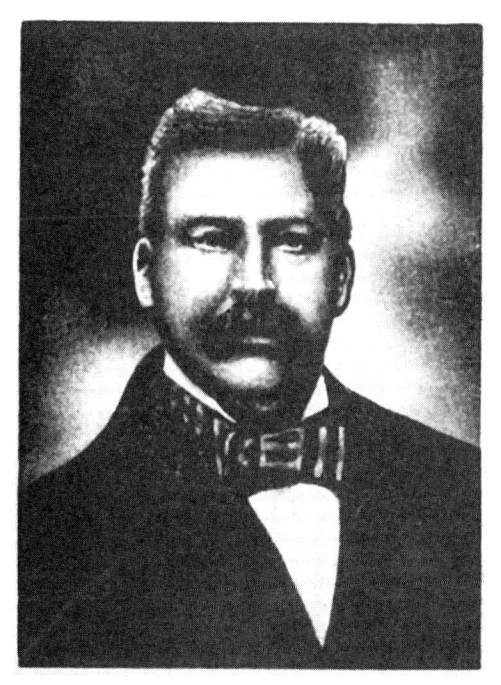

Arthur Timberlake, one of the original NARD Executive Committee members

late if they were seeking cooperation. The PA committee then "retired" from the meeting, and President Hynson continued with the report from the committee on resolutions until adjournment at 4:00 p.m.

There were subsequent attempts to assuage among the strained relations between the three groups. In the break between sessions, members of the executive committee tried to arrange meetings with their counterparts among the NWDA and the PA. Relations with the proprietary group were still a bit strained since the exchange earlier in the day and Hynson was not able to arrange a meeting. But the wholesalers were in a more cooperative mood and the two groups had a productive meeting. They agreed on language for a joint statement regarding price, and President Hynson invited representatives from the wholesalers to sit in the NARD meeting when it resumed deliberations later that evening.

When the delegates reconvened for their next session, Secretary Wooten requested time for personal privilege in order to discuss the new organization's expenses. Wooten noted that the association needed an immediate cash outlay of $1,200 to run the organization's headquarters and estimated that the minimum expenses for the year would be around $2,500. He asked the delegates how they proposed to meet this challenge. Kentuckian Simon Jones immediately announced that he would provide $50 on behalf of the Louisville Botanical Club, and a number of other delegates quickly joined the pledge. In short order, the group pledged almost $600 in voluntary contributions — this in addition to their previously assessed dues. (Financial survival for the new organization often required "passing the hat" for contributions, and association officers for years to come had to chase after the financial wherewithal to support association programs.)

Thus, by October 19, 1898 — a memorable first milestone in NARD history — a collection of delegates from twenty-one states and a wide range of retail establishments reached agreement on common goals. They adopted a constitution with minimum debate, elected a broadly representative group of officers and committee members, agreed on a series of resolutions that expressed their sentiments on a number of issues, and had taken a major step toward cooperation with other interests in the drug trade.

Hynson was in an optimistic mood when he reconvened the delegates at 8:15 p.m. He moved quickly to recognize the two representatives from the NWDA who had accepted his invitation to meet with his group. They were invited to address the delegates, and wholesaler J.C. Eliel responded by saying that since its inception, his organization "has had in mind...the welfare of the retailer." He also warned the delegates "not to expect too much out of your organization and, whatever you do, stand together." He concluded by making a strong appeal for cooperation between the two associations, saying, "We cannot live on the proprietary manufacturers. We can and do live on the retailer...therefore our friendship for you is not so much in your interest as in our own."

But while NARD and NWDA may have reached agreement in principle, the same could not be said for the PA. The NARD Executive Committee could not come to an understanding with its counterpart at PA. After over an hour of fruitless discussions, the executive committee prepared a series of resolutions for the delegates to consider when they reconvened later in the evening. Secretary Prall presented the report for the committee. Reminding the delegates of resolutions passed earlier in the day, he said the executive committee recommended "that we request manufacturers...to restrict the distribution of their goods to the legitimate wholesale dealers as recognized by the Proprietary Committee of the (NWDA) and the Executive of the (NARD)" and "that the prices on proprietary goods to the retailer, should, in no case, exceed $2 for 25 cent items, $4 for 50 cent articles, and $8 per dozen for $1 articles, and all articles in proportion, purchased in lots of a dozen or more."

Prall also reported that the executive committee favored "amending the law under which the stamp act had been imposed." The membership, however, was not united on how the amending should be done. Speaking for one group, M.N. Kline noted that talk about Congress's "intent that manufacturers alone should pay the stamp act (was) speculation." But G.L Hechler countered by saying, "For the past fifteen years we have listened to promises as to what might occur in the future to our advantage if we would only work and not say anything, but...this meeting has assembled in quite a different spirit. We recognize the wholesalers as our friends, but we are not at all satisfied with promises.... We came here friendly; we are willing to (work) with proprietary medicine (representatives) in a friendly and courteous way, but they must make some definite arrangement at this time whereby they will protect us."

Hechler's remarks touched off an extended debate. No one in the group could forge a consensus, and when word came that representatives from PA could not be available for a meeting that day, NARD and NWDA voted to end their discussion and attempt to arrange a meeting with the PA for the next day.

A committee from the PA met with the two other groups on Thursday morning at 10:00 a.m. and discussion on the divisive issues resumed. With respect to the special tax, the joint committee agreed to ask the "Committees on Legislation" of each group to confer and work out a plan to either repeal the law or modify it so that it would work "to the actual advantage of the three branches of the drug trade." On the $2, $4, $8 pricing system, those representing the Proprietary Association said that while they were not authorized to approve it, they were confident that such a plan would be endorsed by their association as a whole.

The distribution issue was another matter. Central to the question was how products were to be marketed. The wholesalers wanted their group to be the sole distributors for all pharmacy products. The proprietary representatives objected, arguing that any plan that did not allow manufacturers freedom to choose their distributors would not be endorsed by their association. NARD members were concerned with getting agreement on two concepts — one, that regardless of the method of distribution, an emphasis be placed on offering "the lowest price possible" to "legitimate dealers" and that, further, both groups also agree not to sell to "department stores or persistently aggressive cutters."

In the close interworking of a small group, the joint committee was able to agree on language for a report to be presented to each association. Confident that they had secured mutual understanding with both the wholesalers and the manufacturers, the NARD delegation returned to their House of Delegates with the document. There, a motion was made to receive the report and commend the committee members for their excellent work.

From all appearances, organizers of this first NARD convention had succeeded in what they came to do. They had reached agreement on the hated war tax and a plan for consistent pricing on drug products. Being together as a retail group created an esprit de corps, and the ability to discuss mutual interests with the manufacturers and the wholesalers gave the community pharmacists an identity. The delegates' somber mood, which had dominated since the convention opened on Monday, gave way to a ray of optimism as the delegates prepared to end their first convention.

After expressing appreciation to the management of the St. Nicholas Hotel and appointing the standing committees mandated by the new constitution, President Hynson adjourned the meeting shortly before 2:00 p.m.

The optimism that buoyed NARD delegates as the meeting wound down was short-lived. While Wooten, Hynson, and others were "tieing up the loose ends" from the convention, word came that the PA representatives to the joint committee wanted to meet again at 5:00 p.m. The request, coming so soon after the original compromise had been reached, gave the NARD party some concern. Their apprehension was confirmed soon after the meeting got under way. The PA group reported that their convention had refused to endorse the joint committee's report. Moreover, the PA leadership took the position that the association could not make a "binding" agreement on its members.

News of the PA's action launched "an animated discussion" with various members of the NARD Executive Committee who expressed their strong displeasure with the PA action. Chairman F.E. Holliday summed up the committee's disposition by pointing out that the convention's proceedings were being sent to some "40,000 retail druggists" throughout the nation, and "if the proprietary manufacturers were willing to have it go on record that they refused to take any action in regard to the monstrous injustice which had been imposed upon the retailer, they might as well make up their minds to take the consequences."

Again, the heated exchange of words in a small group had its effect. Those representing the PA said they would ask their association to reconsider. In the spirit of cooperation, NARD members admitted that "moral support" of the resolution may be all they could hope for — given the procedural rules and tradition of the PA. In any event, the proprietary group promised to have the matter resolved by 9:00 p.m. and invited the NARD Executive Committee and any NARD delegates still in St. Louis to come to the PA session.

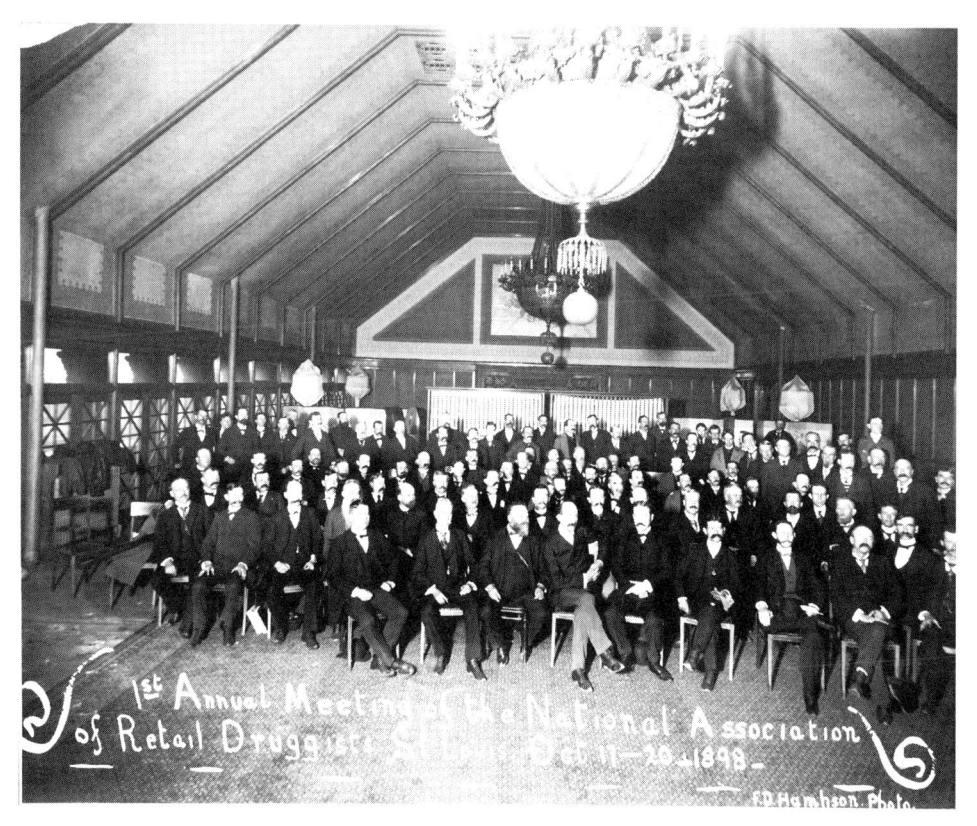

The official photograph of delegates to the first annual meeting of NARD

Wooten, Hynson, Holliday, and other members of the executive committee decided to accept the invitation. When they arrived at the appointed time, E.H. Hance, chairman of the PA, and representatives to the joint committee met them at the door and presented them with a compromise resolution that had just been adopted. The document stated in part:

"At the request of the National Association of Retail Druggists...the (PA) association recommend(s) to proprietors that, wherever practicable, prices to the retailer should not exceed $2 per dozen for 25-cent articles; $4 per dozen for 50-cent articles and $8 per dozen for $1 articles, and all other prices in proportion in lots of one dozen or more.

Wooten and the NARD delegation were disappointed at the "recommend" and "wherever practicable" language, but accepted Hance's explanation that it was all the PA could do — at least for the moment. Chairman Holliday was invited to address the delegates on behalf of NARD. In a hurried conference with other members of the committee, they quickly agreed that he should accept what was being offered and be conciliatory in his remarks. Hance thanked the PA for taking "an important step" in the interest of the retailers and said that when this action was reported, he was confident that members of NARD would feel that "they had accomplished much" of the agenda that had brought them to St. Louis.

In such fashion, the first NARD convention came to a close. The four days had been intense and, at times, the retailers were sharply divided on strategy and by region. But they had never been confused about their purpose, and throughout all the debate, a few principles remained true — a fair price for their products, a reasonable profit for their services, and professional standing among health providers in the retail world. These principles were to prove the bedrock of an association that few thought on its founding would endure a decade, let alone the next 100 years. Such was the spirit of the independent retail pharmacist.

Chapter Two

The First Decade: 1899 – 1908

In Search of Galvanizing Issues: Taking on the "Cutters"

N ARD's first secretary, Thomas Wooten, returned to Chicago from the St. Louis, Missouri, meeting with mixed emotions. The courage and determination the small band of pharmacists had shown was encouraging. But even by the most generous count, the new NARD could not hope to speak for more than a few hundred independents in a field of approximately 40,000 practicing pharmacists. How could the new organization gain enough members to give druggists an effective voice in the health care arena? The new constitution had proudly recognized the office of "Executive Secretary," but without more dues-paying members, the office could be little more than symbolic.

Perhaps the most painful thing was the haughty spirit of the Proprietary Association (PA) in practically daring the retailers to organize. The manufacturers appeared convinced that the retailers could not band together. Even if they should form an association, the PA reasoned, it had not worked before, why should it work now? Wooten was determined that this time would be different.

Wooten's first priority was to build the association membership. Based on attendance at the first convention, the association's strength lay in the Midwest. However, most pharmacists were located in the heavily populated eastern states and gaining their support was critical. Also, in order to be politically effective, Wooten knew that he would have to enlist key pharmacists in the South and on the West Coast. The constitution specified that NARD accept members from "organized groups of independent, retail druggists" and that proved a major asset for adding new members.

Several major cities — including Philadelphia, Pennsylvania, Boston, Massachusetts, Baltimore, Maryland, and St. Louis, Missouri, in addition to Chicago, Illinois — had strong associations. These, coupled with key state associations, provided NARD with the potential to expand its members rapidly. Members of the executive committee committed to work their respective regions, and the strategy paid off.

News of the proprietary group's hard-line response in St. Louis rapidly spread among retail druggists and became a rallying point for NARD. State and city associations readily forwarded dues (25 cents for each member) to Chicago and before the association was five years old, Wooten could boast that NARD represented more than 25,000 pharmacists nationwide. While this represented barely half of the practicing druggists, the number was clearly enough to make NARD an organization to take note of in the world of pharmacy.

Wooten and NARD's inner circle knew that they could not hold a large membership for long without offering them worthwhile services. However, finding something of interest to such a diverse group was not easy. Not only did the membership come from a wide variety of communities spread out over a broad geographical area, but they also represented a variety of business philosophies. Some druggists were located in upscale communities and kept a fairly specialized inventory; others were in small towns and provided multiple services. Some individuals had been attracted to the profession because of their scientific interests, while others were more interested in the retail side of pharmacy.

Wooten and the executive committee members served without compensation. Monies collected from dues and contributions were used for printing and mailing, and all the officers of the association spent a good deal of time away from their businesses.

Communication with the membership was done primarily through "bulletins" prepared by subcommittees of the executive committee or through the trade journals that infrequently reported on NARD activity. Clearly, the new organization needed some rallying point, some program or issue that would grab the attention of the nation's independent pharmacists. But identifying a program or issue that would impress such an independent-minded group was no easy task.

But there was one issue that concerned pharmacists more than any other, it was the matter of price cutting. The unholy alliance among the proprietary interests, the wholesalers, and their pawns in the retail business in support of "discount prices" was a most distasteful practice that NARD had to reckon with and resolve. If the association could not come up with a plan to neutralize the "aggressive cutters," then in all probability NARD would go the way of the previous retail organizations.

The "cutter" issue had been under discussion for some time. As early as 1891, the Association of Manufacturers and Dealers in Proprietary Articles, National Wholesale Druggists' Association (NWDA), and the American Pharmaceutical Association (APhA) had entered into a "Tripartite Plan" in an effort to prevent price cutting at both the wholesale and retail levels. Enforcement of the agreement had been lax, primarily because the APhA was not particularly interested in the retail area, and the plan had not proven effective. Wooten and the executive committee thought they saw potential in reviving the plan and began efforts to do so.

Revitalizing the Tripartite Plan was no easy task. The original agreement had guaranteed the wholesalers a 10 percent profit on most popular proprietary articles. It assumed that retailers would then "hold firmly the retail price" since they too would be assured of "a satisfactory profit." But such was not the case. Both wholesalers and retailers used their profits in one area to offset discount prices in another area and the "cutting" practices continued. A customer shopping at a "cutter store" would ask for an item only to be told by the store's proprietor that the item was "out of stock." The customer was then offered "something just as good for less money" — a substitute. Wooten and other leaders of NARD argued that not only was the substitute inferior in quality, but also its sole purpose for being offered was because it offered greater profits to the vendor.

Wooten and the executive committee first thought that they could make the Tripartite Plan work by educating their membership about the importance of everyone adhering to the agreement. At the executive committee's direction, the secretary prepared a series of "bulletins" pointing out how the plan worked and illustrating how all retailers could make a profit from their stores while still being competitive in the marketplace.

Despite NARD's best efforts, the policy of education had only limited effect. Competition was intense and most pharmacists used almost any tactic to attract customers. The Tripartite Plan, while including a written agreement between the manufacturer and the jobber, did not include a contract between the wholesaler and the retailer. Nor was there any way to trace a particular product after it had left the manufacturer. The concept was more of a dual agreement, with the retailer being left at the mercy of the other parties. What Wooten and the executive committee needed was a plan that would bind each party to the agreement and that could be monitored to ensure compliance.

The price-cutter problem dominated NARD affairs for four years. Wooten tried various approaches to educate the membership and persuade them that even a minimum effort at cooperation would be profitable. A historic breakthrough came on NARD's fifth anniversary. At the annual convention in Cleveland, Ohio, in September 1902, the executive committee presented the House of Delegates with a plan to enforce the Tripartite Plan and they endorsed it overwhelmingly. The new strategy, devised by Executive Committee Chairman Simon Jones, called for the plan to include "a direct contract" with each party and a "serial numbering system" whereby each item of every product in the contract would be assigned a number. The item could then be traced through each step in the transaction — manufacturer to wholesaler, wholesaler to retailer. Individuals who failed to follow the contract could be readily identified by the serial number.

Given this opportunity for enforcement, the executive committee then directed Secretary Wooten to contact the wholesalers and manufacturers and inform them about NARD's new plan. The proprietors had rejected the plan at their annual meeting and Wooten again faced the difficult task of convincing them to cooperate. This task the secretary relished. NARD had been frustrated by the manufacturers on each initiative they had tried to date. But this new plan was different. The direct contract and serial numbering system allowed violators to be clearly exposed and held accountable.

Wooten cautioned the membership to be patient and give the executive committee time to work out the plan. As he noted, our "work...in this connection does not consist in merely 'speaking the word and it is done.'" But he also assured them that "we are going to win out on this" because *"we must have it."* In the meantime, he encouraged the membership to remain loyal to the existing agreement. We must "hold fast to that which we have," he noted, "and get more at the very earliest possible moment." As a warning to those who may be less than patient and cooperative, Wooten said, "it should be

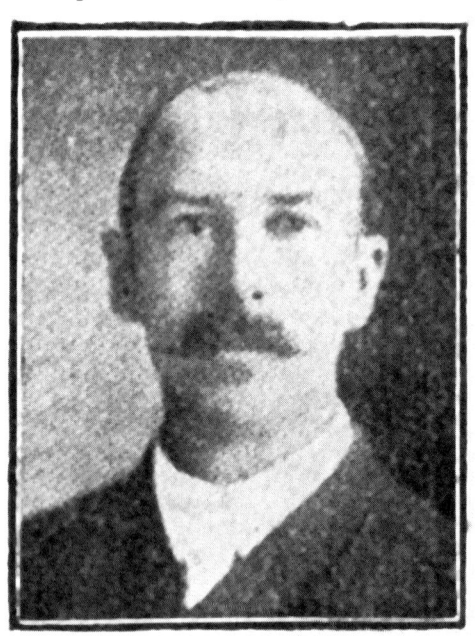

Charles M. Carr, head of the NARD Publicity Department and first editor of N.A.R.D. Notes

distinctly understood that the man or locality that fails to utilize the means that are available *right now,* but instead insists on having means that are *yet to be* brought within reach, places himself or itself, at once under suspicion as a mere *'kicker'* and obstructionist."

The Cleveland convention was important for other reasons. In addition to the Tripartite Plan, delegates also pledged financial support for the executive committee and central office staff. Since the founding convention, financial support for NARD had been limited and irregular, and the association had not been taken seriously by the other trade organizations.

Part of the reason for that lack of respect was the lack of regular communications with the membership. Information was limited to "bulletins" on special topics, direct correspondence, or local contact by members of the executive committee. At Cleveland, delegates approved a recommendation from the executive committee to create a "Publicity Department," which began publishing a weekly newsletter. Previous to this action, Wooten had been forced to produce an occasional typewritten, "information sheet" lacking in professional appearance and consistency.

The new publication, an eight-page printed document called *N.A.R.D. Notes,* was edited by Charles M. Carr. The publication made its first appearance October 18, 1902, and quickly became the central, unifying vehicle of

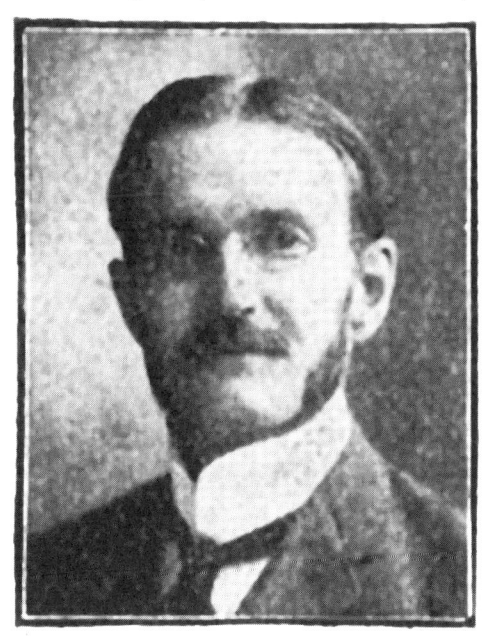

Joseph R. Noel, head of the NARD Organization Department and its field representatives who recruited new members

the association, as well as a formidable voice in pharmacy journalism. Published at the association office at 79 Dearborn Street in Chicago, *N.A.R.D. Notes* was priced at 50 cents, but was included in the price of members' annual dues. Not only did it serve as a regular reminder to members of the association's activities, but it also became the vehicle for publicizing the executive committee's policy decisions and keeping members informed about activities throughout the retail drug trade.

The NARD Publicity Department also worked closely with an "Organization Department" added the previous year at the association's annual meeting in Buffalo, New York. Under the leadership of staff member Joseph R. Noel and assisted by field representatives in key areas of the nation, the organization department was charged with the task of recruiting new members and serving as a "trouble shooter" for the association. The weekly *N.A.R.D. Notes* gave organizers a tangible product to place in the hands of prospective members while also serving as a valuable source of information about association affairs.

The weekly newsletter also gave Wooten the opportunity to target specific policy actions of the executive committee. In the early editions he focused on the issue of price cutting and singled out those companies that supported NARD's position and those that did not. *N.A.R.D. Notes* was hardly a month old before Wooten used its pages to launch a major campaign against the "cutters." Writing in the November 15, 1902, issue, he issued a challenge to the manufacturers. He wrote, "Will you, when specifically requested by the officers of the local associations of retail druggists throughout the country that are affiliated with the NARD refuse all sales to those price demoralizers whom the various manufacturers of *proprietaries* have designated as aggressive cutters?"

In commenting on his open letter to the pharmaceutical houses, Wooten wrote, "The line of demarcation between the friends of the NARD, and the allies of the 'cutters,' is becoming clearer and clearer, and it is the policy of the association from now on to force trading factors of every kind with which the retail druggist has to deal to take a position on the question of whom they serve." He chided those who violated the spirit of the Tripartite Plan through "inadvertence" and noted that the term had been greatly overused since the agreement had been implemented. It was time for the word and the practice to be "retired from active service."

But while Wooten and most of the NARD membership were enthusiastic about the Tripartite Plan, manufacturers were not. In the competitive world of proprietary medicine, individual companies were cautious about taking the first step toward cooperating with the pharmacists. To encourage some response, Wooten prepared a standard contract, or "agreement," for proprietors to use with both wholesale and retail distributors. The agreement was divided into two segments, which included not only standard prices manufacturers agreed to sell to the wholesaler, but also a minimum price below which the wholesaler would not sell to retail pharmacists. Wholesalers violating the agreement were subject to being fined up to $96.00 for each violation, while retailers who sold below the agreed price were charged $48.00 for each violation. Payment in each case was to be made to the manufacturer.

Copies of the agreement were sent to the major proprietary companies in early December. Wooten urged a quick response and pointed out that a similar plan was already enjoying "marked success" in Canada. Adopting such a plan in the United States, the secretary argued, would serve "the death knell of price demoralization and...substitution" and that this was the "best that has ever been devised for protecting proprietaries...."

Wooten's arguments apparently had some impact. Two weeks after the "agreement" forms were sent out, Editor Carr was able to report that "one of the leading proprietary houses of the country has decided to put the...plan in effect soon after the first of the year." He refused to identify the company out of concern that it would "induce cutters to concentrate their buying efforts...to pile up a stock of goods" before NARD's contract system could go into effect. However, he emphasized that "It is up to the retailers...to make the (plan) a success." He noted that "the direct contract and serial numbering movement has progressed to a point where...action of the retailers...is necessary to make the movement a success."

While waiting on details for implementing the new contract plan, Wooten again used the pages of *N.A.R.D. Notes* to urge unity and support for the association. In a strongly worded article entitled the "Future of the Retail Drug Trade," he emphasized that the still fledgling organization was at a crossroads. "If the N.A.R.D. succeeds...it will be to you that future generations of druggists will give credit for the heroic and successful struggle." On the other hand, if retailers failed to seize the opportunity, the secretary warned: "If the N.A.R.D. fails to solve the pressing problems which now confront the retail drug trade, if the movement finally disintegrates and the demoralized conditions that weighed down the trade immediately preceding the formation of the N.A.R.D., or worse, prevail again in the future, the druggists of that day can look back and point the finger of derision and scorn to you and say "Had you done your duty in 1902 and 1903 this calamity would not have overtaken us."

In mid-January 1903, NARD was ready to identify the Dr. Miles Medical Company of Elkhart, Indiana, as the firm willing to agree to the direct contract, serial numbering plan. Miles was not the largest manufacturing firm, but it had a wide-ranging product line and a nerve and liver pill that was one

By their fruits ye shall know them

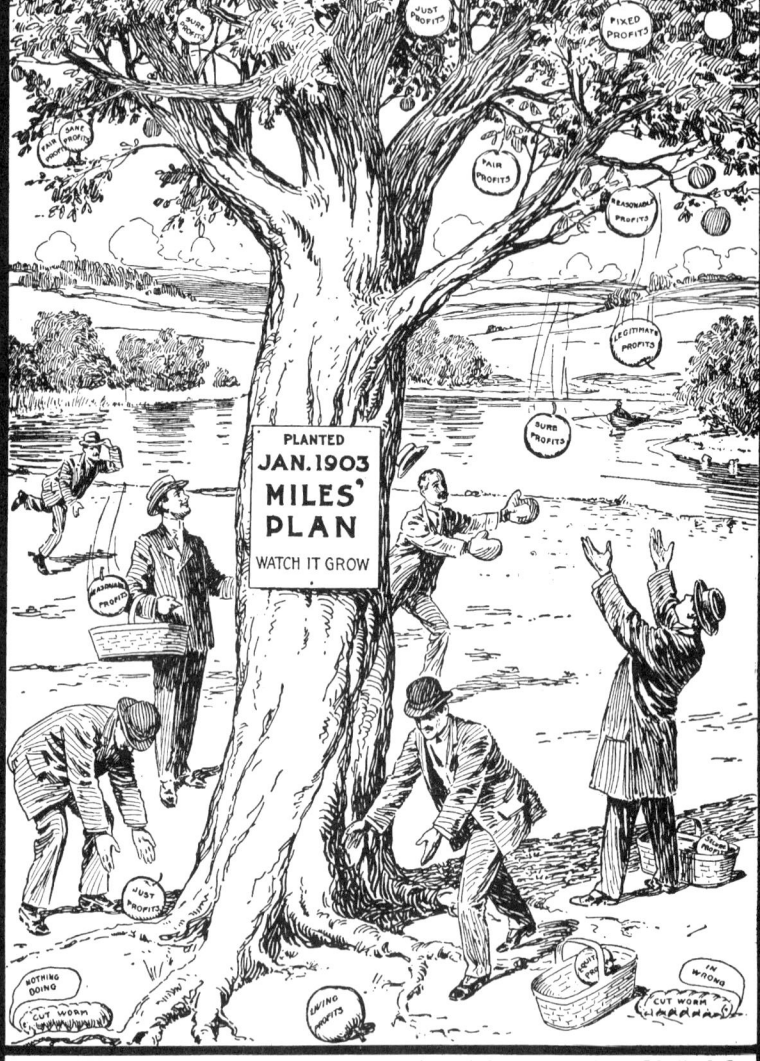

This hardy tree was planted in good soil by the Dr Miles Medical Co. Jan. 19th 1903. — It was blazed and branded "Dr Miles Plan", and thrived from the start, although many wind storms tried to uproot it. This tree continuously bears perfect fruit, which is uninjured by cutworms.

— *From Miles' 1906 Pamphlet.*

of the leaders in its field. It was a start, and as Wooten said in an open letter to the membership, "There is no doubt this system will work successfully if it receives the hearty support of the drug trade." Miles prepared 40,000 copies of the agreement, and NARD agreed to assist in distributing the forms through its local affiliates.

The mechanism for implementing the plan called for individual pharmacists to sign the agreement and return it directly to Miles — each druggist in effect becoming an agent for the company. The signed agreement constituted a contract and could be used in a court of law to prosecute violations — either by individuals or the company. NARD had no direct involvement in the agreement, but obviously enjoyed a significantly increased stature within the pharmaceutical industry as well as with the association's own members. In addition, its members derived benefits under the plan while NARD served as a clearinghouse for promoting it. As Wooten and the executive committee saw it, success with Miles would encourage other manufacturers to join the system and "within a few months all the standard proprietaries will be marketable under this plan."

Quick response was essential for the plan's success. Wooten said the next thirty days would be a time of "crisis," and he urged pharmacists to sign and return the forms quickly before the "cutters" had time to prepare a defense against the agreement. A number of druggists were ready to respond. A week after the agreement forms were sent out, the Miles Company reported that "contracts were coming in so rapidly they were buried under the avalanche." Perhaps more importantly, responses came from "all parts of the country," and company officials confidently predicted success with the plan.

Retail reaction to the Miles contract was encouraging, but before the plan could really succeed the wholesalers, the third party to the Tripartite Plan, had to be also brought on board. The Miles company reported to NARD that the "jobbers" were slow in responding to the plan, and Secretary Wooten placed the matter before the executive committee. Meeting in Chicago in late January, the committee discussed the issue at length, then voted to have Wooten contact his counterpart at the wholesaler organization and arrange a meeting with the latter's proprietary goods committee.

The two committees met the following week in Chicago. A.H. Beardsley, secretary of the Miles Medical Company, also joined the group. The wholesalers were quick to say that their reluctance to join the movement was due to the excessive paperwork involved. Their members handled so much inventory that to keep records on pricing and serial numbering for each item consumed too much time. Beardsley reported that his company had been made aware of that problem, and he presented the wholesalers with a bookkeeping system that he said would reduce their paperwork by 75 percent. He also offered to increase the discounts on Miles products for those jobbers who would participate in the program and agreed to eliminate the clause in the contract that penalized jobbers $96.00 for each violation of the pricing system.

Wooten reported that when the jobbers heard Beardsley's offer they were so "favorably affected...that their attitude was at once radically changed." The meeting ended on a high note with the wholesalers saying they were confident they could now sell the plan to their members. By the end of the month, Wooten was able to report that over half of the wholesale houses had signed agreements with Miles and with more than half of the retailers already on board, success of the program now seemed assured. However, the secretary said he would not be satisfied until a majority of the proprietary houses, and at least 30,000 of the nation's pharmacists, had signed on with the plan.

Four months after its adoption by the House of Delegates, "Resolution C, Manufacturers of Non-Tripartite Goods" now seemed a reality. There were still details to be worked out, and a considerable amount of monitoring of the process, but Wooten and the executive committee now felt comfortable in turning to other matters of interest to the association. Of the issues before them, the most pressing one was the association's financial condition. The

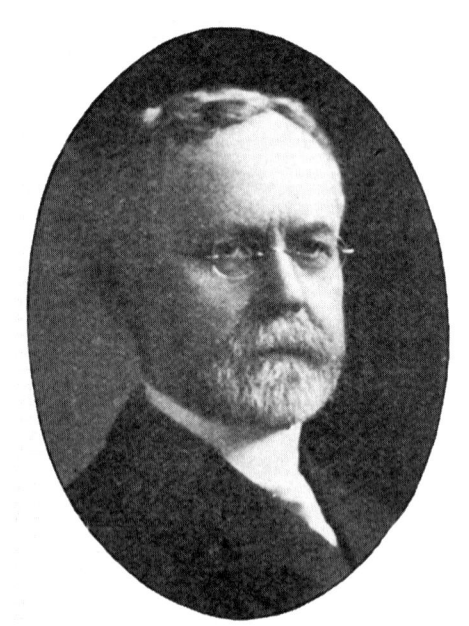

DR. FRANKLIN MILES
Originator of the Miles Remedies.

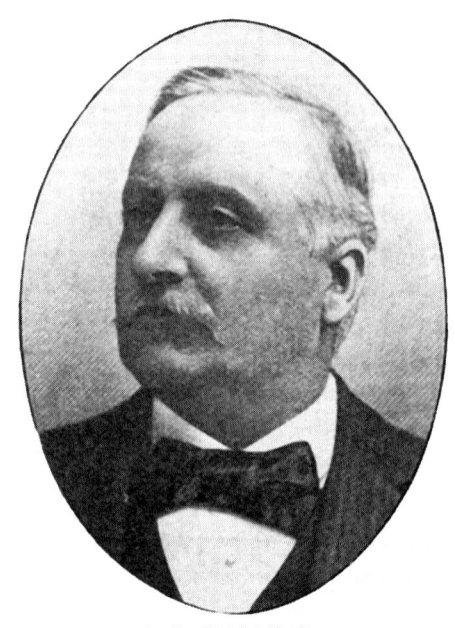

A. R. BEARDSLEY
Treas. and Gen. Mgr. Miles Med. Co.

campaign to implement the Tripartite Plan had been a severe strain on both human and monetary resources, and it was obvious, at least to the leadership, that the organization needed more money.

At the 1898 organizational meeting in St. Louis, delegates set annual dues at 25 cents per member. Those delegates with local or state association experience recognized that such a low fee was a mere token, but with little national experience or record of achievement, it was the most they could hope for. Before the first year was over, Secretary Wooten was forced to curtail activities and ask for donations just to keep the office open. Responding to his plea for a larger operating budget, the House of Delegates increased dues to 50 cents a year. However, even a 100 percent increase in the membership fee did little to change the association's financial conditions. Most pharmacists were reluctant to commit to the new organization until it had established some record of achievement, and even those most sympathetic to the cause were irregular in paying their dues. As a result, the cash flow was uneven at best and uncertain most of the time.

The cumulative effect of inadequate funding began to take its toll on the NARD staff. Wooten found it difficult to initiate any service or program on behalf of the membership, and a growing number of pharmacists began to question if membership in the association was worth the minimal fee. Clearly, independent community pharmacists were facing another roadblock in remaining an organization. As the executive committee prepared for the association's fifth annual meeting in 1902, Secretary Wooten laid his dilemma before them and asked for guidance.

Committee members, particularly Robert Smither (Buffalo, New York) and Thomas Voegeli (Minneapolis, Minnesota), along with Chairman Jones, were particularly sensitive to the issue. In their view, it was time to rethink NARD's strategy for building a national organization. The "cutter" issue was certainly the most pressing in the short term and the secretary was correct in making that the association's top priority. However, in the long run, the organization had to have a solid financial base and a vehicle to publicize its activities. In view of that observation, the group decided to ignore percentage increases for dues and focus instead on how much revenue the national office needed to run an effective operation, including developing a strategy for raising that amount.

According to Secretary Wooten's best calculations, there were approximately 40,000 retail pharmacists practicing pharmacy in 1902. Based on past experience, no more than one-fourth of them would be dues-paying members. The association's actual expenses over the past year were approximately $20,000. Given those numbers, it would take an annual fee of at least $2.00 per member to provide adequate funding for the national office.

The executive committee agreed to recommend the new fee. This, along with the amended "Tripartite Plan" and publication of a trade journal, represented bold moves and stood in sharp contrast to the association's work to date. But in the committee's view, the time had come to "risk success or be doomed again to failure."

Wooten and the office staff recognized that voting a dues increase in the enthusiastic atmosphere of an annual convention did not translate into a larger budget. Collecting was still the key to keeping the association functioning in a orderly manner. However, that task was made somewhat easier with the weekly publication of *N.A.R.D. Notes*. The increase was set to go into effect with the new year, and the secretary prepared a carefully worded appeal for support to run in the first January issue of the publication. Calling on the retailers to "take hold and help," he pointed out that the association was asking for $2.00 for a year's membership: "But what of that? Chicago journeyman barbers pay 60 cents a month, or $7.20 a year...and they are getting in return $5.00 per week, or $260 a year, in increased wages. As the professions go, the barbers do not rank as high as the pharmacists, but they evidently know a business proposition when they bump up against it."

But even the secretary's appeal to professional pride made little difference. New memberships were still slow and dues payments continued to dribble in throughout the year. In almost every issue, *N.A.R.D. Notes* Editor Carr included several reminders to "send in your dues," but with only limited success. By summer, the executive committee was again discussing a dues increase even as they tried to collect on the current year.

The "full-price" contracts and dues issues were matters of top priority, but NARD's national leadership was busy on other long-term projects as well. Perhaps of most immediate importance was a petition drive to reduce the tax on alcohol. To help pay for the costs of the Spanish-American War, Congress increased the tax on alcohol from 70 cents to $1.10 per gallon. NARD took the position that the tax was unfair since each pharmacist already paid a $25.00 revenue tax each year to be a licensed "liquor dealer" and, if not unfair, the tax was excessive and should be returned to 70 cents. Doing so would save retail druggists $1 to $2 million in costs per year.

Congress had a bill to reduce the alcohol tax under consideration, but it was blocked in the House Ways and Means Committee. Wooten was convinced that nothing short of a major lobbying campaign could move the bill out of committee. With executive committee approval, he prepared some 40,000 petitions and mailed them to each state and local association affiliated with NARD. The cost of printing and mailing the petitions placed an added strain on the association's meager budget, but the NARD leadership thought the potential benefits were worth the effort.

CHAPTER TWO — THE FIRST DECADE: 1899 – 1908

Our Goods (Spiritus Frumenti) a Pharmacopoeial Product, Strictly Pure

This is the Fine Old Liquor That You Should Dispense

Every progressive druggist knows the importance of dispensing GOOD whisky. The BEST liquor is none too good for MEDICINAL USE.

You cannot buy better than best—you cannot get more than most. In Old James E. Pepper whisky you get the best liquor distilled—and the most for your money.

For one hundred and twenty-nine years this famous old whisky has been distilled from the same formula. In uniformity, mellowness, fragrant bouquet and sparkling goodness no other whisky compares with

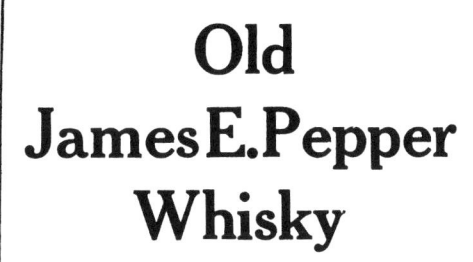

Old James E. Pepper Whisky

The fact that this liquor is conceded to be the best ought to influence you, Mr. Progressive Druggist, to dispense it exclusively.

There is profit, prestige and satisfaction in handling "the standard whisky—by which all other whiskies are judged."

Write us today for liberal proposition to members of the N. A. R. D. Address,

The James E. Pepper Distilling Co.
RECTOR BLDG. CHICAGO, ILL.
Distillery: Frankfort Pike, Lexington, Ky.

No Drug Store Stock Complete Without This Valuable Medicinal Agent

When writing advertisers, just say: "Saw it in our Journal of the N. A. R. D."

Another issue that claimed NARD's attention had to do with licensing trademarks and patents. Specifically, Wooten and the executive committee were concerned about American pharmaceutical companies obtaining patents on medicines manufactured in foreign countries when these formulas or chemicals were in the public domain. The issue that spurred NARD to action concerned the chemical "phenacetin" originally developed by the Bayer Company in Germany. That country, as did most European countries, did not grant patents on medicines "used in the healing arts." However, the United States did grant such patents. The drug sold in Germany for 25 cents an ounce, but was $1.25 an ounce in the United States. While the original intent of American patent laws may have been to encourage scientific investigation, NARD leaders believed that insofar as medicine was concerned, such laws had the opposite effect. In their view, the United States must join those countries who refused to grant patents on articles used in medicine.

Not all NARD activities were this high profile. The central office staff and members of the executive committee worked continually on the "little things" to improve pharmacists' income and professional standing. For example, the trading stamp movement made its appearance soon after the turn of the century as "stamp agents" tried to convince retailers to used their product as an inducement to customers. However, NARD took the position that trading stamps produced unhealthy competition and reduced profits among its members. As Wooten noted, "there is no room in the drug business for any such catch-penny methods."

Sunday closing also became a matter of increasing interest after 1902. Editor Carr commented in *N.A.R.D. Notes* that "druggists are entitled to one day's rest in seven," but NARD stopped short of endorsing this practice as national policy.

In another move to improve the professional standing of its members, NARD worked on a plan to bring its diverse membership into some type of "customary practice" regarding prescription services. Many customers often shopped from store to store seeking the lowest price on a prescription. With the direct contract, serial numbering plan in effect, NARD officials pointed out that pharmacists were now in a position to know what their wholesale costs were going to be and could therefore be more uniform in their own pricing. For an extended period of time, NARD had encouraged its members to adopt what it call "The National Price Mark and Creditor's Bureau System." Wooten explained how that system would work for pharmacists:

"A customer hands you a...prescription and asks "can you fill this and for how much?" Take the prescription immediately behind your prescription case, there consider your customer financially, his probable knowledge of the prescription, the amount of knowledge and labor necessary to compound, then make your price, which is for the entire association. Do not be in a hurry. Write the price in pen or pencil between the first and second lines or items on the prescription and so as not to attract attention. The N.A.R.D. cost mark is:

1 2 3 4 5 6 7 8 9 0
P H A R M O C I S T (sic)

Lastly, write your initials and address on the back of the prescription to direct attention from the true cost mark." In taking such an approach, pharmacists would not only present a more unified front to the public but also increase individual profits as well.

The improved health of the association was best illustrated by its response to an old problem — price cutting — which resurfaced in California during the summer of 1903. The problem began in 1900 in Los Angeles, California. That city's largest pharmacy — Owl Drug Company, locally known as the ODC — with stores also in San Francisco became involved in a price war with other retail pharmacists. NARD sent the chairman of its executive committee to California in an attempt to resolve the conflict. But with limited resources and without an enforceable pricing system, he was unable to get the area's pharmacists to settle their differences. As a last resort, he recommended that the Owl Drug Company be listed as an "aggressive cutter," and the NARD membership was so notified.

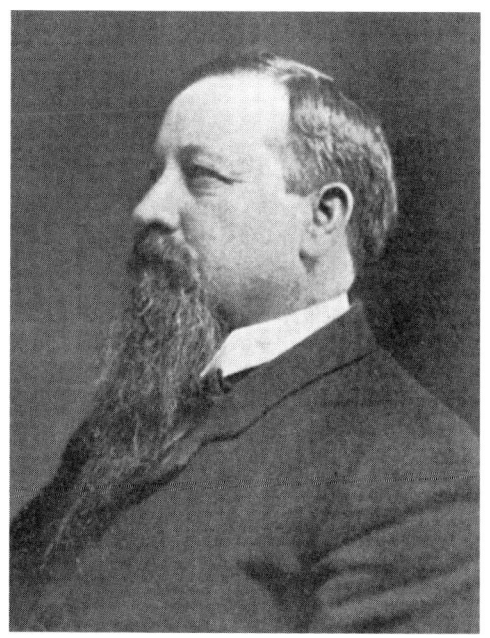

W.B. Cheatham of San Francisco who negotiated on behalf of NARD with Owl Drug

The California situation remained unchanged until NARD reached agreement with the Miles Medical Company on the amended Tripartite Plan. Retailers in Los Angeles, including the Owl Drug Company, agreed to accept the plan and, for a time, it appeared the price war had been resolved. However, in April 1903, the city's retailers learned that the ODC was receiving its inventory from its San Francisco supplier, which had not signed the Tripartite agreement, and ODC was again underselling its competitors.

The situation presented an interesting test case for NARD. Responding to the challenge, the executive committee sent W.B. Cheatham, an experienced and respected druggist, to try again to get cooperation. In an ironic twist of circumstances, he discovered that two large wholesale companies in Los Angeles were shipping their products to Owl Drug in San Francisco, and the latter store was sending the now retail products back to Los Angeles. Cheatham explained that even such indirect action was still in violation of the Tripartite agreement and tried repeatedly to get the wholesalers and ODC to stop the practice. For five weeks he traveled between the two cities enlisting other retailers and wholesalers who had signed the agreement to help persuade the violators to stop their destructive practices. But Owl and its two suppliers would not be deterred.

Losing the "battle" in California helped NARD take a big step toward winning the "war" against cut-rate drug prices. Admittedly, Cheatham had not been able to bring Owl Drug into the fold, but his efforts on NARD's behalf made a lasting impression on retail pharmacists on the West Coast and throughout the nation. Observing the association's methods and realizing the commitment NARD had toward improving their personal and professional standing made a lasting impression on pharmacists and was a major step toward making NARD a permanent organization.

NARD's efforts on the West Coast also earned the association new respect from other professional associations. Officers of the APhA invited Secretary Wooten to speak at their annual meeting. His speech was well received, and APhA delegates responded by passing a resolution urging "the several schools of pharmacy...to include in their curricula a course...to insure that the student is fully capable of properly managing a retail drug business." In addition, NARD First Vice President Lewis C. Hopp (Cleveland, Ohio) was elected president of APhA for the 1903-1904 term of office.

Further evidence of NARD's standing came in early September when the national office received word that President Theodore Roosevelt would meet with association representatives during NARD's annual meeting scheduled for October in Washington, D.C. Access to the president was unprecedented in the organization's nascent history and signaled that it indeed had come of age. Wooten and the executive committee were also convinced that the presidential audience would help motivate delegates to attend.

The leadership's anticipation of a successful convention proved correct. A record number of delegates registered (450) and the esprit de corps was at an all-time high. Being in the nation's capital had its benefits, but most delegates were nearly euphoric as they realized the extent to which the risks they had taken the previous year had paid off. The new publicity department and its publication, *N.A.R.D. Notes,* had succeeded beyond all expectations. As a "propaganda influence" for the association, Editor Charles Carr distributed cumulatively during the year 215,000 copies of the publication, and there were few individuals involved in the manufacturing, wholesale, or retail trades who were not aware of NARD's activities. With 6,000 first-year subscribers, most of whom had paid the 50-cent subscription fee, the publication was largely self-sufficient — requiring only a $600 subsidy in its first year and that was without selling space to advertisers.

The organization department in its second year of operation also had a glowing report. Using maps and charts, Department Director Joseph Noel pointed out the areas of the association's strengths and weaknesses and noted that interest in NARD had picked up noticeably over the past year. He rec-

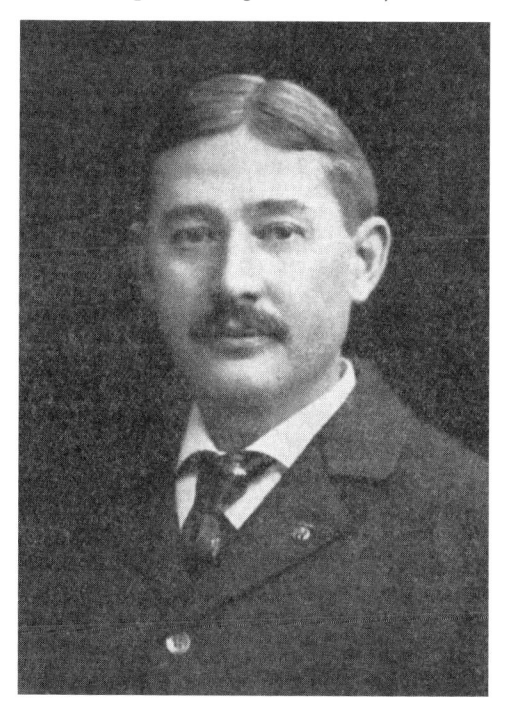

NARD First Vice President Lewis C. Hopp, who was elected president of the American Pharmaceutical Association, 1903 – 1904

ommended, and delegates approved, a plan to organize the nation in "permanent districts" with an "organizer" assigned to each and charged with the responsibility to recruit members and collect dues.

A key strategy in convention programming came on the second day when Secretary Wooten arranged to have representatives from the various proprietary drug companies address the delegates. In preparing for this session, Wooten had flyers outlining the "Miles Direct Contract, Serial Numbering Plan" widely distributed in the convention hall. He hoped to get a commitment from those companies similar to the one the Miles Medical Company had made to NARD.

Proprietary firms sending representatives to the convention included the Chattanooga Medicine Company, Peruna Drug Manufacturing Company, Chamberlain Medicine Company, Lydia E. Pinkham Medicine Company, Paris Medicine Company, Sterling Remedy Company, and World's Dispensary Medical Association. In addressing NARD delegates, each spokesman was careful not to criticize the Miles plan. However, they all "declared their inability to conform their respective business to the provisions until after they have become more fully satisfied as to the plan's merits."

Clearly, there was still a strained relationship between NARD and the proprietary group, but conditions were improving. When A.H. Beardsley of Miles "appeared on the platform, he was given an ovation" and the enthusiasm with which delegates responded to his remarks sent a clear message to the other companies. Wooten's plan to pressure the proprietaries into the contract, serial numbering plan did not work out exactly as he had hoped. But in the coming months, NARD did see a closer working relationship with these firms as many sent regular donations to the national office and purchased advertising space from Editor Carr.

The meeting with President Roosevelt was recorded in *N.A.R.D. Notes,* October 9, 1903, in the following manner:

"A committee was appointed to call upon President Roosevelt Tuesday noon and submit to him carefully prepared papers dealing with the trademark and patent laws as they relate to medicinal compounds. The N.A.R.D. is on record in favor of such amendments as will prohibit the issuing of patents on compounds, but will encourage the patenting of processes instead. The President gave the committee a cordial welcome, listening to arguments (by its members), following which he promised to give our association's proposals careful consideration."

As a first for the association, the visit with the president became the topic of much conversation among the convention delegates. The recreation trip to Mt. Vernon, Virginia, was also a "bonding" event for delegates and gave the leadership another opportunity to build on the concept of teamwork for the organization.

Another first for the convention came in the form of a daily newsletter. Each day Editor Carr produced a "Daily N.A.R.D. Notes" to keep delegates informed about all the proceedings. This "informal update" was particularly helpful as a unifying force and served as a press release to news organizations covering the convention. The final day of the meeting took on "a good old camp meeting, hallelujah time" atmosphere as Executive Committee Member Thomas Voegeli "exhorted" the delegates until "everybody got religion — NARD religion — and the sinews of war to carry salvation to the uttermost parts of drugdom." Voegeli then "passed the hat" and collected $13,252 for the NARD treasury. These funds would serve as seed money for the new year.

Thus, Wooten left the Washington convention with more optimism than at any time since Tillotson had first approached him about organizing pharmacists nationwide. The previous five years had all been "deficit years," and he had to personally loan the association money to keep it solvent. The clerical staff often had to wait to receive their paychecks, and members of the executive committee frequently had to pay their own expenses when doing association business. Now, he had almost one-third of his budget in hand even before the convention adjourned, and the delegates had approved an executive committee recommendation to employ a staff attorney. A fourth professional in the office would reduce the workload and no doubt improve efficiency as well.

The enhanced resources of the national office were soon put to the test. After returning to Chicago, Wooten interviewed several individuals before selecting Joseph W. Errant as staff attorney. Errant was still in the process of "moving in" when word came that the U.S. Commissioner of Patents had reviewed NARD's position opposing existing patent and trademark laws and categorically disagreed with the pharmacists. Patent law had not been at the top of Wooten's agenda, but the vitriolic way in which the commissioner responded caused the secretary to reconsider the issue, at least for the moment.

In writing his opinion, the commissioner gave a reasoned response to each of NARD's complaints. But, in his concluding statement, he wrote that "in each of these cases the commercial plans of the interested individuals appear to have been interfered with, and although in each case suffering humanity was pointed out as standing closely crowded behind their claims, and in whose interest alone the arguments were supposed to be made, the conclusion reached was that it was a commercial proposition and did not require any change of law." The commissioner's tone was as important to Wooten as the substance of his opinion. A national official presenting the association as greedy and manipulative was an affront that could not be left unchallenged. Conferring with the other staff members, it was determined that newly elected NARD President B.E. Pritchard should be enlisted to prepare a response to the U.S. Commissioner of Patents. In a diplomatically worded letter, Pritchard pointed out that the association's position was not a unilateral one, but one supported by APhA, NWDA, and PA as well. He also noted that NARD planned to use its influence to get the patent law revised in the next session of Congress. Errant began work immediately on the revisions.

The patent law controversy served as a good initiation for NARD's new legal department. However, it was only a momentary distraction to the larger concerns of the association. Wooten continued his efforts to persuade proprietary companies to sign contracts with the association and to motivate members to send in their dues. Carr revised the format of *N.A.R.D. Notes* and rearranged the masthead.

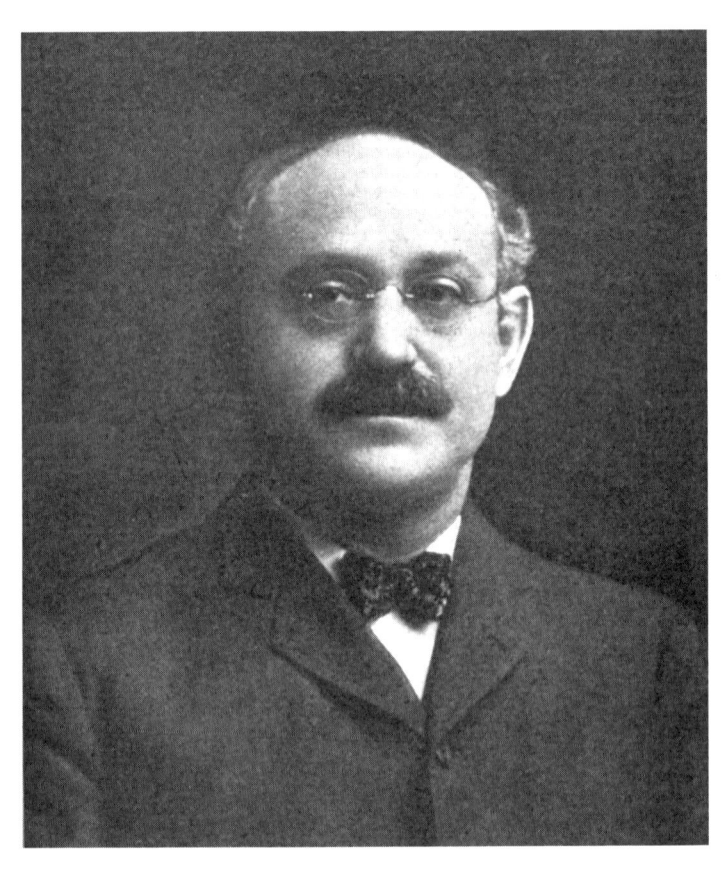

Joseph W. Errant, first legal counsel to NARD

The original publication featured NARD's first motto, "live and let live," centered in smaller type, just below the title. The new look, having bolder, block letters in the title and the motto moving to the last item in the publication data, made its appearance on November 6, 1903. Staff member Noel concentrated on increasing membership and watching for "hot spots" thanks to anti-NARD "propaganda" being disseminated by some individuals and groups opposed to the association.

In addition to patent law revision, Errant inherited a new legal problem soon after the new Congress convened in January 1904. Senator McCumber filed a "pure food and drug" bill that defined drugs as "any substance intended to be used for the cure, mitigation, or prevention of disease." In NARD's opinion, this definition was much too broad and would "produce endless controversies, widespread trouble, and frequent injustice."

The new bill was particularly objectionable because the association had previously endorsed a bill introduced by Senator Hepburn that defined a drug as "all medicines and preparations recognized in the United States pharmacopoeia for internal and external use." This definition was "comprehensive...easily understood" and had the support of the other "drug interests."

Errant prepared a petition pointing out the differences between the two bills. Both President Pritchard and Secretary Wooten signed it, and the document was mailed to the leadership of the U.S. Senate. Ironically, NARD's support for pure food and drug legislation brought the organization into conflict with some members of the proprietary association just as it appeared the two groups were moving closer together in their business dealings.

Other matters requiring Errant's attention in his first legislative session for NARD were the continued efforts by the association to reduce the tax on alcohol, a new series of bills to assist parcel post deliveries, and a House proposal to "prevent unfair and dishonest competition." None passed in that session of Congress, but Errant spent most of the winter and spring in Washington to monitor the bills' progress.

The parcel post bills caused Wooten to revise some of the association's priorities. Since its inception, NARD had philosophical differences with "mail order houses" and department stores including pharmaceuticals in their product line. (This was a harbinger for many more battles in subsequent decades to be waged against mail order pharmacy in all of its trappings.) The bills in question provided a major subsidy for the United States Postal Service to deliver "parcels" to rural areas of the nation.

As Wooten saw it, "the mail order system...and its triumph means the ruin of the retail interest of the country." The "rural free delivery," as critics were calling the bills, gave mail order firms a major advantage in the marketplace, and Wooten was convinced the association must take a strong stand against the legislation. He placed the matter on the agenda for the executive committee's spring meeting. The group subsequently reiterated its opposition to "mail order pharmacy" and promised to work toward defeating the bills in Congress.

Another item Wooten asked the executive committee to consider at its spring meeting was the matter of drug companies and wholesalers selling to physicians. Since its founding, NARD had "walked a tight rope" in its relationship with the medical community. Community pharmacists had to have the support of local physicians if they were to see any profit from their prescription department.

But physicians were still in the formative stage of their profession, and most were quite interested in maximizing their profits as well. Drug manufacturers routinely sent new products to physicians in an effort to encourage them to prescribe their use. The temptation was great for the physician to not only prescribe, but also dispense drugs directly to the customer. (This

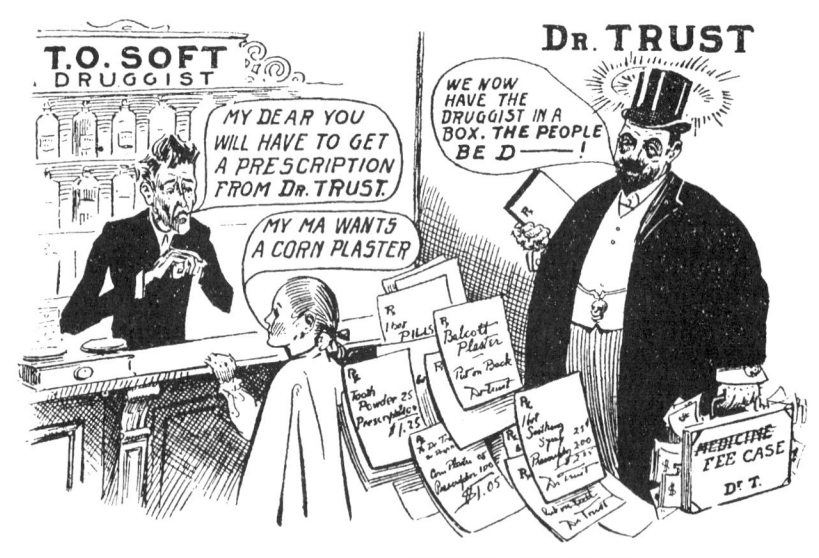

RESULT OF THE CLEVELAND BILL.

Any Person, Druggist or Pharmacist other than a Licensed Physician who prescribes or compounds for, or furnishes to any person any medicine or drug without a written prescription from a Licensed Physician, is guilty of a misdemeanor. This Act shall take effect immediately.

Legislation supporting physician dispensing was a constant battleground for NARD

issue proved to be a long-standing crusade that NARD was to wage on behalf of its members.)

Both NARD and the American Medical Association (AMA) officially opposed physicians' dispensing prescriptions. However, as Wooten pointed out, there had been too much "looseness in the matter of pharmaceutical houses and jobbers selling (to) physicians direct." Members of the executive committee agreed with that assessment and voted to have Editor Carr research the issue and list the "offenders" each week in *N.A.R.D. Notes.* Such action was minimal, but lacking legislation to adequately separate the two professions, it was the best the NARD leadership could hope for at the time.

The "dues issue," however, continued to be of concern. Collections were up over the preceding year, but still far below what the executive committee and staff thought they should be. The leadership was divided over how to deal with the problem. Some thought the association should place more emphasis on the organization department, while others supported a plan for the secretary to make a "direct mail" appeal to individual pharmacists.

After much discussion, it was decided that a pilot project should be launched in two states — one northern, one southern — with a direct mail solicitation for dues. Secretary Wooten was asked to write a personal letter to every pharmacist in those states, encouraging them to join NARD by sending their dues directly to national headquarters. The venture was expensive, but the costs were offset by the "large amount of missionary work...done" in promoting the name of the association and its accomplishments before the retail druggists' community.

Wooten selected Michigan and Alabama for his solicitation. He sent 1,400 letters to the former and 900 to the latter. Over the next six months, "an even 100 replies" dribbled in from the 2,300 letters, containing $42.50 in dues. It cost $84.73 to prepare and mail the letters — a loss of $42.23.

The small return from the direct mail campaign was disappointing enough, but as Wooten later reported to the association, "there were only a few recipients...who seemed to be really impressed" with the effort. In addition, the correspondence campaign led to only four new local organizations being formed and only 19 requests for information about how to organize. In Wooten's view the campaign had been a total failure, and he recommended that the association return to field representatives sent out by the organization department. (The use of field representatives and their one-on-one access to potential members in the regions they served proved to be the most effective form of membership acquisition in the coming decades.)

On other matters, NARD created a new "Honorary Membership" category; reiterated the association's opposition to druggists using "trading stamps"; asked that "wholesale druggists...hold a strict rein over wholesale grocers," when it came to supplying them with proprietary drug products; and urged retail pharmacists to consider installing "slot telephones" in their stores for the public's use.

In the months preceding the 1904 annual meeting scheduled for October in St. Louis, Editor Carr used the pages of *N.A.R.D. Notes* to educate pharmacists about issues and policies important to the association. At regular intervals he printed articles about the prescription department in the local store; the profits pharmacists could realize from a "slot" (i.e., customer pay) telephone; the relationship with physicians, wholesalers, and drug manufacturers; progress on the Mann (Patent-Trademark) bill; the need for members to pay their annual dues; and a variety of "helpful hints" designed to help the retail pharmacists realize greater profits.

Secretary Wooten used his office to emphasize pharmacy as a profession. The national mood of "progressivism," with its emphasis on political, social, and economic reform, placed the spotlight on professionals and small businessmen, and Wooten wanted to take advantage of that.

In public speeches, letters, and "circulars," Wooten urged pharmacists to exemplify that reform spirit and build the reputation of the profession. But, he argued, pharmacy's image was not helped when individuals engaged in "aggressive price cutting" and "product substitution." Such practices created "suspicion in the public mind" as to the product's integrity and the druggist's commitment to quality service. The secretary suggested that retailers could overcome this suspicion by adopting a price schedule, such as the Miles plan, and consistently adhering to it.

NARD's sixth convention opened in St. Louis on October 10, 1904. The near euphoric spirit that had characterized delegates at the last annual meeting had waned a bit, but the tempo was still upbeat. More than 800 members presented credentials as official representatives. Many of those had been present at the association's inaugural meeting and could not help but compare the current mood in St. Louis with that in 1898. Certainly, the association had made great strides, at least in the last two years. But there was still much to be done.

For Wooten and the executive committee the overriding issue continued to be finances. Increasing the dues from 50 cents to $2.00 had allowed NARD to expand its services, but failure of the "correspondence campaign" to add to the membership was an indication that more organization was necessary. The organization department was the most expensive account in the national office, but without it, the association had small prospect for growth.

In its regular pre-conference meeting, the executive committee decided to ask the membership to increase dues again — to $4.00. Some members of the executive committee worried that such a large percentage increase might cause a drop in membership, but when John Straw, chairman of the finance committee, presented the idea to the delegates, they approved the increase by a unanimous vote.

In addition to the dues increase, the executive committee also considered two other revenue-producing proposals. One was to endorse a "fire insurance company," chartered specifically for pharmacists as one of the first forms of group insurance. Members of NARD would purchase this insurance through the association with a percentage of the premiums allocated to NARD. The other proposal was to authorize the publicity department to sell advertising space in *N.A.R.D. Notes*. The executive committee accepted the insurance proposal, but fearing a product ad in the association's official publication might imply endorsement, the committee decided against selling advertisements.

Significant among the other business items at the convention was agreement to amend the constitution to allow the executive committee to "have charge of all business with full authority to act in the interim between annual meetings." Accepting that change represented an important step in NARD's development. Not only did it reflect a level of confidence in the national leadership, but it also allowed the association to respond to policy issues in a timely fashion.

Entertainment continued to be an important part of the annual meeting. Developing an identity as an organization among a group of "indepen-

---

N. A. R. D. NOTES

THE "LITTLE GIANT,"
Only Seventeen Months Old.

N. A. R. D. NOTES

Two Editions—Official Publication of The Retail Druggists' Great National Organization—Member of the Chicago Trade Press Association.

March Circulation, 62,126 Copies, larger than that of any other Drug Trade Journal in the World.

NO ADVERTISING ACCEPTED.

An early promotional ad for N.A.R.D. Notes. Later in the decade, advertising was accepted in the publication as an important source of revenue.

dents," particularly when they came from all sections of the nation, was a challenge. But activities away from the "business sessions" perhaps did as much as anything to draw druggists together and give them a sense of common purpose. The St. Louis World Fair organizers had declared Friday, October 14, as "Druggist Day" and that, coupled with other "outstanding entertainment" provided by the St. Louis area pharmacy association, developed a great sense of camaraderie among the delegates.

Wooten left the second St. Louis convention with another sense of accomplishment. Getting a significant increase in membership dues, authority to make policy decisions without waiting for the next annual meeting, and reestablishing the importance of the organization department were significant gains. That six additional proprietary companies agreed to support some form of the "direct contract" plan was a bonus.

The last half of NARD's first decade of existence was a time for solidifying its base of support. Traveling to Boston in September 1905 for the seventh annual meeting, delegates were struck with the "harmony and confidence" that permeated the meeting. The editor of the onsite "Pharmacy Bulletin" called the convention "the most placid, the least dramatic and sensational of the conventions thus far held; it was intensely enthusiastic and resolute, not a discordant or even a dissenting note marring the impression of harmony and union."

There were reasons for such feelings. The direct contract, serial numbering plan was working well, and the income it generated allowed the national office to provide more services to the membership. For the first time since the organizational meeting, NARD was self-sustaining and financially sound. Delegates readily agreed to increase the subscription price for *N.A.R.D. Notes* to $1.00 and Wooten told the membership the national office expected to spend about $100,000 on behalf of NARD causes in 1906.

The new year saw community pharmacists continuing to rally behind their national association in the wake of a tragedy. In April, a massive earthquake hit the San Francisco area causing damage of disastrous proportions. Wooten called a special session of the executive committee and gained their approval to set up a special "earthquake fund," and editor Carr published a special "California Relief Edition" of *N.A.R.D. Notes* to appeal to the membership for help, saying "'To Live and Let Live' should stimulate every druggist to action."

In addition to the central fund at NARD headquarters, a number of pharmacists used various approaches over the next several months to appeal to citizens in their local areas. The tragedy had a unifying effect on retail pharmacy as a profession as thousands responded to the call for help. By September when delegates gathered in Atlanta for the annual meeting, the fund had grown to almost $40,000 and funds continued to come in even a year later.

The association's eighth year of operation also saw another unifying factor. Wives of NARD members, who had informally met during the Boston meeting, reconvened in Atlanta to officially organize as an auxiliary group. Chartered as the "Women's Organization of N.A.R.D. (W.O.N.A.R.D.)," the group announced its purpose was "to unite more closely the families of the druggists...in bonds of sympathetic union."

The need for such an organization was best expressed by founding President Emma Gray Wallace. In addressing the first meeting, she noted, "the strenuous conditions which now govern the drug trade, the incompetency of drug store help and the fierce competition which demands the constant attention of the druggists (to such an extent) that he forgoes every social pleasure." It was time for "some organization which would promote the brotherhood and sisterhood of the profession." The group was officially recognized by the NARD House of Delegates and given a place on the convention agenda to report their activities.

The women's organization symbolically recognized subtle changes occurring in NARD. The early conventions had been largely attended by men and focused on business. However, as the health of the organization improved, the agenda shifted to include more time for social activities. This in turn led to a growing number of wives and children accompanying the men and attending the annual meeting as it became a major event for the host city.

Another first occurred at the 1906 Atlanta convention when 125 of the charter members from the St. Louis meeting formed an "Old Guard" organization. According to a brief statement printed in *N.A.R.D. Notes,* "the object of this organization is to encourage social relations at the annual meeting." Having a group of "alumni" was further evidence that NARD was coming of age. Editor Carr gave his endorsement to the group and commented, "May the 'Old Guard' live long, laugh much and wax fat and strong."

The feelings of goodwill extended well after the convention. However, a small cloud of doubt appeared amidst the optimism not long after the new year got under way. In April 1907 the U.S. Court of Appeals in the Sixth Circuit ruled that the direct contract plan violated the Sherman Antitrust Act. Wooten and the executive committee met soon after the decision was handed down and decided not to rush to judgment as to its consequences. The decision was appealed, and legal counsel Errant gave the executive committee a briefing as to the number of times the plan had been upheld. Chances seemed good that the case would either be overturned or remanded for clarification.

In the meantime, other plans went forward. The association continued its healthy growth and the various departments at headquarters seemed to have found a secure, even comfortable level of operation. Even news that most of the drug companies were canceling their participation in the direct contract plan did not seem insurmountable.

Indeed, there were many things over the past couple of years for which the association could be justifiably proud. That it had survived so long was an accomplishment in itself. Putting in place a national organization of some of the nation's most independent retailers and developing a name identity was significant. NARD's emerging political power, particularly its role in shaping the Mann Patent Bill and the Pure Food and Drug Law, were also something of note. Most of all, the organization was solvent, independent, and respected (even feared) in the drug trade. Wooten and the executive committee prepared for the ninth annual meeting with a high degree of enthusiasm.

The convention opened at the Congress Hotel's Orchestra Hall in Chicago on September 19, 1907. A special arrangement of J. Winchel Forbes's concert march "Live and Let Live" was performed by the Johnny Hand Orchestra for more than 2,000 delegates and guests. It was a festive occasion and the spirit continued through two days of meetings.

Delegates were particularly impressed with a new "Pharmaceutical Exhibition" hosted by the drug manufacturers. This was a new feature for the convention, and pharmacists were impressed at being able to see the latest pharmaceutical and store merchandise displayed in thirty exhibits by the largest drug companies. The more adventuresome could also take an automobile ride around the streets of Chicago — thanks to the local arrangements committee who had secured seventy-four vehicles for the activity.

From canvassing state delegations and talking with individual pharmacists, Wooten and the executive committee believed the time was right for an aggressive legislative campaign in the coming year. Rather than wait for the Supreme Court's decision, the association would chart its own course on matters important to the membership. Soon after the convention was concluded, the leadership began to plan a strategy.

Part of the new approach was to neutralize the negative publicity the association had received from the direct contract decision. In a series of articles to the membership, Wooten, Carr, and Errant denied, as had been charged, that NARD was a trust and that the direct contract plan was in any way a restraint of trade. The trio recognized they could not make their opinions binding, but at least they could educate the membership. As Carr editorialized, "The pharmacist's rights as a professional and business man must be recognized and respected, and through our offensive and defensive efforts, he is going to come into his own."

Unfortunately, the ambitious plan never really got under way. The lack of a contract led to a new round of intense competition in most sections of the country. The cooperative spirit began to fade a bit, and dues to the national association were among the first to suffer. Some pharmacists dropped out of the association because they were afraid they might be held personally accountable in the antitrust decision. The cash flow at headquarters slowed to a trickle, and members of the executive committee had to take out personal loans to continue the work of the organization. The low point came in early summer when the association was forced to give up its office space at 79 Dearborn Street and move to less expensive accommodations in the city.

Legislation and most other issues were lost for the year as the executive committee wrestled with finances and worked to curb negative publicity about the association. Secretary Wooten also decided it was time for him to retire and he told the executive committee of his plans at the mid-year meeting in May. Wooten had an attractive job offer in California where he had family, and the prospect of facing another battle over funding the association was more than he wanted to face. From the time of his announcement, until the convention opened in September, the executive committee spent more time talking about transition than about new legislation or member services.

The tenth annual NARD convention opened in Atlantic City, New Jersey. A spirit of uneasiness and some tension characterized the meeting. Some pharmacists blamed Wooten and the NARD leadership for the direct contract decision, others resented the negative publicity the association had received, and the jockeying for leadership positions limited the spirit of fellowship and goodwill that had been present in past meetings.

In addition to Wooten, Simon Jones, who had been chairman of the executive committee almost as long as Wooten had been secretary, announced his retirement at the end of the meeting. Both men were afforded a cordial reception, but the "prolonged applause," which typically greeted and interrupted their annual reports, was missing. The differences among the delegates became apparent when the nominating committee recommended the annual slate of officers. Typically, the committee's report had been "rubber stamped" by the House of Delegates — but not this time.

When the official slate of twelve nominees (six officers and six committee members) was presented, delegates immediately recognized that five of the nominees were from the current Nominating Committee. Six more on the slate were presently serving on the Resolutions Committee.

Murmurs of opposition immediately rose from the floor. One delegate from New Jersey openly complained that "he had never seen such politics played as in this convention." Another suggested that the nominees were not "loyal N.A.R.D. men." Secretary Wooten was moved to address the delegates and urged them not to "make too radical change in the management of the association's business affairs." Outgoing Chairman Jones felt compelled to offer an alternate list of nominees — rejecting all but four of the original slate.

Supporters of the nominating committee's recommendation protested that Jones's action was "unusual," but when the vote was taken, the Jones slate was elected.

Key among Jones's nominations was Thomas H. Potts who won the position of secretary by some 40 votes (out of 270 cast) to replace Wooten. Potts, current president of the association and a long-time active member in the Philadelphia Association of Retail Druggists, was fully informed about NARD's status and needed little orientation to replace Wooten.

The fight over electing officers was not the way Potts and most of the delegates wanted to remember the first decade of NARD's existence. In many ways, however, the disagreement was typical of the association. An independent-minded, culturally and geographically diverse group had seen the first decade as a struggle to keep focused. As Wooten said, the organization was in better condition than it had been ten years earlier, and he was confident that Potts could continue to move the association forward.

CHAPTER THREE

THE SECOND DECADE: 1909 – 1918

Economic Forces Reshape the Marketplace

*T*he selection of Thomas Potts as executive secretary facilitated an easy transition at NARD headquarters. Having served as president of the association, he was quite familiar with how the office worked and he knew the personnel on a first-name basis. Potts had attended the St. Louis, Missouri, meeting that established the organization and had been an integral part of the association's activities since that time. He also had extensive experience with the the Philadelphia Association of Retail Druggists.

These credentials were important because Thomas Wooten's shadow still loomed large over NARD. While Potts inherited a different organization, one thing remained constant — that of raising enough money to keep the association afloat and in business. Fortunately, the tenth convention, while acrimonious at times, did adopt two measures that contributed greatly to the organization's future financial success.

One measure was the delegates' decision to allow *N.A.R.D. Notes* to accept advertising. While the executive committee had approved advertisements in the "Pre-Convention Edition" of the publication each year, members had made a distinction between the special edition and the regular publication.

Editor Charles Carr had been lobbying for some time to gain approval for advertising and had even prompted the publicity committee to recommend such action at the 1908 convention. But that action was set aside by the resolutions committee whose members feared that advertising would force the association to compromise its independence. Carr revived the idea at the tenth convention and assured delegates that the publication would be quite selective in its choice of advertisers. This time the measure passed.

The new *N.A.R.D. Notes* or "Greater Notes," as the publication was dubbed, proved an instant success with both advertisers and members of NARD. The increased income also came at a critical time for the association. Carr was able to report more than a $13,000 surplus in his account at the Louisville, Kentucky, meeting and profits continued to build in succeeding years. Perhaps of equal importance, advertising helped NARD begin to develop a professional relationships with manufacturers that repeatedly paid dividends in promoting association issues.

A second key decision at the Atlantic City, New Jersey, meeting in 1908 involved keeping the organization department intact. This department, consisting of General Organizer Frank C. Ulrich and eight to ten field workers, was the most expensive item in the NARD budget. It came under intense scrutiny whenever a financial crisis developed. There continued to be a widely held view among some in the association leadership that direct mail solicitation for dues collection was more cost-effective. However, while Wooten had disproved that theory with a pilot project in Michigan and Alabama, it was an idea that died slowly. The argument was revived at Atlantic City, but delegates voted to retain the department.

Ulrich was forced to reduce his field organizers by two in 1909. But by focusing just on "dues paying members," aided by the new look in *N.A.R.D. Notes* (the name was changed to *The Journal of the N.A.R.D.* in 1913) and the "bulletins" produced by the secretary and executive committee, field work-

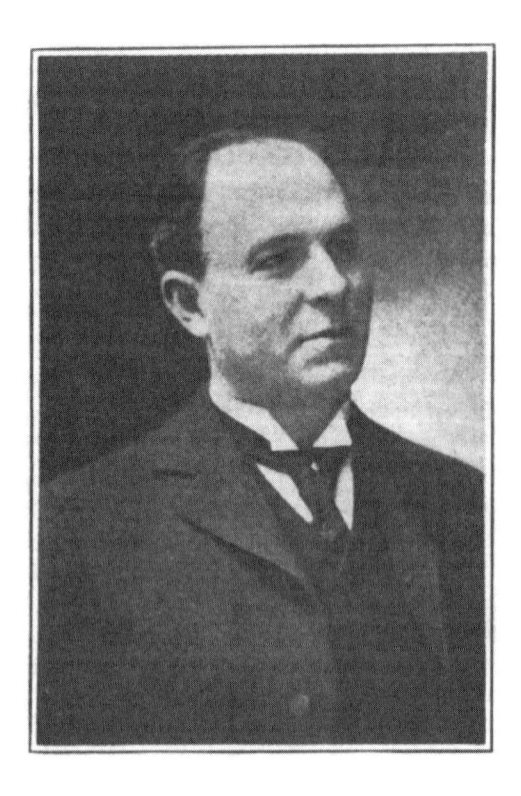

Thomas H. Potts, NARD Executive Secretary, 1908 – 1917

ers were able to effectively promote the association to retail druggists and thus gain an even greater measure of support. This approach, in Ulrich's words, "gives the dues paid member something the other fellow cannot get. Self-interest helps him to see the necessity of helping to maintain the National Association."

At the Louisville meeting in 1909, Ulrich reported a surplus for his department of over $20,000. Speaking to the delegates, he said, "Those who are experienced in association work know that if it were not for our field representatives interviewing druggists throughout the country, acquainting them with the work which is being done and is being planned for the future and thereby keeping them in line, the association's present condition, financially and numerically, would be very different from what it is."

Ulrich's point was well taken. The value of the organization and publicity departments was not in what each cost the association, but in developing and extending NARD's presence and purpose to a wider audience. Of more immediate consequence, profits from these departments allowed the headquarter's staff to move back into the Dearborn Street office space they had been forced to vacate the preceding year.

Secretary Potts kept a fairly low profile in his first year in office. Fortunately, for the first time in several years, there was no pressing legislative issue, and he could concentrate on the organization's infrastructure. Beyond finances, there were two areas that he felt needed special attention. One was repairing the professional image of community pharmacy that had been damaged by the adverse publicity surrounding the court decision on the direct contract plan. The other was developing a closer relationship with the American Medical Association (AMA).

Calling upon members of the executive committee and utilizing the services of the new "Propaganda Committee," he set out to educate pharmacists, physicians, and the general public about NARD's strong commitment to professional standards in the drug industry. Using the 1908-1909 officer corps, particularly President William S. Elkin Jr. and Executive Committee Chairman Charles F. Mann, NARD representatives traveled to most of the major cities to meet with physicians. Their message was not only a strong commitment to drug standards as defined by the United States Pharmacopeia and National Formulary digest (USP and NF, respectively) but also, as Chairman Mann said, "to get physicians back to the so-called first principles in prescribing."

This strategy had a measure of success, at least temporarily. President Elkin noted at the Cincinnati, Ohio, convention in 1909 that "the past year has...seen more get-together meetings of druggists and physicians than have ever occurred before." The NARD team was confident that "the active propaganda work (brought) the physician and pharmacist into closer relations" and that the "evils of self-dispensing and counter-prescribing" would be, if not eliminated, greatly reduced.

An unstated but clear purpose of NARD's leadership was to establish the association as more than a retail organization. Indeed, a defining purpose in the association's original charter as an organization was to stifle a patent medicine industry that was out of control. Being a major player in defining drug standards not only was important professionally, but it also had obvious retail advantages as well.

To be recognized, however, Potts and the NARD leadership realized that NARD must have a seat at the decennial USP convention. Since 1830 when Congress established the USP, this organization had met every decade to review and approve drugs for the National Formulary Digest. Participation in the discussions was limited to those organizations that were incorporated and actively involved in the drug/health care industry at least five years prior to the decennial meeting. The ninth USP convention was scheduled to meet May 1, 1910, and Potts wanted NARD to be there.

In an effort to earn a place at the USP convention in May, the propaganda committee since the NARD Louisville convention the previous September had kept a steady flow of information about the professional (pharmaceutical) aspects of the retail trade, which led NARD to become quite confident that it would be admitted to the convention.

But to the leadership's dismay, NARD was denied membership in the ninth USP convention. Although the source of opposition to retail pharmacy's participation was cloaked behind a committee recommendation, individuals close to the convention's inner workings indicated that the AMA was a primary opponent to the "retail trade" being part of the "scientific" discussions. Potts and the officers appealed to the convention as a whole, but were again refused. Neither APhA nor the key manufacturers came to NARD's defense.

The USP incident proved quite embarrassing and upsetting to the leadership. Chairman Mann called the action "unjust and unwarranted," but also said that it was pointless to "attempt to analyze the motive." Instead, he suggested the association should plan for the future and be even better prepared for the next USP convention. President Huhn said the action "has helped the association more than it was hurt" because it violated the principle of "fair play and a square deal" and the denial helped pull NARD together.

Other issues of concern to NARD in its second decade included the relationship between mail order houses and the U.S. Postal Service, Sunday closing, "slot" telephones, a price protection plan to replace the Tripartite Plan, the emergence of chain stores as an economic threat to independent retail pharmacists, the continuing pattern of physician dispensing, and a variety of federal legislation.

In this decade, mail order became an old issue in a new package. The association had opposed practices employed by the mail order houses since its inception. But early in 1910 a new dimension was added. Representatives of the nation's agricultural interests joined with the pharmaceutical mail order industry and persuaded Congress to consider "parcel-post" legislation.

Combining mail order with a free, or greatly reduced price, delivery system was threat enough to NARD. But when "itinerant drug vendors" joined the mail order team, the whole scheme became intolerable. President Henry B. Guilford called on his fellow community pharmacists to take note of the danger, saying "very strong efforts should be made to suppress this evil. The

A Modern Business Pharmacy; Its Good Points

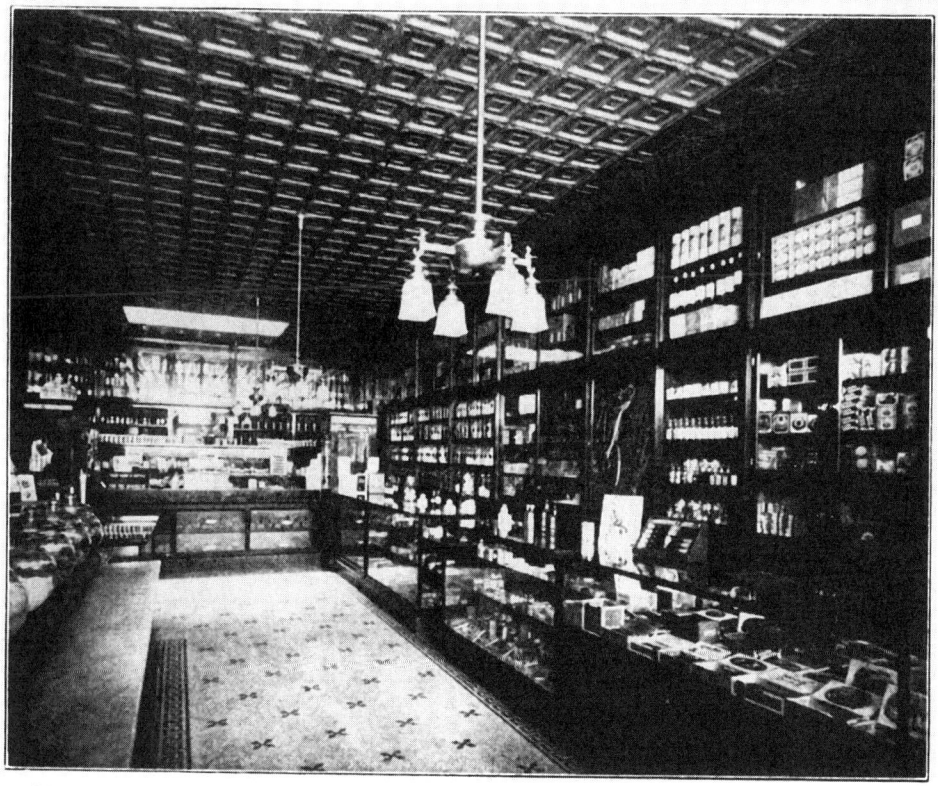

Pictured above is a 1910 NARD member store interior, a new feature of N.A.R.D. Notes, The Journal of the N.A.R.D., to help members become better merchandisers.

mail order houses...who have a large trade on their fancy goods and toilet articles are now beginning to appoint walking house-to-house agencies for the sale of these drugs and pharmaceutical preparations."

Despite NARD's concern, Congress considered several legislative proposals designed to subsidize freight rates on parcel post. The language that emerged with the most support came in an amendment to the Post Office Appropriations Bill. It gave the Postmaster General broad discretionary powers to assign shipping rates. In the original bill it was a flat rate without regard to the distance a package was shipped.

NARD opposed parcel post in any form and particularly opposed the single rate. Lacking support to defeat the full proposal, NARD moved to amend the bill and have the rates at least fixed by zone. NARD Legislative Committee Chairman William S. Richardson and Secretary Potts organized a telegraph and letter campaign to members of the Senate Post Offices and Roads Committee and succeeded in getting the amendment included in the final bill.

This "half a loaf" was hardly grounds for celebration at association headquarters. NARD's goal had been to defeat the entire measure. However, in characteristic fashion, the leadership put the matter behind NARD for the moment and moved on to other issues.

Another issue was a standard "Sunday Closing" policy that became a repeated concern for delegates to annual conventions. Almost everyone favored reducing the number of hours spent at the store during the week and particularly closing the store altogether on Sundays. The women's group (W.O.N.A.R.D.) strongly advocated that position and *The Journal of the N.A.R.D.* regularly ran testimonials about the value of having a day away from work. An article in the publication from an anonymous writer explained the situation this way: "I saw my father pass into an early grave. Our home hardly knew his presence. He was a stranger. He was always at the store. He came home after we had retired and left before we were up. He never tasted the joys of life that count. He never had time for a hobby. He became a mere machine."

Secretary Potts was sympathetic to the issue and said, "it is one of the most important matters we have to discuss at this time." However, he and the executive committee consistently maintained that Sunday closing was a local matter and had to be worked out among the community pharmacists.

The readily available slot telephone in the pharmacist's store was another issue NARD left to local proprietors to resolve. The issue emerged when improved technology allowed the Bell Telephone Company to provide commercial customers with a "slot" or pay telephone. Most community pharmacists had a long-standing tradition of allowing the public free use of the store

CHAPTER THREE — THE SECOND DECADE: 1909 – 1918

Sharpening Up for the Fray

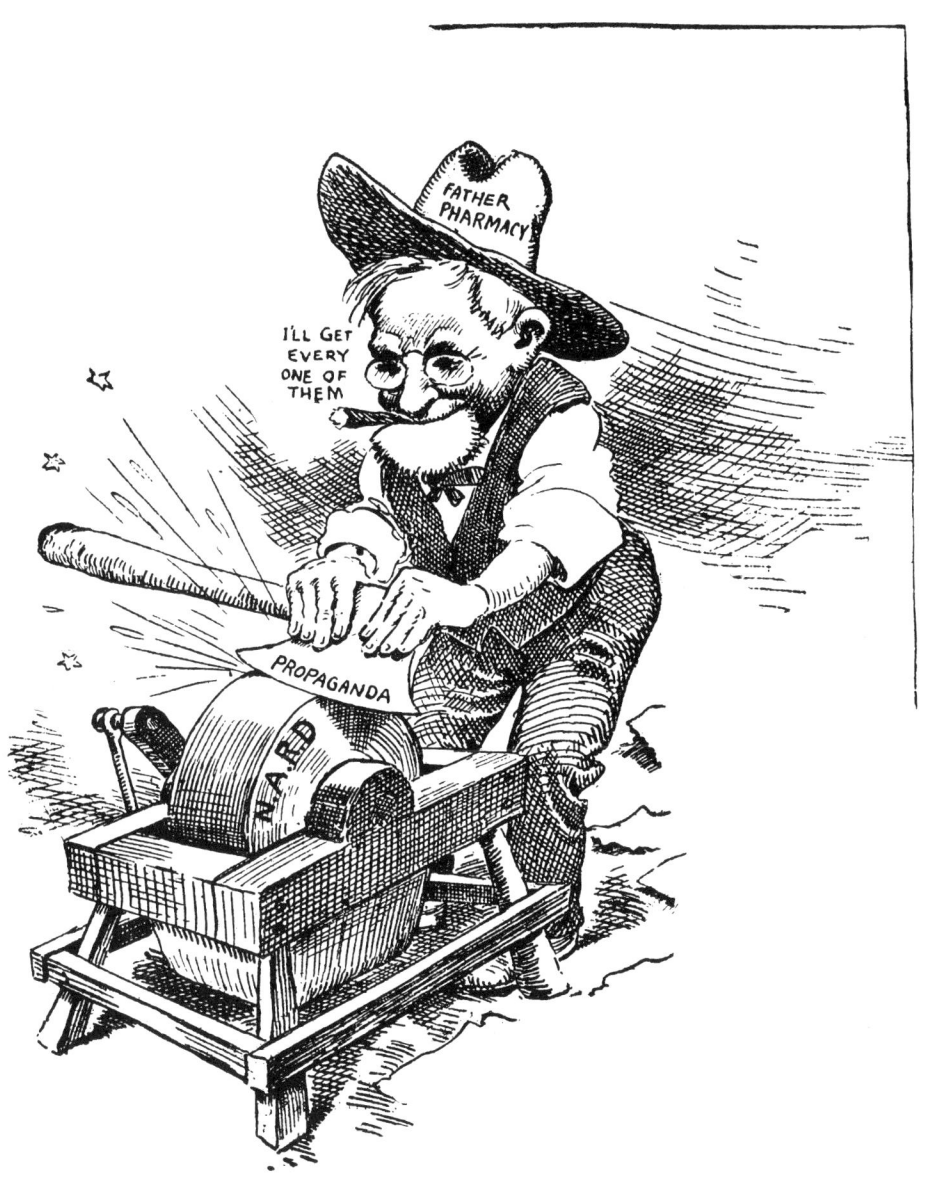

NARD's Old Father Pharmacy put a "keen edge on Propaganda," saying "legitimate pharmacy in action means decapitation for all Prescription Products which are committing high crimes and misdemeanors against honesty and efficiency in pharmaceutical and medical practice."

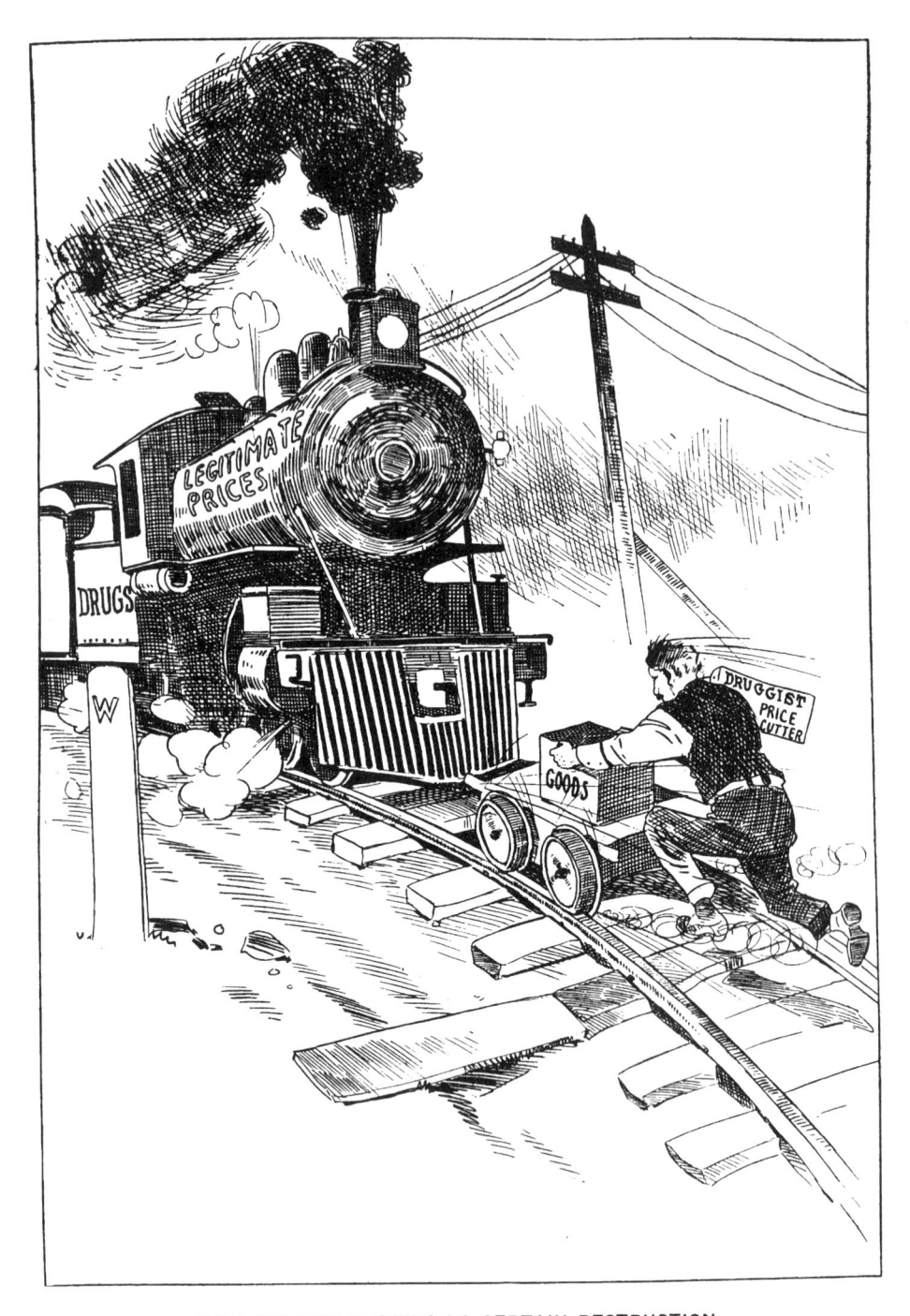

THIS FELLOW IS GOING TO CERTAIN DESTRUCTION.

This Cut Typically Illustrates the Danger in Which the Price-Cutter Constantly Finds Himself.

telephone. This practice frequently worked to the detriment of the store when callers tied up the phone and prevented customers from calling in orders. Many "customers" also came into the store only to use the phone.

This new "customer pays" phone was coin activated and kept the "store phone" available for business purposes. NARD became interested in the slot telephone because of its possibilities of earning money for community pharmacists. Under Wooten's leadership, the executive committee had gained approval from the House of Delegates to form a "Telephone Committee." The committee was charged with the responsibility of researching the phone issue and keeping the membership apprised of advantages and disadvantages to pharmacists providing that service to their customers.

William Bodemann of the Chicago Apothecaries Association was appointed chair of the new committee. He began an energetic campaign to point out the advantages of the service and urged all community pharmacists to adopt it. However, not all druggists shared Bodemann's enthusiasm. Before the slot telephone became widely available, some worried about its impact on "competition" and whether or not it would be cost-effective.

A corollary issue derived from the wide variance telephone companies charged for installation of slot telephones and the rebate paid to pharmacists for providing the service. Some pharmacists received as little as five percent of the revenue generated by the phone, while others were paid as much as twenty percent.

The association was repeatedly asked if it could develop standard criteria to serve as a guide for retailers. But other than keeping members informed about the practices related to the service and using persuasion with the Bell Telephone Company as to consistency in its rebate practices, a series of executive committees over a twenty-year period could not develop a standard policy for all of the membership. By 1920, the technology had become so widely used that the members' concerns became moot.

The association also continued to focus on emerging marketplace factors that would affect the business practices of community pharmacists in this decade and decades to come. In one instance, after the Tripartite Plan was declared unconstitutional, a number of community pharmacists became interested in "cooperative buying" as a price protection measure. The executive committee reviewed several cooperative buying proposals between 1908 and 1910, but did not find a way to make the concept an association-sponsored program similar to its sponsored insurance program launched the previous decade. In the words of President Charles Huhn, NARD was concerned about "running amuck of legal restrictions" and was reluctant to enter into another agreement. Instead, the leadership encouraged pharmacists to establish local buying clubs that would be sensitive to community interests.

While not opposing cooperative buying, NARD leaders cautioned local retailers to carefully monitor their practices. Unless the pharmacists did so, they could easily become a mere front for "jobbers" and manufacturers to pass on a particular product line without real consideration for their customers.

The House of Delegates at the 1911 convention in Niagra Falls, New York, passed a "mandatory resolution" instructing the executive committee to develop a new price protection plan. At its December meeting, the committee

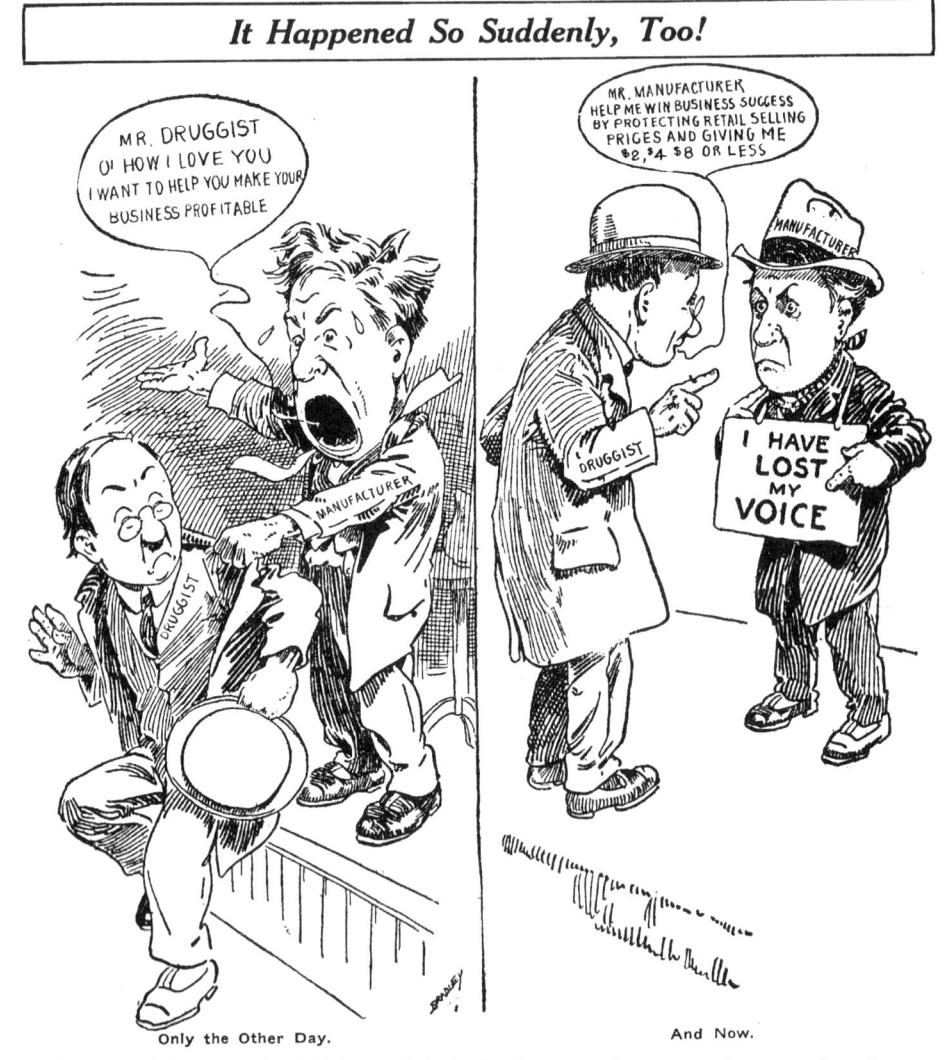

An editorial cartoon in 1911 noted the lack of support from manufacturers for price standardization.

responded. Enlisting the services of special attorney Frank H. Freericks and soliciting the help of former Executive Committee Chairman Simon Jones, a major architect of the Miles Medical Plan, the group developed a proposal that combined some of the Miles Plan's serial numbering approach with a system developed by druggist John Boehm of the Chicago Retail Druggists Association.

The modified Miles-Boehm Plan was based on a "coupon system." Retailers signed no contract but bought inventory through their normal suppliers. Manufacturers agreeing to participate in the plan printed discount coupons to accompany their respective product line. After receiving this merchandise, the store owner simply collected the coupons and returned them to the manufacturer and received credit toward the next order or a cash reimbursement.

Freericks took the proposed plan to Minnesota Senator Moses Clapp, chairman of the congressional Senate Interstate Commerce Committee. Clapp introduced the bill in May 1912 and held hearings, but was unable to get enough votes to get it out of committee.

Further bad news came during the fall session of the U.S. Supreme Court. While not issuing an opinion directly involving NARD, the court reaffirmed lower court decisions prohibiting "the fixing of resale prices through common channels of distribution." Outgoing President Henry W. Merritt told NARD members that they should not expect help from the courts on price protection and that it would be "idle to speculate on a change in the attitude of the court by a change in its personnel." Even if President Woodrow Wilson did have the opportunity to appoint new members to the court, Merritt said that "he (the President) will take care that the appointee shall be thoroughly anti-trust in his opinions" and that the high court's interpretations would not change.

Rather than wait for a new court, Merritt urged his fellow pharmacists to take the initiative and develop their own plans. He offered three possibilities. One was cooperative buying. A second possibility was purchasing items within the boundaries of the pharmacists' host state and thus avoiding the rules of interstate commerce. A third plan, buying on consignment from the manufacturers, was the concept embodied in the Clapp bill. Merritt was still hopeful that NARD could keep that proposal alive.

Although it was not yet apparent, the issue of price protection was assuming a larger scope. In 1913, a group calling itself the American Fair Trade League emerged. This collection of "manufacturers, retailers, and laymen" was committed to price standardization. In this organization, NARD found a valuable ally, and while it would take more than two decades to produce results at the national level, the wait was more than worthwhile.

Secretary Potts and his colleagues were equally concerned about "the Chain Store." This new marketing device made its appearance soon after the turn of the century and in the words of NARD President Charles Huhn, it had the potential to turn retailing "into a mighty war unless the means to checkmate the inroads on protected and unprotected goods be adopted." But finding a means to counter the growing popularity of chain stores was difficult because these stores had enormous purchasing power in the wholesale market.

While NARD wanted to follow its "live and let live" motto, the competitive practices employed by chain marketers made "living" all but impossible. As a first strategy, members of the executive committee decided to enlist the drug companies and wholesalers in a front-line defense. As Chairman Mann noted, "If the chain-store disease spreads, it will annihilate neither the jobber nor the manufacturer, but the tendency will be to reduce the number and handicap business progress for the remaining to a extent hitherto unknown." Through the subtlety of understatement, NARD hoped to convince their partners in the drug trade that the chain store was a bigger threat to them because they had more to lose. (The NARD argument proved to be unpersuasive as the chain store movement gained momentum and status within the pharmaceutical community.)

Relations between NARD and AMA remained stained over the physician dispensing issue. By the turn of the century, drug manufacturing became more complex, and the public placed an increasing emphasis on "pure food and drugs." Leaders of NARD did not think that physicians were adequately informed about the variety of drugs and their various interactions that could endanger public heath.

Physician dispensing was particularly problematic in the area of habit-forming drugs. In an editorial in *N.A.R.D. Notes* shortly after the 1910 convention, Editor Carr criticized the practice and noted that "the reckless dispensing of habit-forming drugs by physicians is responsible in most instances for the army of 'dope' fiends which curse our land." Some pharmacists wanted to push for immediate legislation that would prohibit physicians from dispensing their own prescriptions.

In a sharply worded resolution by the House of Delegates during the 1913 convention, the delegates declared that "physicians who choose to be their own pharmacists shall furnish their patients with prescriptions for all remedies applied, just as they would if the prescriptions were to be dispensed by licensed pharmacists, and that in case of fatal termination where physicians have dispensed their own medicines, the local health officer and not the dispensing physician shall certify to the cause of death." While obviously lacking opportunity to enforce the measure, it nevertheless represented a

CHAPTER THREE — THE SECOND DECADE: 1909 – 1918

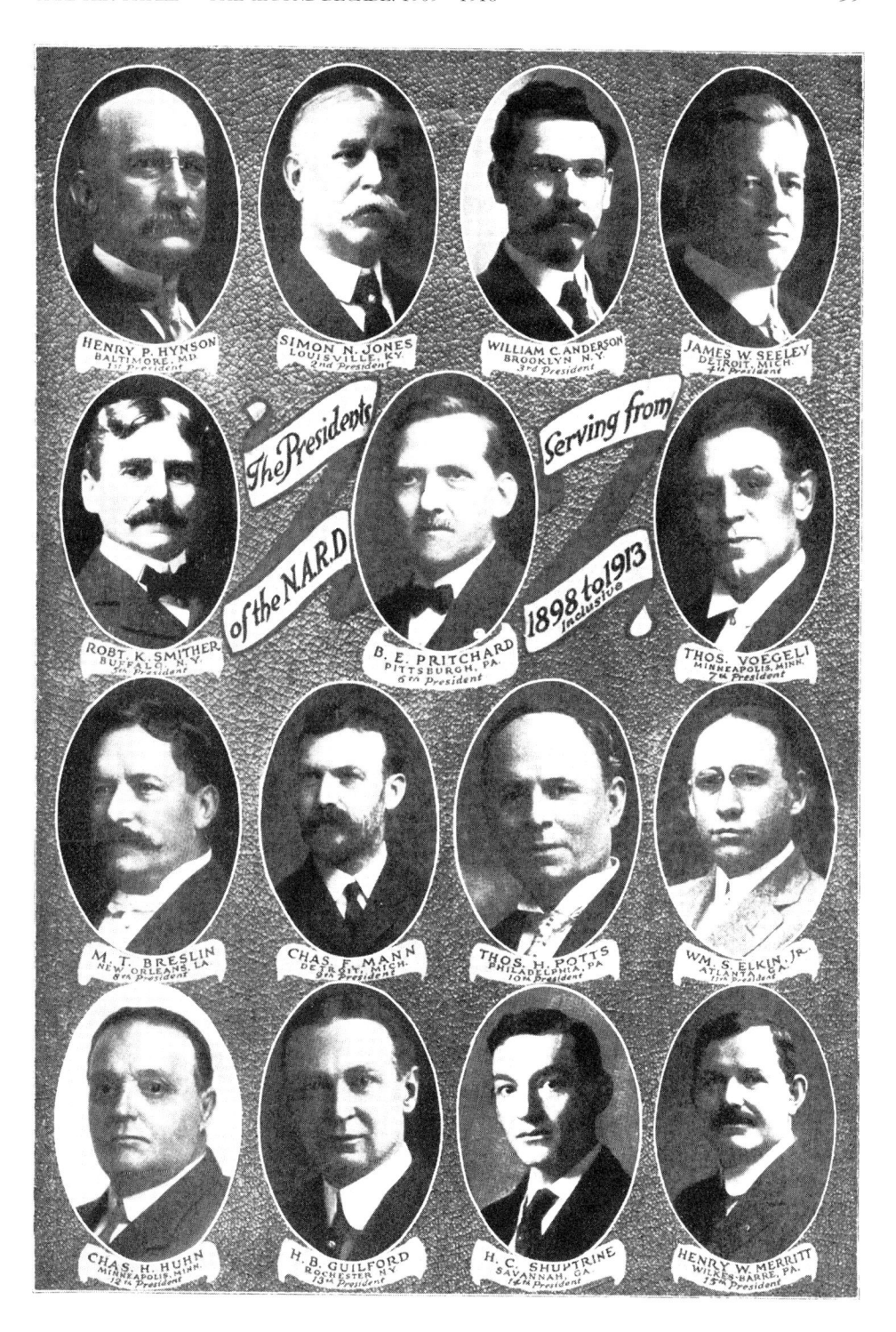

widening gulf that even the leadership of NARD and AMA could not readily bridge.

Other professional alliances were also under strain. Although the American Pharmaceutical Association (APhA) had never made retail pharmacy a priority among its leadership, membership, or policy-making bodies, most NARD members still held out hope for a mutual alliance between the two organizations. The two groups held various joint meetings, invited association officers to address one another's conventions, and talked regularly about their common interests and needs.

But former APhA President J.H. Beal may have summed up the relationship best in a speech to the 1911 NARD convention on the matter of NARD and APhA cooperation. He said, "Frankly, I do not believe that the American Pharmaceutical Association could perform its own work...if it should attempt to perform your work in addition, and speaking with equal frankness, I do not believe that the National Association of Retail Druggists could succeed half so well in its chosen line of work...." Thereafter, for a variety of reasons, some personal and some professional, the two organizations maintained a fraternal but distant relationship.

Perhaps it was coincidental that when APhA revised its constitution in 1912, it allowed affiliated associations to send only three official delegates to APhA's annual convention. NARD revised its own constitution in 1913 and reduced APhA's official delegation from five official delegates to three.

As the new century reached its teen years, a new set of issues began to appear on the NARD agenda. One was sales of alcoholic beverages in community pharmacies. To maximize profits and in some cases stay in business, an increasing number of local pharmacists began to stock beverage alcohol as part of their "front-end" business. The NARD leadership and House of Delegates condemned such practices and called upon all pharmacists to refrain from stocking or selling non-medicinal alcohol.

Drug addiction also became a problem for a growing number of Americans. By 1914, the U.S. Congress had taken note of the issue and several congressmen had introduced legislation to respond to the problem. One piece of legislation — the Harrison Interstate Anti-Narcotic bill — garnered NARD's attention.

In its original draft, the bill placed tight restrictions on pharmacists by requiring them to keep detailed records on prescriptions involving narcotics. That provision was acceptable, but NARD leaders argued the same language should apply to physicians. AMA strongly opposed such restrictions, and both the NARD and AMA lobbied hard for their respective positions. But while the physicians had support from dentists and veterinarians, NARD had to fight the cause alone. Charles F. Nixon, chairman of the association's legislative committee, noted with some bitterness that even representatives from the APhA "had not upheld the (NARD view) for the interest of the retailer." Others felt the National Chamber of Commerce had not been supportive of NARD's position and that the association should cancel its membership in the chamber.

The matter was still unresolved when delegates gathered in Philadelphia, Pennsylvania, for the 1914 NARD convention. President James Finneran said that "If...the physicians succeed in killing that bill, then we must not fail in having the responsibility for such failure placed where it belongs — on the physicians." But the physicians were able to amend the bill and delete language requiring them to keep records of their prescriptions.

Executive Committee Chairman Charles Huhn sent a telegram to President Wilson urging him not to sign the amended bill, warning that "it encourages the illegitimate distribution of narcotic drugs...(and) weakens the whole structure of the bill." Unpersuaded, President Wilson signed the bill into law.

The battle over the Harrison bill convinced many delegates that NARD needed a full-time attorney in Washington, D.C. The battle also reopened a fracture in the membership that always lay just below the surface. There were those in the association who favored a public policy approach to solving problems — one that focused on rules, regulations, and penalties for violations. Another group believed that solutions to the association's problems were in the marketplace where the forces of competition in an open market could have full play. A centrist group saw value in both approaches, utilizing elements of each. Typically, this group led the organization. However, in times of crisis, those in the middle had to choose sides.

In 1915, the association was at one of its crossroads. The executive committee's failure to come up with a plan for price protection, and being overpowered on the Harrison bill, brought delegates to Minneapolis divided in spirit and less than confident in their leaders. A symptom of this unhappiness surfaced early in the convention when two resolutions were introduced and passed. The first resolution called for the "incoming President (to) appoint...a special committee of five members, none of whom shall hold any other office in the association, to whom all suggestions received from individual members and affiliated organizations during the next year shall be referred."

The second proposal called upon the association to appoint "a special committee...(to shape a) clearer definition of the duties and limitations of the legislative committee" and to make the appropriate changes in the NARD Constitution to reflect those changes. Circumventing the executive committee and redesigning the responsibilities of a key committee were strong indications of an incipient rebellion. But in the open sessions called to debate these and all other resolutions, it was clear that members wanted "redress" more than "revolution." Specifically, delegates from Iowa and Ohio felt that they had been overlooked for leadership positions in the association. Selected groups from New York and Pennsylvania felt that their views had been misrepresented in the debate on whether or not NARD should withdraw from the National Chamber of Commerce. Responses pro and con to these positions went on for hours. But the debate was therapeutic for the membership. In the course of the debate, it became clear that most were motivated out of a desire to strengthen NARD and not for personal ambition.

By the time delegates gathered in Indianapolis, Indiana, for the 1916 convention, the discontent of the previous year had been largely forgotten. Most pharmacists were more concerned about the persistent war in Europe and how long the United States could steer a neutral course. The war had disrupted the shipment of a number of supplies, particularly drugs, and the uncertain business climate weighed upon everyone's mind.

President M.A. Stout took note of the conditions in his presidential address and commented, "At the present time soda fountains and lunch counters are taking the place of the prescription department in a great majority of the stores in cities, while in the smaller cities and towns the drug store is a variety store because of competition by dispensing physicians, wagon peddlers, and others."

Overall, the tone of the meeting was upbeat. The executive committee responded to the mandate of the House of Delegates and retained Eugene C. Brokmeyer as a staff attorney assigned to Washington, D.C. Samuel C. Henry, the immediate past president, was appointed chairman of the legislative committee and an auxiliary legislative committee was created with one member from each affiliated state.

Still, the war clouds dominated the meeting. By the time the nineteenth convention assembled in Cleveland, Ohio, in 1917, the United States was in the war. Domestic legislation was all but forgotten, and all members of NARD focused on how the association could assist in the war effort. Potts and members of the executive committee were particularly interested in getting a "Pharmacal Corps" established in the Army. This organization, in President Robert J. Frick's words, was "to secure proper recognition for the pharmacist in the army," and would "improve the pharmaceutical practice in the army, navy, and public health service."

Creating the corps required special legislation. Samuel Henry, chairman of the legislative committee, and the association's attorney, Eugene Brokmeyer, persuaded Congressman Edmonds to introduce the Edmonds Pharmaceutical Corps bill, but it failed to pass in both sessions of the Congress. Henry said it was because there was an "apparent lack of cooperation on the part of the various individuals and organizations logically interested in such a movement." The war ended without the corps being established.

The inability to get the Pharmaceutical Corps bill passed was a serious blow as evidenced by another anti-industry development that emerged soon after the convention. With the demands of the military conflict becoming more acute, federal officials were forced to decide which industries qualified as "essential" to the war effort. That decision was lodged with the Council of National Defense, and that group looked to the Medical Department of the Army and Navy for guidance.

NARD was not represented on either body and, predictably, did not make the "essential industries" list in the drug field when that group was identified. Instead, the Defense Council named "drug and pharmaceutical interests that manufactured and distributed drugs and medicines for the army and navy as essential." All other groups in the industry were classified as nonessential.

Potts and Executive Committee Chairman Fenneran protested this decision "to the point of being called unpatriotic," but their action paid off. The council reconsidered its initial action and agreed to seek broader input into its decision-making process. In recognition of NARD's complaint, Professors James H. Beal and Charles H. LaWall, along with Charles J. Lynn of the Eli Lilly & Company, were added to the council's "medical advisory committee."

While none of the appointees was an active retail druggist, each was well known to NARD and quite acceptable. Having these men as part of the policymaking process caused the council to reconsider its original decision and also include "drug and pharmaceutical interests which serve the civilian population" on the essential industries list. Having this classification allowed NARD members to be given a priority for receiving "raw materials and finished products" for the duration of the war.

For its twentieth convention in 1918, NARD returned to the South. President Walter Cousins called the delegates together in New Orleans, Louisiana. Except for Atlanta, Georgia, the association had not met in the South. NARD leaders were quick to point out the need to do more "organization" work in the area, particularly in the larger cities.

The unfinished war in Europe still overshadowed the proceedings. President Cousins noted "the drug market has been unsettled and in a state of chaos for the past year," not to mention the shortage or unavailability of certain supplies. But Cousins also said "probably the most serious problem that has come to the druggist as a result of the war is the shortage of efficient help." In many instances, help was simply not available and pharmacists had to all but sleep at their store. Perhaps of more long-term importance was the new price of labor. Competition from defense industries forced labor costs up while reducing the number of hours worked.

In an ironic turn of events, NARD had to defend its members against charges of violating the Harrison Narcotics Act. A congressional subcommittee monitoring compliance with the law noticed records showing that 35,000 gallons of paregoric had been sold in just three months to fifteen states. Congressmen Raney and Moore called upon the association to explain the increased activity.

New Legislative Committee Chairman Frank Stone and attorney Brokmeyer met with the congressional subcommittee and pointed out that the fifteen states in question had a population of over 20 million. Brokmeyer asked Congressman Raney if the records showed why the medicine had been prescribed. When Raney said no, Chairman Stone responded that it was therefore impossible for the association to determine how it had been used.

Stone also used the opportunity to point out to the congressman that according to the Internal Revenue Commissioner's reports, "the number of physicians who had violated the Harrison law was much larger than the number of druggists."

The last half of the decade were years of transition for NARD. Changes in the central office and increasing age of the charter members began to have an impact on the annual meetings. For the founding fathers, attendance at the convention resembled a family reunion. But over a period of fifteen years, the combination of lifestyle and failing health began to take a toll and many stopped coming to the annual events. Labor problems and travel arrangements caused by the war also contributed to this group's declining attendance.

In addition to "the old guys" dropping out, changes at headquarters also charted a new direction for the association. Charles Carr, the founding editor of the *N.A.R.D. Notes/Journal*, resigned in 1914. His replacement, Hugh Craig, continued Carr's excellent work, but he too resigned in 1918. But the biggest change came in 1917 when Secretary Potts resigned to enter private business in Detroit.

Potts had been equal to the task of filling founding Secretary Thomas Wooten's shoes. Under his leadership, the association had significant growth in membership and budget and became a strong voice in national politics.

New Secretary Samuel Henry also came from Pennsylvania. As a past president and chairman of the legislative committee, he was thoroughly familiar with the association. But he was not one of the "guys at the beginning." His election signaled the beginning of a new generation of pharmacist leaders and perhaps a new direction for NARD.

CHAPTER FOUR

THE THIRD DECADE: 1919 – 1928

Prohibition and Retail Pharmacy: The "Great War" in the Marketplace

*T*he Great War was still raging when NARD finished its convention in 1918, but the end of the conflict was in sight. The German government asked for an armistice and peace negotiations began in January 1919. Like most Americans seeking a return to a normal pre-war existence, NARD leaders began planning for "reconstruction" as the profession and the nation adjusted from "total war" to peace-time conditions.

Secretary Samuel Henry and incoming President Charles F. Harding lobbied federal officials to give druggists an early discharge from the military. Almost 10,000 community pharmacists had enlisted in some branch of service and their skills were sorely missed in most communities. That need was further compounded when a national influenza broke out just as the war was ending. This "Spanish Influenza" became an epidemic and was a factor in allowing many pharmacists an early release from military obligations.

Beyond the public health crisis, the domestic economy took a jolt from the abrupt end of the war. The uncertain business climate prompted President Harding to tell pharmacists that "it is (my) firm belief that never again will drugdom return to 1914 or prior conditions....we are living in a new era." Fortunately, the unsettled conditions did not last as long as some predicted. By late spring, the economy had begun to recover and NARD experienced a resurging interest in association affairs.

When retail druggists met in Rochester, New York, in 1919 for their twenty-first convention, Secretary Henry reported an increase of more than 1,000 new members from the previous year. The rapid increase in membership presented a bookkeeping problem for the staff at headquarters. As part of the association's contribution to the war effort, the House of Delegates had approved an executive committee recommendation to waive the membership fee for pharmacists inducted into military service. But the rapid demobilization following the war made it hard to keep up with the veterans' new status with respect to their association dues.

Perhaps as important as the increased membership was a new spirit of cooperation that permeated the meeting. Executive Committee Chairman James Finneran noticed this and told the delegates "the great world war taught...many valuable lessons, none of which we venture to say stand out more prominently than the necessity of organization and cooperation." Few realized how much that "organization and cooperation" would be put to the test just months after the convention adjourned.

The challenge came from a new plan for "national prohibition," a matter that had been at issue since before World War I. NARD had repeatedly adopted resolutions and editorialized in the *Journal* about its opposition to pharmacists selling alcohol as a beverage. However, the association had spoken out just as forcefully about the necessity for using alcohol in a variety of medicinal preparations — using formulas from the U.S. Pharmacopoeia and the National Formulary Digest. The former position was frequently ignored, the latter was consider a professional necessity, and the whole matter became a divisive wedge in NARD's membership.

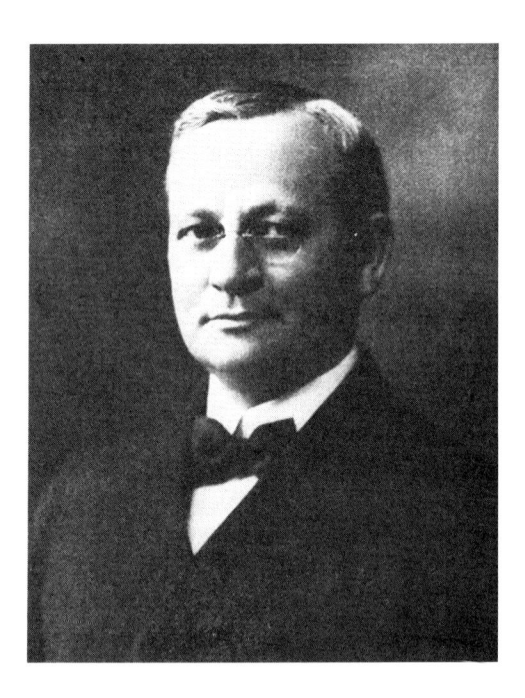

Samuel Henry, NARD Executive Secretary, 1917 – 1933

The near crisis situation in the association began at 12:01 a.m., Saturday, January 16, 1920. On that date, a century-long crusade reached fruition when beverage alcohol was prohibited everywhere in the United States. Approved by the U.S. Congress as the Eighteenth Amendment to the Constitution on December 18, 1917, and ratified by three-fourths of the states by January 16, 1919, the amendment was slated to go into effect one year after ratification.

The amendment mandated that "the manufacture, sale, or transportation of intoxicating liquors within, the importation thereof into, or the exportation thereof from the United States and all territory subject to the jurisdiction thereof for beverage purposes is hereby prohibited." Enforcement provisions for the amendment were contained in the National Prohibition Act of 1919, commonly known as the Volstead Act in honor of its sponsor, Representative Andrew Volstead of Minnesota.

While the act was being drafted, NARD leaders became most concerned with that provision of the act known as Regulation No. 60. This provision related to the "manufacturing, sale, transportation, importation, exportation, delivery, furnishing, purchase, possession, and use of intoxicating liquors" and placed the community pharmacist as the gatekeeper to help enforce the provision.

Henry, still new in his position as NARD Secretary, was ready to ask the NARD membership to abandon the measure if it meant that the burden of enforcement fell on his group. After repeated attempts to block Regulation 60, Henry and the executive committee led the various groups in organized pharmacy — including the American Pharmaceutical Association (APhA) and the National Wholesale Druggists Association (NWDA) — to adopt a resolution opposing the concept of pharmacists "dispensing intoxicating liquors." NARD also endorsed a resolution adopted by the American Medical Association (AMA) that said in part that "alcohol was not a medicine."

Representatives of the alcohol industry countered NARD's efforts by arguing that there were various "legitimate uses" for their product, particularly in medical preparations, food recipes, and religious ordinances, and that such a provision must be left in the bill.

Volstead and his colleagues drafting the bill were sympathetic to the arguments advanced by both NARD and the liquor interests. They sought ways to accommodate the necessary needs for alcohol while still keeping it under control. But to most staff members working on the bill, regulation could best be done at the point in distribution where the product reached the public.

For medicinal purposes, that point of contact was typically the neighborhood drugstore. Consequently, despite NARD's appeal, the rules for enforcement were drafted placing a special responsibility on the retail pharmacist. In deference to the liquor industry, "medicinal alcohol" was kept in the bill, but such alcohol was to be prescribed by physicians and dispensed by pharmacists.

To placate those who feared "medicinal alcohol" as a loophole, the bill provided for strict controls and a vigilant inspection system. But as Henry and his colleagues predicted, the burden for that inspection fell on their

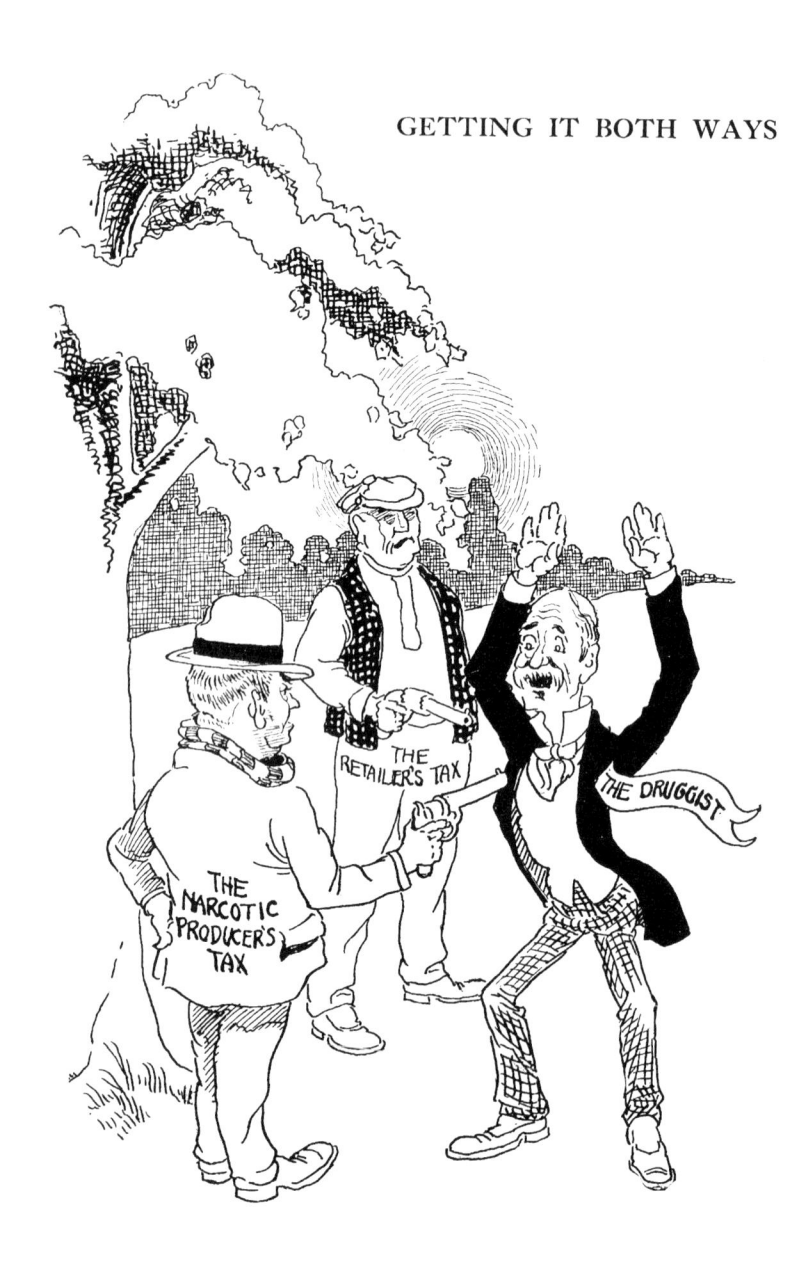

GETTING IT BOTH WAYS

industry. Both physicians and pharmacists were subject to unannounced visits from prohibition agents who had wide discretionary powers for enforcement.

To obtain medicinal alcohol, an individual had to first contact a physician, be examined, and be diagnosed as needing such medication. The physician then wrote the prescription on a special sequentially numbered form that also included the name of the pharmacist chosen to fill the prescription. Physicians were limited to prescribing a maximum of one pint of medicinal alcohol per ten-day period per patient.

The enforcement act required pharmacists to annually apply for a license to sell alcohol for "medicinal purposes," post bond equal to the amount they anticipated selling in the year, and pay a special franchise tax. This qualified one as a "retail liquor dealer."

For all prescriptions that included alcohol, the pharmacists had to make a record and keep a separate file showing each patients's name, the physician writing the prescription, and the quantity dispensed. This information was reported by the 5th of each month to the Collector of Revenue at the Bureau of Internal Revenue.

Another odious aspect of the enforcement act, which caused NARD to speak out against it, was the strict control over liquor wholesale houses — at the pharmacists' expense. Orders for alcohol had to be placed in quadruplicate, and the druggist was required to keep a record of all "intoxicating liquor...received." Moreover, one could only obtain a maximum of four and seven-eights gallons with each order.

There was no limit to the number of times an order could be placed, but the extensive recordkeeping and the threat of spontaneous inspection by revenue agents caused many pharmacists to resent the system intensely. Not only did every liquor transaction have to be recorded, but also the collective summary had to be reported to the Collector of Revenue by the 10th of each month. The object of such reporting was to allow enforcement agents to see how much alcohol a pharmacist bought and dispensed through prescriptions in a given month. The druggist had to account for any discrepancy between the two amounts.

Pharmacists responded to this recordkeeping in a variety of ways. Some refused to do all the paperwork and simply did not fill prescriptions requiring alcohol. Most resented the "bartending" appearance imposed by the system and decried the decline in "professionalism," at least in appearance. One pharmacist complained, "I'll be hanged if I'll turn bartender just because the Government decides to put the saloons out of business." During the first month the law was in effect, less than five percent of the nation's pharmacists filed for a liquor permit.

But the lure of sales, particularly lucrative profits, was simply too much for many pharmacists. As one druggist noted, "Let me assure you that it will be very much worth his while to the man who makes that decision (to use medicinal alcohol)." Another said that he could "boost his prices for liquor to make up for the discomfort and the red tape." But he also mentioned that should anyone do that he would "cease being a druggist and gain the reputation as a bartender."

Some pharmacists initially refused to stock medicinal alcohol. But even that action did not entirely remove the retail pharmacy profession from the appearance of a saloon keeper. As the public became more conscious of prohibition's impact, many turned to alcohol substitutes. Numerous druggists soon saw their toiletry department decimated as individuals expressed an abnormal appetite for bay rum, perfumes, and toilet water in general — anything with even a small amount of alcohol.

Henry, Finneran, and the rest of the NARD staff found themselves in an awkward position as the full impact of the new regulations began to take hold. As a professional association, it was necessary for the association leadership to encourage the membership to act as "good citizens" and comply with the law. Henry, in an editorial in the *N.A.R.D. Journal,* noted that "whether or not national prohibition is desirable is no longer a subject for discussion. The question has been definitely settled." At the same time, he readily admitted that the method of "conducting the retail drug business, at least insofar as dispensing alcoholic liquors and preparations are concerned," had been materially altered.

But while the question may have been decided, interpreting the act's many provisions was not so clear. Volstead's intent — to prevent the sale of any alcohol preparation, medicinal, toilet, or otherwise, if it was to be used for beverage purposes — was not in dispute. But who was to determine how the preparation was to be used? Clearly, the legislation intended for the seller (i.e., the pharmacist) to make that determination, even though such a decision potentially brought his professional ethics into sharp conflict with his proprietary interests as a retail businessman.

For a number of pharmacists, the retail argument won. Numerous schemes to circumvent prohibition made their appearance, even before the law became effective. A favorite activity involved "bogus whiskey" made from denatured or wood alcohol. The NARD staff regularly warned its members to be on guard for such activity and to report anyone wishing to purchase either of these items without a prescription to enforcement authorities.

Rather than try to figure out whether these products were legal or not, NARD advised pharmacists to use common sense and know that if they as the sellers had reason to believe wood or denatured alcohol were going to be used for beverage purposes, they indeed would be in violation of the law.

CHAPTER FOUR — THE THIRD DECADE: 1919 – 1928

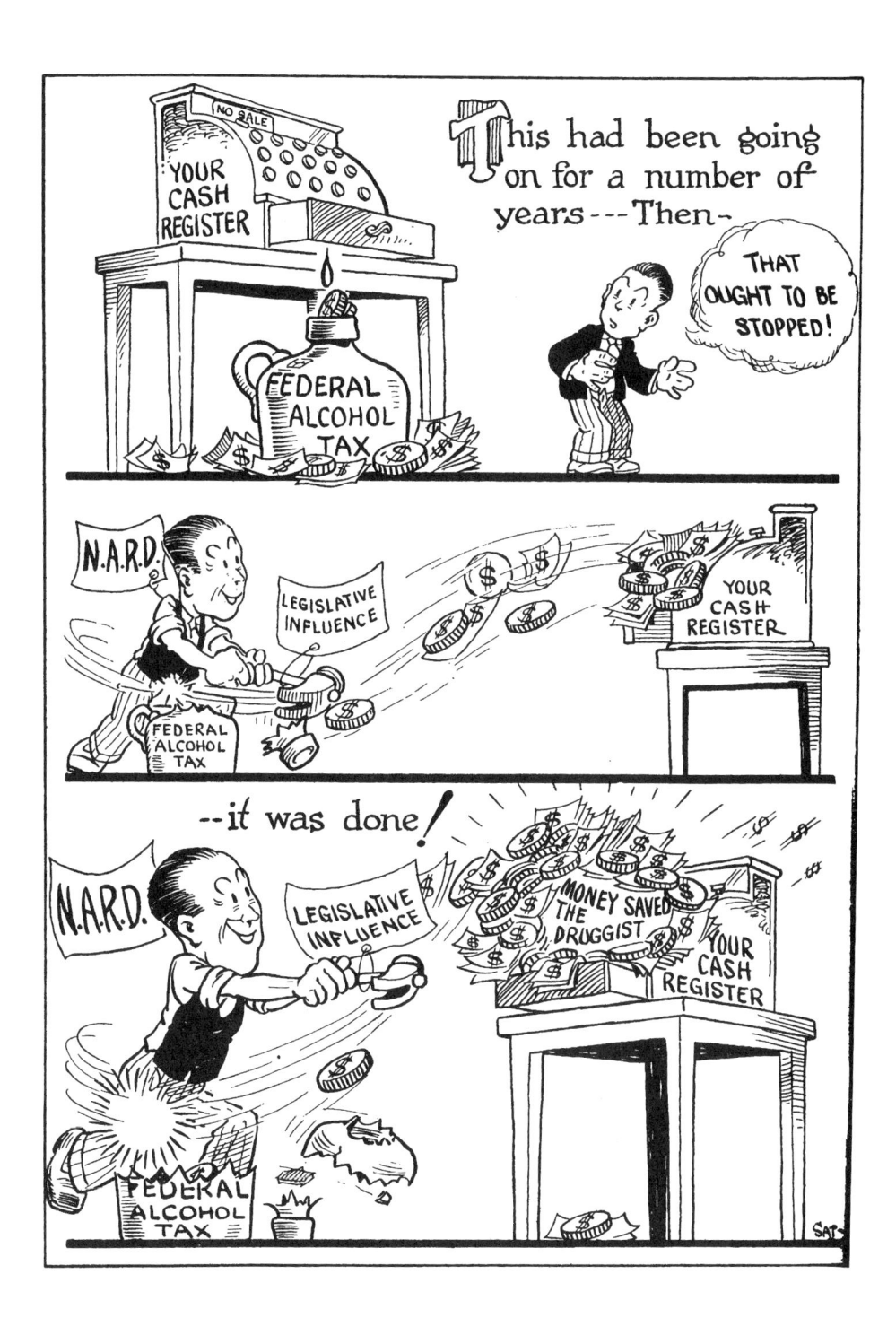

The wood and denatured alcohol issue was yet another instance where pharmacists' professional ethics and proprietary interests came into conflict. In addition to their intoxicating properties, both wood and denatured alcohol products were poisonous and extremely dangerous to human life if taken internally. However, the same products were widely used in a variety of ointments, balms, and salves and obviously had many side benefits as well. The crux of the matter came down to intended use and that often placed the pharmacist in a delicate situation, not only judging the intent of the customer, but also as a health care provider and retailer in choosing between the professional and proprietary side of his business.

Association officials tried to influence the thinking on this issue by expressing "absolute faith in the integrity and law-abiding character of the retail druggists" and telling government officials they could "count upon (pharmacists) of the nation to do their part honestly and conscientiously in carrying out the law." But there was mounting evidence that the "official position" was losing ground.

Another dimension to enforcement had to do with maintaining an inventory of "liquors on hand." To comply with this provision, pharmacists were required to identify all forms of alcohol by name and quantity as of January 16, 1920, the date the Volstead provisions went into effect. This inventory was to be done on special forms supplied by the IRS and filed with the district revenue collector within ten days. Ironically, despite the law's rigorous intent, the IRS had not printed the official forms when the law took effect. To compensate for this mix-up, pharmacists were granted a delay until the summer when the forms were finally distributed.

Indeed, it was the inconsistencies between the letter of the law and the actions of its enforcement agents that gave NARD officials the most concern. Before the law was two weeks old, Henry wrote an editorial sharply critical of the initial enforcement and commented that "we are led to the conclusion that at least some of our present public officials do not fully comprehend either the law or its regulations."

The "red tape" of documenting so many practices that had been routine for generations was particularly bothersome to retail druggists. For example, the IRS ruled that pharmacists were required to apply for a retail liquor license in order to dispense medicinal alcohol. This was particularly galling. Alcohol had been an essential ingredient in the practice of pharmacy from the profession's inception and pharmacists always kept a supply on hand. Requiring them to obtain a license was an insult to their ethics.

Speaking for the membership, Secretary Henry complained that it appeared to him that "the purpose of the prohibition law was to legislate the saloon out of existence and to legally establish the drug store as its successor." This he strongly denounced and pledged to "throw down the gauntlet and enter upon the battle...in defending the honor and decency of the pharmacists of the nation and the drug business as a whole."

Despite NARD's strong rhetoric, the IRS stood firm with its requirement on liquor licenses and by June some 57,000 pharmacists had formally filed an application to become a licensed dealer in alcohol. But again, enforcement officials were not prepared for the response to their ruling, and IRS state bureaus became hopelessly backlogged in trying to process the high volume of requests. Such bureaucracy gave the NARD yet another reason to decry the policy.

Haggling with the IRS over the proper forms and reporting deadlines was only part of the problem facing NARD in the early months of prohibition. New types of drugstores made their appearance just weeks after the law went into force and made a mockery of the professional neighborhood pharmacy.

In Chicago, Illinois, one type of new store was the "Talcum Shop" where a "talcum powder druggist" equipped with a "box or two of talcum powder for window display and, in NARD terms, "an inexhaustible supply of whiskey" for medicinal purposes opened for business. Assisted by physicians who cooperated by writing prescriptions to be filled at the new stores, the talcum shops became saloons fronting as pharmacies, much to the chagrin of NARD and those pharmacists who followed both the spirit and letter of the law.

The chain drugstore also became another scheme to circumvent the enforcement act, at least in some cases. In this model, a proprietor bought the building and/or inventories of various retail druggists, employed a licensed pharmacist to operate the store and apply for a retail liquor license. With a license in hand, the pharmacy could then dispense "medicinal alcohol," assuming there was a physician who was willing to write a prescription to such a store.

Finding a cooperating physician to write prescriptions for "medicinal alcohol" was not difficult. Less than six months after the law had gone into effect, Hubert Howard, federal prohibition director of Illinois, reported that Chicago area physicians had written over 500,000 prescriptions for whiskey. Of that number, he estimated that at least 300,000 were spurious. As quoted in a local newspaper, Howard said that "investigations from my office have brought to light many evasions." He noted that one physician admitted that "when my regular patients come to me famishing for a drink of whiskey, I seek for symptoms on which I can hang a prescription, and generally find an excuse for a pint."

In another case highlighted by the director, a doctor who was bedfast and unable to visit his patients wrote 200 prescriptions in two days. Howard's office discovered the practice when the physician's wife came to get a new book of prescriptions forms.

Alerted to potentially fraudulent actions, Howard and his staff reviewed all the prescription stubs of Chicago's 3,000 physicians. It was then they discovered the vast numbers of scripts. They also quantified the prescriptions and that added to their suspicions of fraud. For example, one physician had prescribed an "ounce of whiskey three times a day as a cure for insomnia" and on the stub next to it wrote an order for "a pint of whisky to be taken in identical doses as a remedy for fainting." Other suspicious practices included 354 prescriptions for bronchitis, 162 for grip, and 167 for general debility. Several others fell into the category of curious, including one prescription for senility, one for eyestrain and headache, and one for ptomaine poisoning.

Officials at NARD watched these developments with a growing sense of concern. Long at odds with the physicians over their respective roles in the health care field, the prospect of doctors cooperating with saloon keepers fronting as pharmacists, even if only occasionally true, was a serious problem.

Beginning as early as February 1922, NARD officials complained about the physicians' role in prohibition enforcement and urged its membership to be alert to schemes for obtaining alcohol illegally. Henry again addressed the issue in a sharply worded editorial and commented, "It...behooves every druggist filling such prescriptions (involving alcohol) to thoroughly satisfy himself that the physician issuing them has the legal right so to do."

All of NARD's protests about the professional deterioration of pharmacy and medicine went unheeded by local and federal authorities — and by many in its own membership. The aforementioned physicians were never charged with fraud, and numerous pharmacists ignored the advice of their association. The temptation was just too great and the loopholes too many to put professionalism over commercialism.

The "noble experiment" of national prohibition continued until 1933. It was an admitted failure even to its original supporters and died an ignoble death. Officials at NARD were not among the mourners. NARD never supported the role that retail druggists had been assigned in enforcing prohibition and thus they were relieved it was over. The official position made no apology in saying that, in the association's opinion, prohibition had been "decidedly detrimental to the drug trade," and it was time for it to be over.

The issue of prohibition, "medicinal alcohol" prescribing and dispensing, and the retail pharmacists' ambivalent role in it dominated this decade. However, there were other issues, some familiar and ongoing from the perspective of the association staff and membership, that required response.

CHAPTER FOUR — THE THIRD DECADE: 1919–1928   75

Of keen interest to delegates at the twenty-second convention in St. Louis in 1920 was the announcement that retail pharmacy had been accepted for membership in the upcoming tenth U.S. Pharmacopoeia (USP) convention. Having been embarrassingly shut out of the last convention, Secretary Henry told the delegates that "it is...a real pleasure to be able here to record the fact our efforts met with success, our representatives being seated in the convention and taking part in the proceedings."

The association also found itself, like its members, flush with a nascent healthy postwar economy, a booming growth in membership, and a healthy financial balance sheet. While government regulations continued to be a common topic of discussion, most wartime controls had expired and the new administration of President Warren G. Harding appeared less inclined to impose new restraints on the business community.

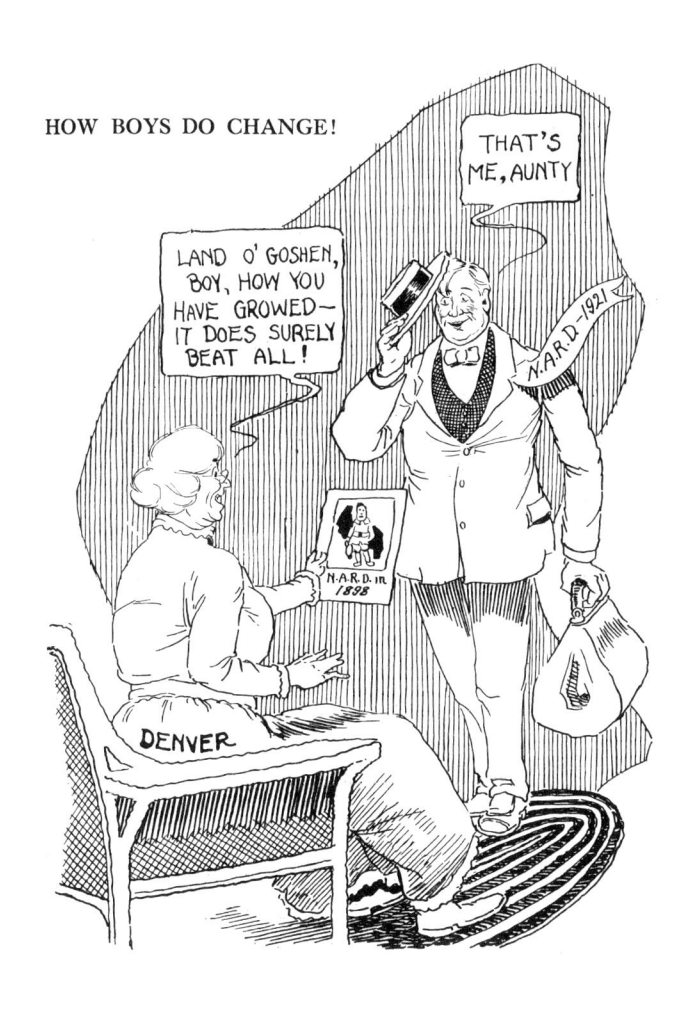

The continued increase in membership was reflected in the "many new faces" at the convention. The transition from the "founding fathers generation" to the "Great War generation" was becoming more evident. Founding President Harold Hynson died in 1921 and second president, the acknowledged "grand old man of NARD," Simon N. Jones died in 1922. Jones's passing was mourned perhaps as no other in the association's history. The 1923 executive committee established a scholarship in his honor at the Louisville (Kentucky) College of Pharmacy as a tribute of his service to NARD.

To the surprise of many, business conditions earlier in the decade did not continue to improve as predicted. When pharmacists came to Detroit, Michigan, in 1922 for the twenty-third NARD convention, their mood was more subdued than in the recent past. President Ambrose Hunsberger noted the "contraction in the general volume of business" and attributed it to "the unsettled political and economic situation in Europe" and "numerous prolonged and extensive labor controversies" in America. In view of the circumstances, he told the delegates that "it behooves (us) to watch the situation carefully...and maintain full control of the three 'overs' — over-head, overstock, and turn-over."

The slow down in business activities led to the reappearance of an old NARD nemesis, "price cutting." This time, however, the nemesis was a bit more subtle. Manufacturers began to provide discounts for "quantity buying," and chain and department stores began to take advantage of the opportunity. Chain store growth had plateaued in the years immediately preceding the Great War, but experienced a resurgence in the 1920s.

Another indirect approach to price cutting was a tactic known as "cooperative advertising." In this instance, in return for quantity buying, the manufacturer paid for the costs of local advertising. NARD Executive Committee Chairman Julius H. Riemenschneider complained about this practice in the *Journal* and urged community pharmacists to make their views known to their local suppliers. He noted that "87 percent of the merchandise sold in drug stores is sold in the smaller, individual stores," and he suggested that manufacturers "consider more carefully the good will of the smaller independent retailer."

It was a bit ironic that the price cutting issue resurfaced on the eve of NARD's twenty-fifth anniversary. While the matter had never really gone away, NARD had been successful in neutralizing its more pernicious aspects. But the extended time without a price maintenance agreement allowed the practice to revive.

NARD returned to Boston, Massachusetts, for its "silver anniversary," meeting in the Mechanics Building in 1923. One of the features of that meeting was introducing seventeen of the charter members from the 1898 con-

CHAPTER FOUR — THE THIRD DECADE: 1919 – 1928

vention, including Thomas Wooten, the first executive secretary. Perhaps the significance of the twenty-fifth meeting was the measure of progress the association had made over the years. Without question, price cutting continued to be a problem; relations with the physicians were strained over prohibition; the relationship with APhA, though not strained, was distant; the mail

THAT SITE FOR THE PRICE-MAINTENANCE BILL

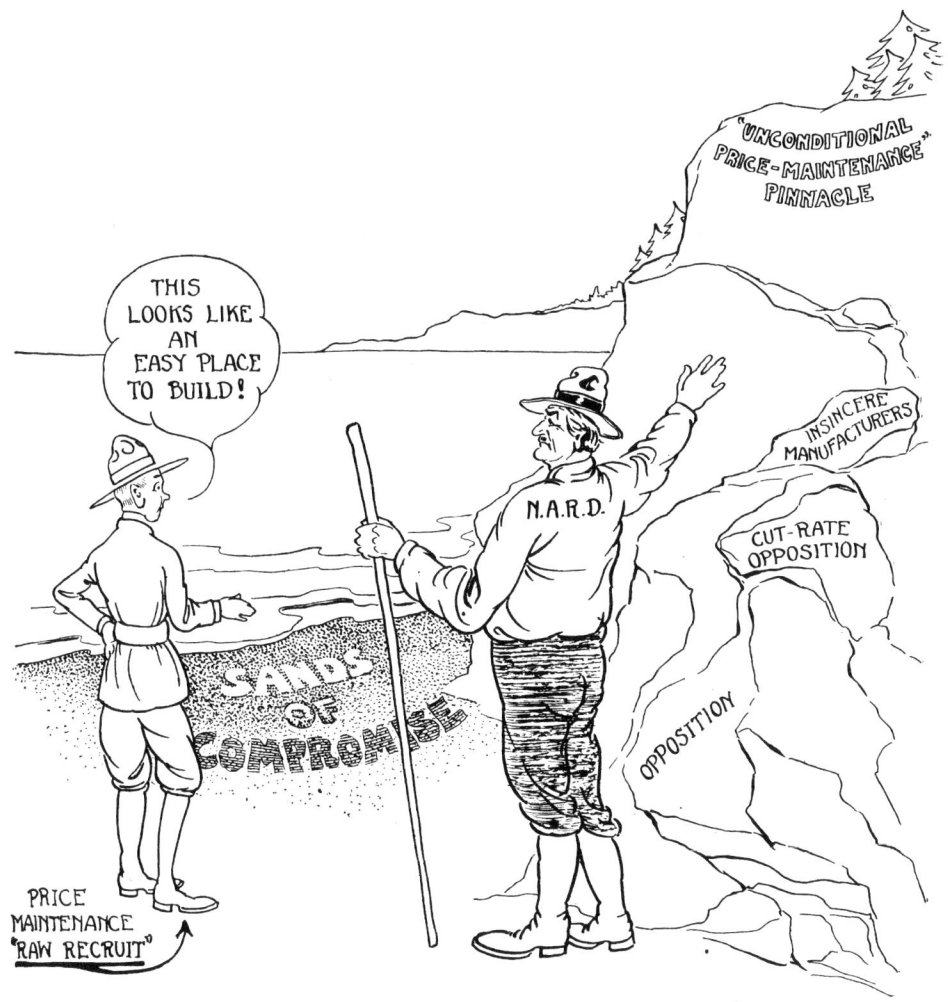

N. A. R. D.: "It's a harder climb, son; but it's building on a rock!"

order/parcel post issue had been replaced to some degree by the chain store movement; and Sunday closing was still a local matter unevenly observed.

But in a number of other areas NARD had made substantial progress in its first twenty-five years. This was particularly evident in the financial health and the widely based membership. The association also had widespread acceptance and respect in the drug industry. Membership in the National Drug Trade Conference, the National Chamber of Commerce, and the decennial USP convention gave NARD professional standing.

As further evidence of its development, the House of Delegates authorized the executive committee to secure a permanent headquarters building for the association. President Curtis P. Gladding strongly supported the idea, telling the delegates "at no time in our history has the druggist occupied a more conspicuous position or been charged with greater public responsibilities." It was believed that an NARD building would be a fitting tribute to the association's quarter century of growth.

Surprisingly, the resolution for a permanent building touched off a lively debate among the delegates. Some of the discussion was procedural — whether the decision should be a committee or a convention decision; other discussion was more concerned with substance, such as the site of the building. A number of delegates voiced the opinion that if the association moved to a permanent building, it should be in Washington, D.C. Ultimately, convention members agreed to leave the decision to the executive committee. (The decision regarding a permanent home for the association was finally cemented in the foundation of its own building in Alexandria, Virginia, near the nation's capital nearly sixty years later.)

During the 1920s — with the debate about prohibition, the multitudinous bureaucracy that had been built around its odious enforcement requirements, and the heavy taxes forced upon the use of alcohol ever escalating — NARD's leadership from year to year worked to marshal the members in widespread support for political action. For example, President Frank T. Stone exhorted the membership in 1926 to work to ensure "more pharmacists in public office. The cause of pharmacy needs leaders on the floor of the national Congress."

President Samuel C. Davis in 1927 continued a similar political theme at the twenty-ninth convention in Kansas City, Missouri. What is meant by "druggists in politics," he asked rhetorically, "it means...the druggist must become active in practical politics in order to get in a position to demand and obtain his rights. He must not be afraid to discuss the questions of the hour with his customers."

In 1928, NARD met for the first time on the West Coast. Gathering at the Whitcomb Hotel in San Francisco, California, delegates heard President

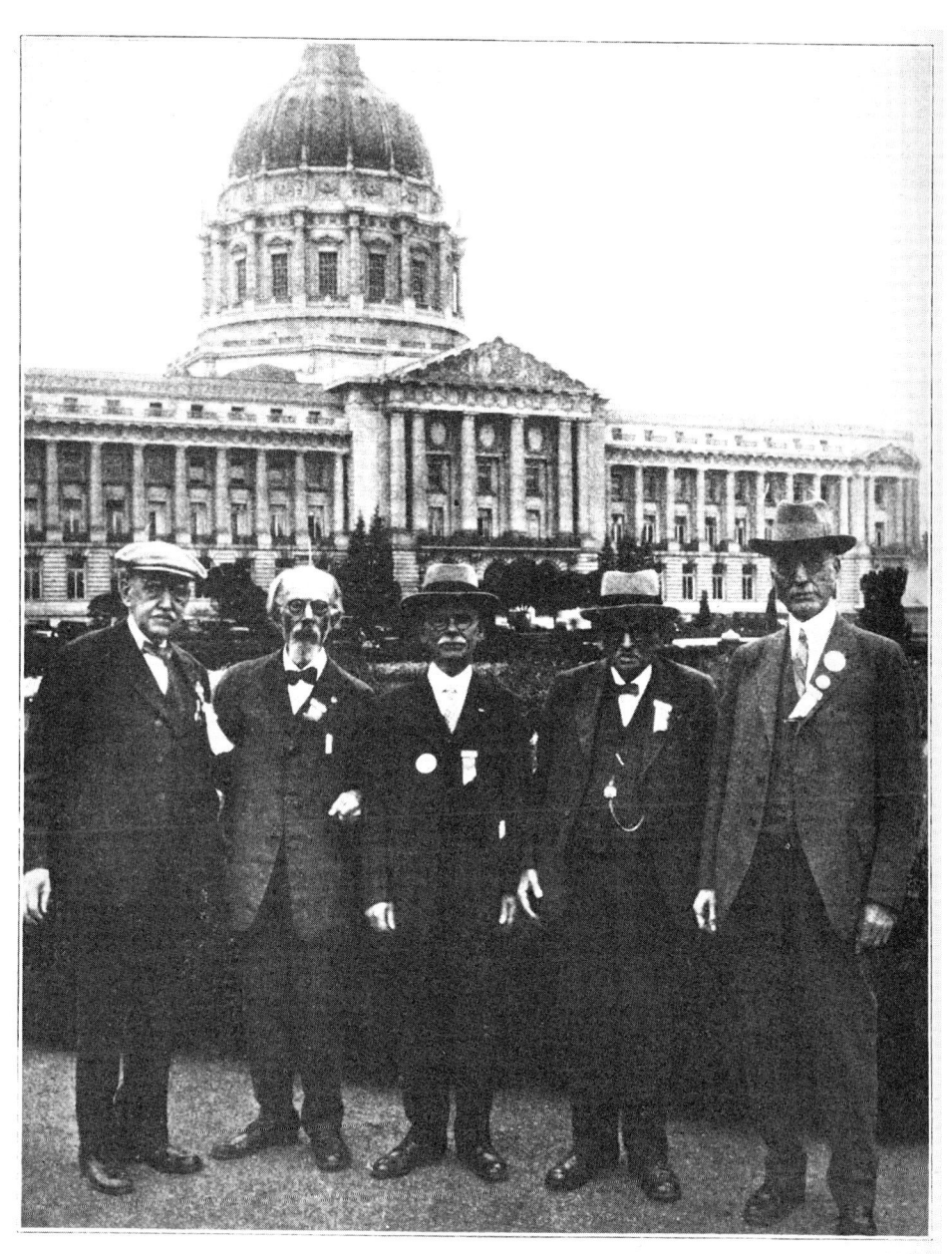

CHARTER MEMBERS OF THE N. A. R. D. WHO WERE PRESENT AT THE SAN FRANCISCO CONVENTION. FROM LEFT TO RIGHT: FRED MEISSNER, LAPORTE, IND.; WILHELM BODEMANN, CHICAGO, ILL.; JOHN LOWE, BOSTON, MASS.; WILLIAM BAUM, DANVILLE, ILL.; THOMAS STODDART, BUFFALO, N. Y.

From The NARD Journal, October 4, 1928 — San Francisco convention coverage

William A. Oren move the political discussion to the state level. Noting that retail druggists in a number of states were "taking an active interest in practical politics," he commented that "this may be regarded as one of the most encouraging signs of the time." He continued, "I urge the formation of permanent political organizations in each state, beginning with a county unit."

The "Great Crash" of the stock market was still a little more that a month away when the delegates assembled for the thirty-first NARD convention in Minneapolis, Minnesota. The delegates at the convention showed no evidence of being anxious about existing economic conditions. President Denny Brann used his time to talk about the changing nature of the drug industry.

He noted that the major mail order houses had begun to open retail outlets and that the chain store movement was losing some of its momentum. He also warned delegates about a new marketing scheme called "quantity of merchandise," whereby a manufacturer sold goods to "hospitals, civic, and government institutions, at a price less than the druggist is forced to pay for similar products." President Brann held out hope that federal legislation would soon be passed to limit such practice. (This issue of price discrimination served as a talisman of NARD's political activity for the remaining decades of the 20th century.)

The decade of the 1920s was a bit paradoxical for community pharmacists. The dominate presence of regulations related to prohibition and illegal narcotics was frustrating to the point that some druggists left the profession. Also the rapidly shifting demographics, farm to city, worked a hardship on many pharmacists in rural America. The inability to reach agreement on any price maintenance program hurt as well. Early in the decade, the chain store interest moved so aggressively that many independent pharmacists sold out to these syndicates rather than compete with them.

A survey taken by a trade organization in 1923 illustrated the emerging influence of the chain store movement. According to that report, there were some 52,304 drug stores in the nation. Of that number, 2,014 stores were affiliated with 327 chain organizations (a chain was defined by the survey as organizations operating three or more separate stores). The average number of stores per chain was 6.1, however, 263 stores were operating under the name of a single company. Surveyors estimated that two-thirds of all retail trade was being done by independently owned stores and the volume of sales was approximately $1.25 billion. The average business done by each retail drug store was between $24,000 and $25,000 annually with an inventory ranging from 8,000 to 13,000 items.

From that survey, it was apparent that community pharmacists were competing quite effectively and enjoyed the rising tide of prosperity during the 1920s. NARD benefited from the prosperous times as well. For example, it took the association over twenty years to amass its first $100,000 in assets; but it earned its second $100,000 in less than half that time. By the end of the decade, NARD's budget was running above $200,000, and only the old guard could remember the days when the House of Delegates "passed the hat" to collect operating money for the coming year.

The 1920s brought a number of changes to the association. One change came in 1921 when delegates at the Denver convention voted to change the motto from "Live and Let Live" (adopted at the 1898 convention) to "Live and Help to Live." The resolution committee in making this recommendation said "the N.A.R.D., through its executive officers, is devoting time and energy, to so mold business conditions that every retail druggist in the United States will be afforded the opportunity to live — thus exemplifying the religious faith of the Good Samaritan."

Another change in the decade was the recognition that an increasing number of women were becoming pharmacists. President F.R. Peterson commented on this in his address to the 1925 convention, noting that "it is estimated there are now between 22,000 and 23,000 women engaged in operating or clerking in the drug stores...twenty-five years ago there were probably less than 50 of the fair sex who had chosen pharmacy as a career."

In language characteristic of the day, Peterson continued his tribute to women in the profession. He said, "we welcome the sweeping scientific advances (that) have contributed to the elimination of the household drudgery of the old days and released women to larger fields of usefulness such as our professions. We invite *pharmasisters*...to become active members in the great retail druggists' association and help us with the aid of their innate refinement and culture to build up a spirit of 'One for All and All for One.'"

Innovations in the decade included two annual promotions — one on "First Aid Week" and the second on "Pharmacy Week." First Aid Week began in 1922 after delegates at the Denver convention adopted Secretary Henry's recommendation that the association do so. Henry had been approached by officials from the Johnson & Johnson Company who wanted to run a national advertising campaign with support from the retail druggists. The promotion began with the Johnson & Johnson Company placing ads in newspapers throughout the nation urging consumers to "Try The Drug Store First" when buying the advertised products. The association designated the third week in March as "First Aid Week," in coordination with the promotional campaign, but also stressed that the window displays were open to products from all companies. The first week was so successful that "First Aid Week" became an annual event.

Pharmacy Week was established in 1924 by action of delegates at the Memphis, Tennessee, convention. Delegates recommending the concept identified the second week in October for the special emphasis and urged NARD members "during that week (to) display in one or more of (their) windows chemicals, pharmaceuticals or apparatus that will impress on the public mind the fact that the pharmacist is not merely a merchant but also a member of a profession that should be highly respected." That recommendation resulted, in part, from a study commissioned by APhA. The report concluded that "after two and a half years study, we have positively determined that pharmacy is a profession and not a trade."

The association also showed remarkable stability at headquarters during the decade. Secretary Henry completed his twelfth year in 1929, and there was little turnover in the headquarters office. But this stability may also have been a symptom of a silent problem. When *Journal* Editor Craig had resigned in 1918, Secretary Henry had taken over the editorial duties. When Henry made that decision, the association was in a budget crunch and that personnel move seemed the prudent thing to do. However, he continued as editor throughout the decade. Considering that he also had supervisory responsibilities for the field workers (Secretary Potts had moved the organization department under the Secretary's supervision before World War I, also in an economy move), it was apparent that the secretary's office had a heavy work load.

Obviously, the secretary had too many responsibilities. The *Journal* and the field workers were time-consuming, and as the association increased in size and complexity, there simply was not time enough to accomplish all the office's commitments. The executive committee frequently complimented Secretary Henry for working nights and on Sunday when in reality steps should have been taken to lighten his work load.

The *Journal* was one indication that too much work was assigned to one office. The front cover did not change in appearance throughout the decade and it changed only slightly during this period of time in layout and design — despite the 1920s signifying the first age of mass culture with an emphasis on media and public relations. The publicity department continued to more than pay its own way, but it also failed to reach its full potential.

Even so, NARD ended its third decade on a high note. The approaching "Great Depression," in some respects, presented an even greater challenge to NARD and its membership than prohibition, but the association was in a better condition to face the new crisis, although no one could have anticipated the great challenge that lay just ahead.

CHAPTER FIVE

THE FOURTH DECADE: 1929 – 1938

"Great Depression" Yields a New General and a Great NARD Victory: The Robinson-Patman Act

The "Great Depression," painful though it was for those experiencing it, yielded a long-term advantage for NARD. The extreme business conditions that followed the stock market crash in October 1929 changed a number of political leaders' attitudes about the role of government in the economy and made possible price maintenance legislation (or fair trade practices, as they were to be called in future decades). For more than a decade, NARD members had worked for laws to eliminate the evils of price cutting, but to no avail. But after the crash of the market, public and private leaders alike actively searched for solutions to the collapse, and one approach gave NARD the opportunity to make its mark for fair business practices.

That circumstances were to be different in the new decade was evident within weeks after the thirty-first convention adjourned. One of newly elected President Thomas Roach's first responsibilities was to attend a national business conference in Washington, D.C. The U.S. Chamber of Commerce (formerly the National Chamber of Commerce) had hastily called a meeting to "survey national business conditions" and discuss possible solutions.

But, as President Roach listened to representatives from the other trade organizations talk about deteriorating conditions, he realized that his own group was not experiencing the same kind of decline. Indeed, as the year progressed, it became apparent that independent retail pharmacists were not yet in an economic crisis as so many of the other industries seemed to be. In reality, Roach spent most of the year on traditional issues that had been before the association for some time.

One of those continuing issues concerned legislation to establish a system of price maintenance. In the early 1920s, Pennsylvania Representative Clyde Kelly introduced a bill to allow manufacturers to set the retail price for their "trade-marked" or "brand-name" products before such goods left the factory. The bill stayed in committee most of the time, but did generate support from Kansas Senator Arthur Capper late in the decade and improved its chances for passage. Capper-Kelly came to be known as NARD's bill to establish control on retail prices. But NARD could not get it passed. Lobbyists for the department and chain store interests and representatives from the wholesalers either kept the measure bottled up in committee or delayed its coming up for vote when the bill got out of committee.

On another traditional issue, the chain drugstore, NARD had more success. Actually the slowdown in growth for chain drugstores was not so much NARD's doing as it was a factor of the economy. Much of the chains' expansion had been driven by credit, and the decline in market conditions caused many banks to reduce or refuse loans for new mortgages. Some trade publications suggested that sales would decline in chain-operated stores by as much as 25 percent before the year was over and that profits might decrease as much as 50 percent. While NARD leaders took no pleasure in others' failures, they did see an opportunity to improve their own circumstances. President Roach said he thought the times may be a "blessing to the independent druggist" because it "forced him to keep a clean store, his merchandise in stock in better shape and displayed in an attractive manner...things vital to his business."

By annual convention time, the business trends for the year had been established. Sales and profits for chain-owned stores were down almost 50 percent, but community pharmacists reported only a 10 to 15 percent decline. When delegates gathered at Atlantic City, New Jersey, in 1930, President Roach told them "the independent druggist...has largely regained his confidence...and given anything like a decent location and sufficient capital, he, with his own personal effort, is more than a match for the chain store." Roach was so confident that a new era was dawning for community pharmacists, he predicted that "the last twelve months will go down in history as a time when chain stores reached their zenith, and also the time when the public as a whole finally awoke to the fact that the continued domination of the retail field by chains would eventually spell economic doom."

Executive Committee Chairman Julius H. Riemenschneider echoed a similar theme in his address to convention delegates. He encouraged his colleagues to take advantage of the times and "out compete" the chain stores. He admitted that "to be successful one must have a well-lighted store with merchandise arranged on counters and shelves in such a manner as to command the attention of prospective buyers." He continued, saying "it is becoming more and more apparent that successful retailers are paying more attention to the selling end of their business than the buying end...concentrating energies on selling profitable items."

CHAPTER FIVE — THE FOURTH DECADE: 1929 – 1938   85

Secretary Samuel Henry reported that "despite the dark clouds that have hovered over and about the business world," the association had been "particularly fortunate" and was on "solid financial footing." This was due primarily to "a surplus this organization has succeeded in acquiring through long years of patient toil and pursuit of sound business policy." He noted that over the years he had sometimes heard criticism about having a surplus in the treasury, but perhaps now delegates could see "the wisdom of maintaining a substantial balance to meet any unforeseen contingency (so that) the task to which the association has been dedicated is carried on successfully without fear or favor."

In many respects it was business as usual at the thirty-second convention. Henry fully expected the economy to turn around in the fall quarter and this view seemed to prevail among the delegates. In other matters of business, the House of Delegates approved "purple and gold" as the association's official colors and agreed to make "Pharmacy Week" a permanent event. Secretary Henry also reported that founding Secretary Thomas Wooten had died in February and that his successor, Thomas Potts, had been seriously ill. Despite that bad news, the convention ended on a note of optimism for the upcoming year. A resolution urging the executive committee to hire an editor for the *Journal* was all but overlooked in the closing day's activities.

The economy did not turn around in the fall quarter and even community pharmacists began to feel the pinch. New NARD President Julius H. Riemenschneider reported that by the end of the spring quarter, volume among independent stores was "down as much as 25 percent in some areas." Even so, he maintained that the "retail drug business...has fared better than any other business." So that they would continue to do so, he urged association members to adjust their businesses to reduce operating costs even if it meant working more hours. He assured his colleagues that the association "stands as solid as the Rock of Gibraltar."

As the depression lengthened into its second year, the competitive forces of the marketplace began to surface in a variety of ways. By convention time, the NARD staff had had an opportunity to chart several of these activities and Riemenschneider decided to make "unfair trade practices" the centerpiece of his presidential address. The association returned to Detroit, Michigan, in 1931 for its thirty-third meeting.

In speaking to the delegates, President Riemenschneider warned them of a practice known as "allowances" where for either advertising space or other service, "manufacturers gave a pharmacist 'an allowance' that permits him to sell below your costs and still make a profit." Riemenschneider called that an "unfair trade practice," as he did another tactic called a "combination." In this instance, "a companion item is given away in connection (combination) with a sale." According to the president, this violated traditional sales rules because "the druggists of the country have been (taught) that to become better merchants they should suggest and sell companion items." But now, "millions of dollars worth of merchandise (are being) given away instead of being sold."

The depressed economy also brought community pharmacists a new form of competition. Called the "pine board store," this business practice began

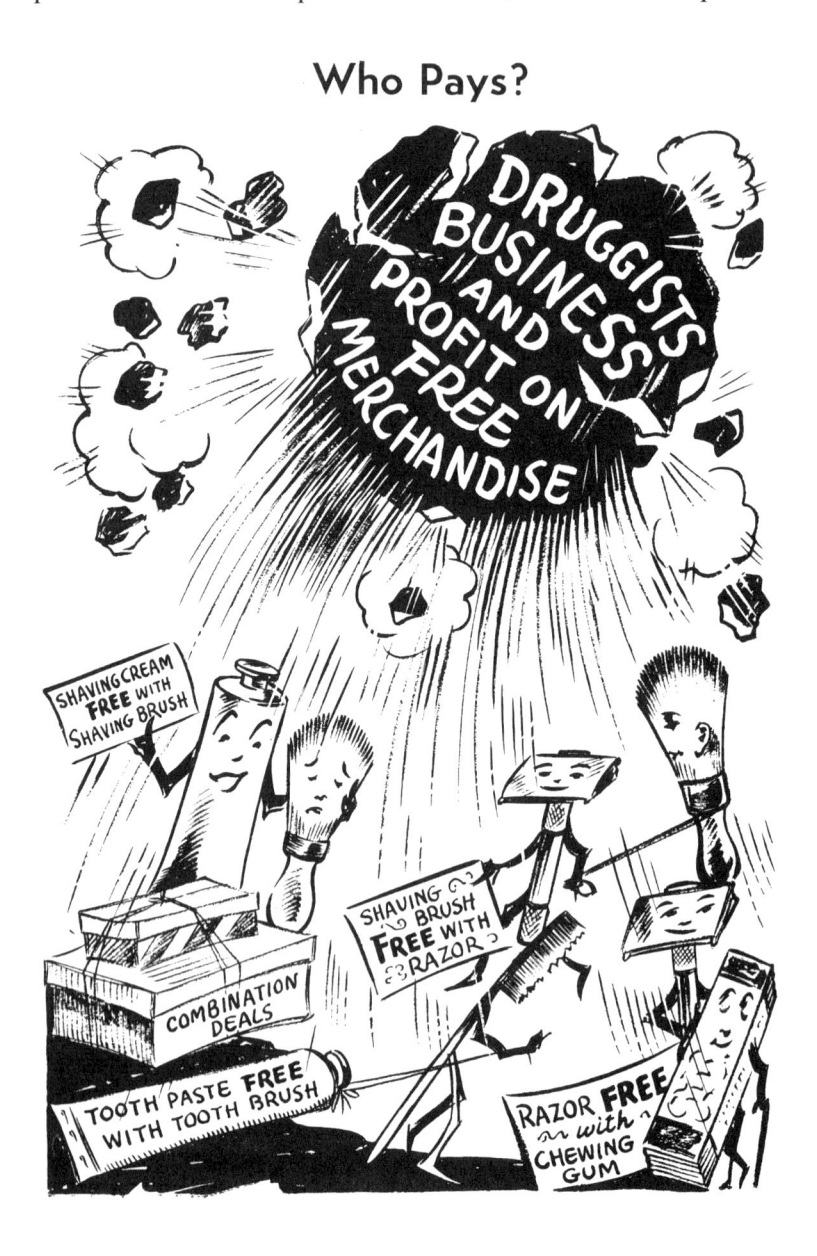

Who Pays?

on the West Coast and gradually extended its influence across the nation. It featured a well-financed "silent partner" who entered economically depressed areas of a community and bought an existing pharmacy or sometimes opened a new store. Being in a "low rent district," employing "cheap labor," and buying large quantities of merchandise (and usually getting an allowance), the pine board store was extremely price competitive. Riemenschneider called the practice "predatory price cutting" and said it was a national problem.

The growing "unfair" trading schemes proved to be a cloud with a silver lining. President Riemenschneider saw it first and told the delegates "as 'big business' is now beginning to feel the pinch of cut-throat competition, perhaps Congress will take heed and enact some form of legislation that will be of some relief in our case."

As a first step, the House of Representatives passed the Capper-Kelly bill, but it died in the Senate without being brought to a vote. Still, getting even one legislative body to approve the measure was a major step toward legalizing a price maintenance agreement. As a consolation prize, word came just before convention time that the state of California had passed a state price maintenance law, a junior Capper-Kelly bill as it was called. While it only applied to that state, the concept was important, and NARD began to work more closely with other states to get similar legislation.

The 1931 NARD convention delegates needed to hear some good news because the annual report from Secretary Henry identified a couple of major problems. First, the bank the association had used in Chicago, Illinois, for twenty-six consecutive years closed its doors on June 17. Fortunately, the executive committee had negotiated a loan with the bank "to tide over an emergency" and when the bank closed, the association's cash account was simply transferred to offset the loan balance. On real estate accounts, NARD was not so fortunate. Rent payments on all the association's property were slow in coming and, in two instances, tenants defaulted on their mortgages. Not only did NARD lose income, but it also had the added burden of finding new tenants.

When Henry finished giving his report, the delegates gave him a standing ovation. That action belied a growing spirit of uneasiness among the delegates that hovered just below the surface throughout the meeting. In addition to those who had traditionally disagreed with the secretary's financial strategies, others wanting a more aggressive response to the depressed conditions questioned the association's "business as usual" approach. Thomas Stoddart, a charter member and active in the "old guard," responded by saying, "there are many financial institutions in this country that would be glad to have Mr. Henry (as) secretary of their organizations at double the salary he is receiving from N.A.R.D." The strong fraternal spirit of the previous decade was being put to the test. The convention also brought news of Leonard Tillotson's death. The passing of the "father of NARD," coupled with Secretary Wooten's death the previous year, was symbolic for those looking more to the association's future than its past. The more traditional members were encouraged in that the executive committee rejected a motion to change the name of the organization to the "National Association of Retail Pharmacists," but clearly, the association was approaching another threshold.

That the association was in transition became evident in the leadership style of the new president. John A. Dargavel, a young activist in the Minneapolis Association of Retail Druggists, was among those who wanted NARD to take a more proactive approach toward the depressed business conditions and the price maintenance issue. The new style was quickly demonstrated in the executive committee's post-convention meeting. The only agenda item of substance concerned the association's official representative in Washington. Eugene Brokmeyer had been filling that role on a part-time basis since 1915. Dargavel and some on the new executive committee wanted to make the office full-time and establish NARD's presence on Capitol Hill. Others on the executive committee were concerned about the added expense and questioned the timing of the move. A few members also felt loyalty to Brokmeyer and questioned if he would be comfortable in the new role. But as the discussions developed, it was clear that those favoring change were in the majority. The executive committee voted to terminate Brokmeyer's contract with a thirty-day notice and accepted bids for a full-time legal counsel in Washington.

At its second meeting, in November 1931 at NARD headquarters, the executive committee revisited again the issue of a Washington representative for NARD. Only one person, W. Bruce Phillip, had expressed an interest in the Washington position. In addition to his law degree, Phillip was also a pharmacist, active in both NARD and the American Pharmaceutical Association (APhA). He also had a large insurance business in California. In his interview, Phillip urged the executive committee to commit to the Washington office for a minimum of four years and said that he needed a salary of at least $7,500. The executive committee was reluctant to make a four-year commitment to a new office, given the "current conditions," and voted to offer Phillip a three-year appointment with an annual budget of $10,000 — $7,500 in salary and $2,500 in office expenses.

Another indication that NARD's style was changing came in a new look to the *Journal*. For almost fifteen years the cover and format remained largely unchanged. Beginning with the January 1932 issue, the new *Journal* changed from a weekly to a biweekly publication, the design was altered to include a more "modern" cover, and the page size was increased. Secretary Henry continued to serve as editor, and the executive committee again urged him to "look around" for at least an assistant if not a full-time editor.

When Congress reconvened in December, Congressman Kelly reintroduced the Capper-Kelly bill and NARD made ready to fully utilize its new Washington office. But with 1932 a presidential election year, and with the economy still not responding to efforts to stimulate its growth, it was difficult to get action on most legislation. Declining revenues forced Congress to make new funding proposals a top priority, and the price maintenance issue faded to the background.

NARD leaders had carefully prepared for the Capper-Kelly bill, but soon found themselves involved in a fight over a general sales tax bill. Early in January, an administration-sponsored bill to raise the general sales tax by 1.5

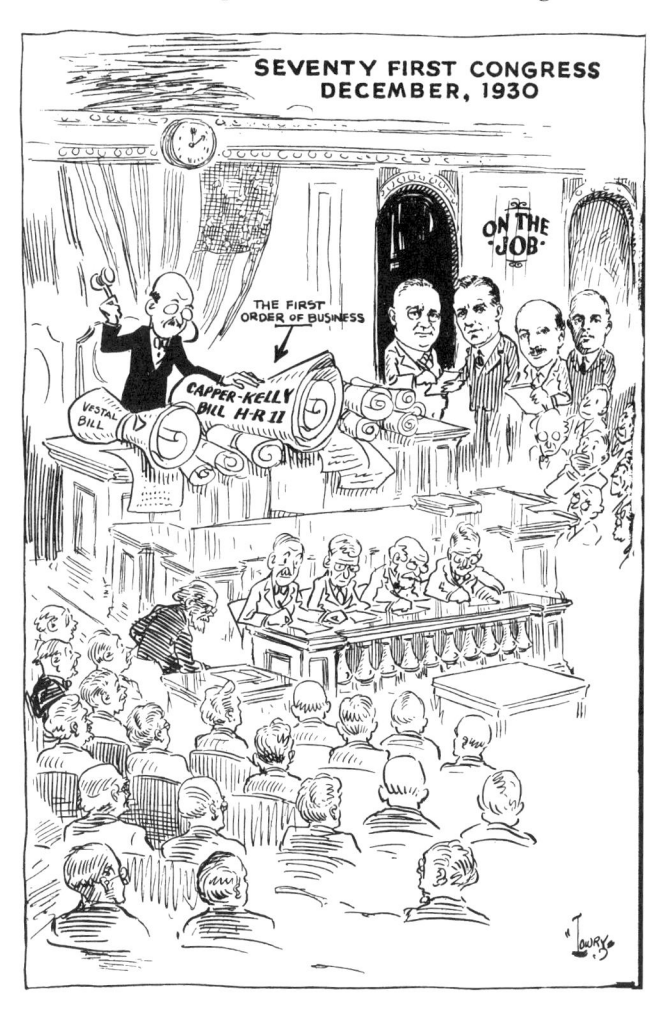

percent was introduced in Congress. Since delegates to the 1931 convention had passed a resolution opposing any sales tax increase in any form, Henry, Dargavel, and Chairman Hunsberger spoke in opposition to it. As hearings on the bill progressed in subcommittee, the sales tax was amended to substitute a 5 to 10 percent tax on designated articles. For pharmacists, those items would be cosmetics, dentifrices, and some soda fountain products. When it was apparent that the tax bill would get a favorable recommendation, NARD leaders supported the 5 to 10 percent tax rather than risk passage of the lower, more general sales tax.

The higher rate was adopted, causing NARD's leaders to be criticized by some in the membership for supporting such a high tax. Dargavel defended the leadership's action on the basis that "pharmacists are a great deal better off under the present taxation plan than if a general sales tax had been passed."

Despite the influence of a presidential campaign, the economy did not improve in 1932. By some reports, the volume of sales among independent pharmacists was down another 20 to 25 percent over the previous year and the stress of hard times was again reflected at the annual meeting.

The thirty-fourth convention returned to Boston, Massachusetts. Attendance was down from previous years due in part to the economy and to the distance in traveling. In addressing the delegates, President Dargavel noted the changes made in the *Journal*, explained the decision to expand the Washington office, and explained why the NARD leadership supported the new tax bill.

Dargavel also gave an update on the Capper-Kelly bill, which still languished in Congress. The reason it had not passed, in his opinion, was because "the druggists were of divided opinions as to the (bill's) material benefits." He said in his travels to the state associations, he had heard all manner of "misinformation and propaganda spread by those who desire the failure of its enactment." He lectured the delegates about the importance of a united front and said, "I cannot comprehend why the druggists throughout the country will believe the stories put out to deceive them and refuse to rely upon the integrity and honesty of the officers...who are fighting for this piece of legislation."

But President Dargavel reserved his strongest language for "unfair trade practices." He said the time had come for the association to call manufacturers into account for their "secret allowances" and "rebates," including refusing to allow those who engaged in such practices to advertise in "the *Journal* or exhibit at the Convention drug show." For Dargavel "the time has come when the sheep should be separated from the goats and the pussyfooting ended. Manufacturers who are willing to help the retailers should be commended and every possible effort should be made to cooperate with them in the sale of their merchandise. Those who are unwilling to maintain a fair sales policy should be condemned and put where they belong."

When Dargavel finished his speech, he received an ovation that Samuel Henry, as editor of the *Journal,* wrote "was undoubtedly one of the outstanding demonstrations of the convention." Thomas Stoddart, who had attended every convention, said it was "the best and ablest" he had ever listened to and asked the delegates to stand and give the president "three rousing cheers." Other delegates echoed a similar theme and some asked that the speech be reprinted and circulated to "every retail druggist in the United States." Clearly, the soon-to-be-retired president had struck a responsive nerve with the delegates.

The executive secretary was not among those cheering. When it came his time to address the convention, Secretary Henry was in a defensive mood. The association's financial picture was bleak, and he had not been able to pay all the organization's bills for the year. He explained that the association had sunk into this condition for three primary reasons. First, a large number of checks sent in for dues payments were returned unpaid because the bank of issue had closed its doors. Second, NARD traditionally relied on local asso-

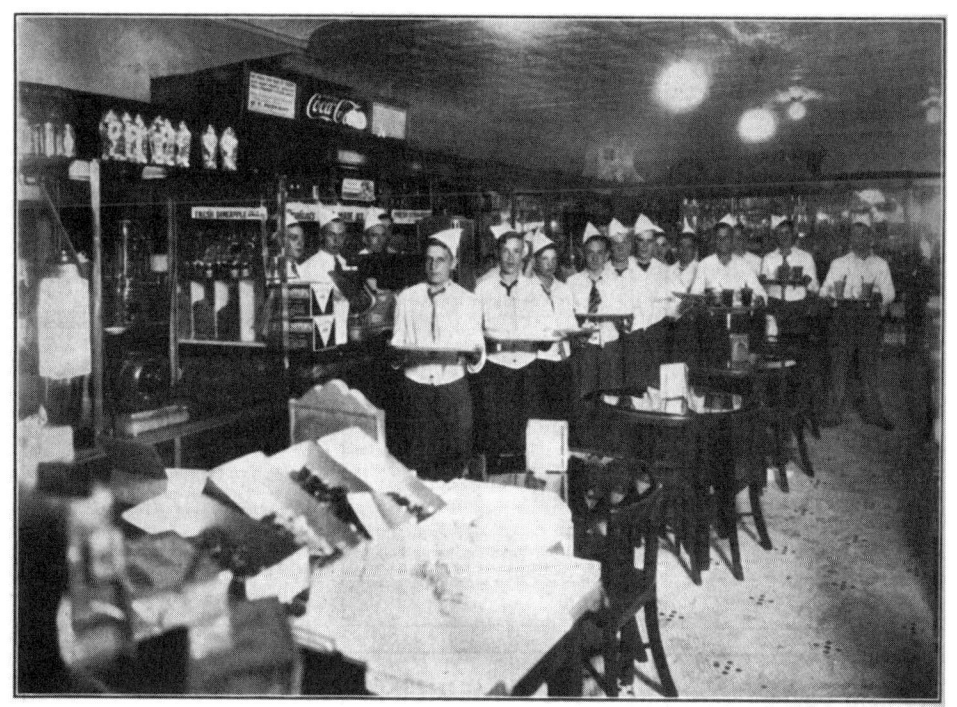

The interior of a modern drugstore of the 1930s with an emphasis on the fountain business

ciations in the larger cities to collect all dues from members and pass along the appropriate share to the national office. Dues collection from this area was the association's "heaviest loss." Finally, Henry noted that "defaulted interest on mortgages held by the N.A.R.D." had not only deprived the organization of income but also cost more to make legal settlements.

In addition to losing income, the association had also incurred some additional costs. The new Washington office had not been included in the budget adopted at the 1931 convention, and the fight for the Capper-Kelly bill cost more than had been anticipated. He tried to answer his critics by saying, "what has become of those men who, but a few short years ago took exception to the association accumulating any surplus at all?"

But the sharpest demarcation between the secretary and the activists in the convention had to do with the *Journal*. He noted that he was not in sympathy with those who wanted the publication to "assume a more militant attitude in dealing with questions that arise from day to day." He reminded his readers that "Some years ago the *Journal,* or *Notes* as it was then called, did follow a decidedly militant course hurling accusations in all directions apparently on the identical theory now being advanced to the effect that one accused of wrongdoing should first be clubbed into insensibility and reasoned with only when he regained consciousness...." He concluded, "Your secretary-editor cannot bring himself to accept any such theory as either sound, constructive or honorable, nor do I believe that it expresses the will and desire of the membership in this splendid organization."

How the delegates responded to the secretary's speech was not recorded. However, President Dargvel announced that the secretary had an announcement to make, and Henry came back to the podium to say: "I am here to say to anyone in this room this morning that if anyone knows, or thinks he knows, or has reason to believe that I have ever accepted $1, or any other valuable consideration from any source whatever in the fifteen years I have served as secretary of this association, that man owes it to you, as members of this organization and to me, to make his statement in open meeting."

When no one came forward, the secretary concluded his statement and was given a standing ovation. A number of delegates spoke in his defense and "deplored the insinuations" that had been cast upon the office. President Dargavel said he was confident that "any fair-minded, intelligent member of the association that knows Secretary Henry would not put any faith in any insinuation that his office has not been properly conducted." Dargavel also voiced displeasure with "the politics that were being played." Delegates ended that session with a rising vote of confidence in the secretary.

The thirty-fourth convention concluded by adopting a record number of resolutions. Included among them was one in support of Secretary Henry that read, "We consider his services to be of inestimable value to our association and indulge in the hope that he may continue to function in his present capacity for many years to come." There was also a resolution to "endorse our president's words...all that independent retailers ask of manufacturers is fair and square business dealing under the motto 'equal privileges to all with special privileges to none'."

All was not well in the leadership of the association, and problems surfaced in the new executive committee meeting just hours after the convention adjourned. John A. Goode had been elected the new president. While in past years he had served on the executive committee, in the year preceding the 1932 convention he had neither been on the executive committee nor an officer — the traditional steps to being nominated to the office of president.

The post-convention meeting of the new executive committee was traditionally for purposes of organization only. After each officer took the oath of office, President Goode called for nominations to chair the executive committee. F.R. Peterson nominated Ambrose Hunsberger, the incumbent chairman. Goode, after asking Thomas Roach to temporarily chair the meeting, nominated John Dargavel. When the vote was called, Peterson and Roach voted for Hunsberger; Goode, C. Fred Wright, and new member Charles

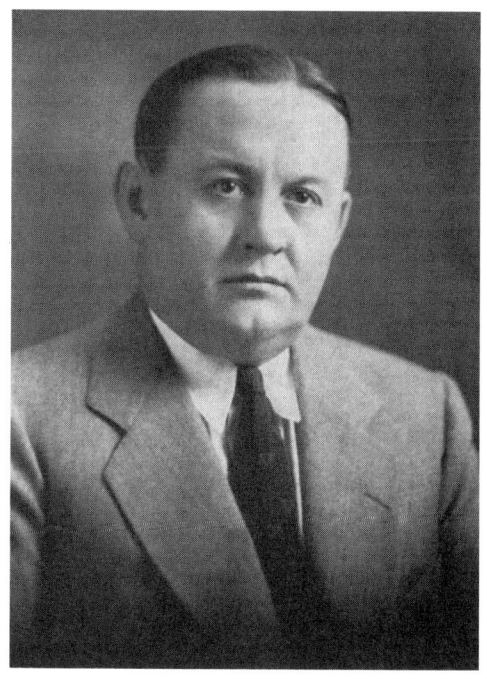

John W. Dargavel, NARD Executive Secretary, 1933 – 1961

Ehlers voted for Dargavel. Hunsberger and Dargavel did not vote. Hunsberger then moved to make Dargavel's nomination unanimous and the executive committee proceeded to routine business. But matters were far from routine in NARD. Within a month of the convention, a major disagreement developed between Secretary Henry and Chairman Dargavel over the secretary's official position with the executive committee. The NARD Constitution defined the secretary's role as one of voice but not vote in the committee. However, on items requiring official action when the convention was not in session, the secretary, by tradition, prepared a written motion and mailed it to each member of the committee with a return ballot. Results of the vote were also announced by mail. Dargavel objected to this practice, and the issue became a matter of "heated discussion" at the executive committee's regular November meeting.

Before the meeting was over, additional items, including the method of auditing the association's accounts and a new editorial policy for the *Journal*, became the object of disagreement between the secretary and members of the committee. President Goode appointed an independent audit team to review the association's accounts for the past four years and in June, the executive committee hired George A. Bender, a Minneapolis journalist, to be the new editor of the *Journal*.

Relationships within the NARD leadership remained strained throughout the year. A sense of formalism replaced fraternalism and camaraderie as the executive committee prepared to respond to the membership's needs. With the change in presidential leadership, the Capper-Kelly bill was dead. Congress prepared for a "New Deal" from President Franklin D. Roosevelt and were all but overwhelmed by the "100 Days" of legislation unleashed by the Roosevelt "Brain Trust."

The initial contact between NARD officials and staff members of the Roosevelt administration was cordial. Goode, Dargavel, and their colleagues were impressed that the new administration seemed to understand the plight of the small businessman and were perhaps even sympathetic to the independent retailers. From these and other meetings, the administration fashioned the National Recovery Act (NRA) and pushed it through Congress as part of the 100-Day package. In theory this bill replaced the price contract features of the Capper-Kelly bill with more comprehensive provisions affecting prices, wages, and conditions of the small businessman. However, the key to making the bill work was in obtaining "industry-wide" agreement on a "code of fair competition."

Throughout the summer, Goode, Dargavel, and legal counsel Bruce Phillip worked with other representatives from the drug industry and administration officials to develop a code for pharmacy. But after the industry submitted five draft proposals, including one prepared by NARD, the Roosevelt staff decided to write the code by themselves. They were still writing when the NARD convention opened in September 1933 in Chicago, Illinois.

The thirty-fifth convention was reminiscent of 1898 in tone. President Goode and Chairman Dargavel reviewed their activities on behalf of the association as their predecessors had done. However, according to George Bender's reporting in the *Journal,* while Dargavel was reading his report, "a tense silence hung over the convention hall, mutely evidencing the serious determination of the delegates present that the association's affairs should be rectified and the organization placed upon a firm basis that would permit it to go forward to achieve the greatest good for all."

Another tense time came when the nominating committee made its report on the last day. Noticeably absent from the slate of candidates was Samuel C. Henry. Conspicuous by its presence was John W. Dargavel as secretary. Henry was nominated from the floor, but he asked that his name be withdrawn. The committee's slate was then elected by the House of Delegates. Bender wrote, "Convention Orders 'New Deal'" for a headline and the association began a new era in its history.

Dargavel, newly elected President Monte L. Powell, and new executive committee Chairman Harvey Henry realized that nothing would end controversy like success. Consequently, they moved actively to pick up the fair trade issue. The year of internal strife and the advent of a new presidential administration had hampered slightly the association's focus, but before the year was ended, NARD was back in the fight for fair prices. By that time, the NRA representatives had worked out a Fair Trade Code for the drug industry, and President Roosevelt signed it into law on October 22, 1933.

The NRA Code created an advisory committee, the National Retail Drug Code Authority, and allowed a maximum of two members from each branch of the drug industry. The executive committee appointed Secretary Dargavel and Immediate Past President John Goode to be NARD's representatives. But overall, the code was a disappointment for NARD. It did not contain NARD's original recommendation for a price contract and did not sufficiently control the possibility for price cutting.

Dargavel reminded the executive committee that the code had been "handed to us by executive order of the President," and the association had no input into its final form. Still, it was of some value to retail druggists in that it prohibited "selling below a manufacturers' list price." The secretary pointed out that this was the first time in retail history that such a law had been put in place, and with the Drug Code Authority advising administrators, he was confident pharmacists would gain more benefits from the code being in place.

The executive committee also worked hard on increasing membership. Hard times had reduced the number of paid field workers to two and several others worked part-time or on a commission basis. Secretary Dargavel suggested using the *Journal* to promote membership with a target goal of 35,000 members by the end of the year. Editor Bender began an energetic campaign for "35 in 34" and kept the idea before the membership for most of the year.

Militancy became the word of choice for the NARD officer corps in 1934. The intensity of the leadership to not only overcome the immediate internal crisis, but also fashion a long-term strategy to ensure fair trade practices began to be transferred to the membership. Bender noticed this new attitude while covering the thirty-sixth convention meeting in New Orleans, Louisiana, in 1934. In his words, "militancy was the keynote of the convention...druggists in twos, fours, dozens, and throngs, displayed an intensity of purpose and determination to achieve their aims."

President Monte Powell told the delegates the association had "broken out of its rut" and had "adjusted to the changing business conditions." Chairman Harvey Henry emphasized that NARD continued to be the champion for "fair trade laws," while also opposing "price discrimination," and it would push for those measures even as the Roosevelt administration worked out the details of the National Recovery Administration.

Secretary Dargavel reminded the members that "a year ago you demanded a new deal" for the association. With the association showing a significant increase in membership, an independent audit certifying that all bills had been paid, a surplus in the treasury, the new and improved *Journal,* and a closer working relationship with the state associations, he felt confident the leadership had largely succeeded in meeting that mandate. For the coming year, he proposed a three-pronged emphasis: "a comprehensive and well-defined legislative program, an aggressive and definite arbitration policy between retail druggists and their suppliers, and a plan to assist members operate their stores efficiently and profitably."

Perhaps it was the lavish entertainment provided at the New Orleans, Louisiana convention or the signs of progress in the association, but whatever the reason, the strained relationships of the past year were largely forgotten. There were few floor debates on the various committee recommendations, and the slate of officers for the new year was elected unanimously. Harvey Henry moved from the executive committee to become the new president and in the post-convention meeting of the officers, Charles Ehlers was elected chairman of the executive committee.

As the new committee previewed the year ahead, the NRA code enforcement on fair business practices appeared to be the major issue. The legal

CHAPTER FIVE — THE FOURTH DECADE: 1929 – 1938   97

technicalities were complicated, and Secretary Dargavel believed the association needed better leadership in the Washington office. He and several of the officers had become upset with staff attorney Bruce Phillip because he had failed to stay focused on NARD affairs and was frequently unresponsive to issues the executive committee considered priority. After some discussion, the executive committee voted to accept the secretary's recommendation and terminate Phillip's contract. Reopening the position for new applicants,

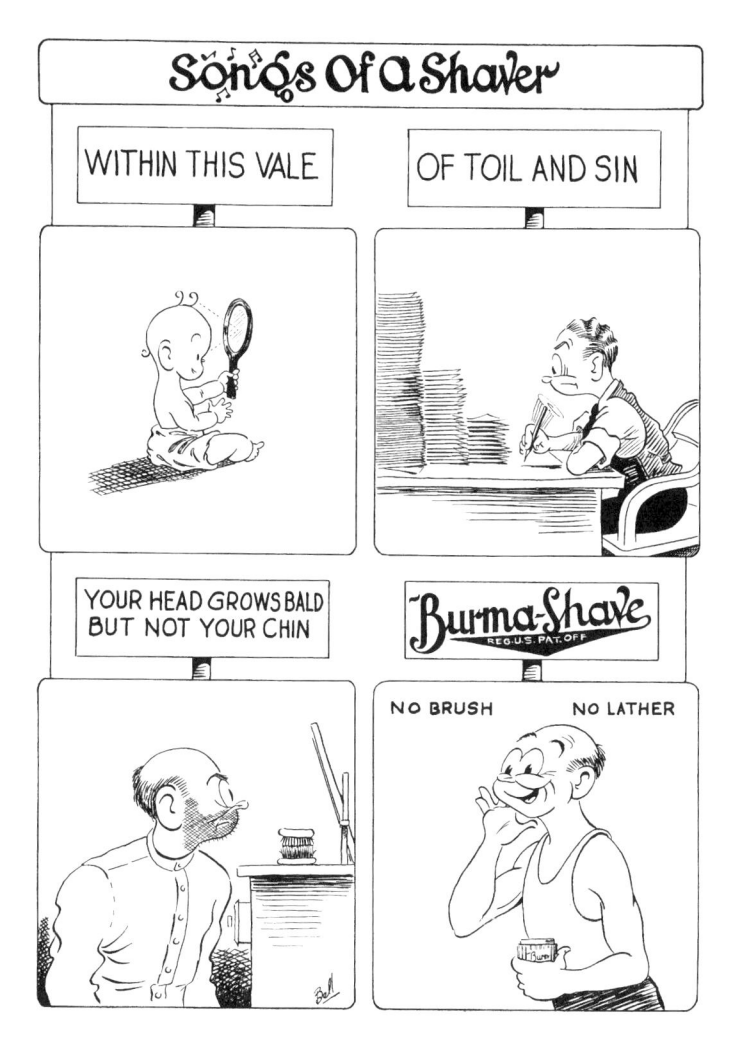

A familiar advertisement and product of the 1930s

the executive committee chose Rowland Jones, Jr., a pharmacist and lawyer from South Dakota. Jones had served as secretary of the South Dakota Pharmaceutical Association, and he came from a family of pharmacists.

As Dargavel and his colleagues prepared to lobby Congress about their needs, word came of a powerful retail group being organized to do battle with the Roosevelt administration's NRA codes, fair trade laws, and any other measure that allowed public agencies to interfere with the marketplace. Calling themselves the American Retail Federation (ARF), these power players allegedly represented the largest retail establishments in the nation, and they were determined to silence all efforts at standardizing price and labor codes. Contacting the major news outlets, officials with the ARF let it be known that their belief in "self-help" was to be preferred over governmental interference in the retail sector — particularly as it had been expressed thorough the NRA trade codes. In their view, even the near-crisis atmosphere of the depression decade should not alter the fundamental laws of a market-driven economy.

According to information released to the press, ARF organizers argued that "there is no single authoritative group to speak for retailers," and since retailing was the "third largest (industry) in the country," they should be organized. Moreover, membership was to be "open to all merchants, whether large or small," and the organization would focus on "cooperation with government and other agencies participating in movements for the promotion of general prosperity...of the United States."

Dargavel and the executive committee were not willing to accept such rhetoric. In a highly publicized telegram to NRA Code Administrator Gen. Hugh Johnson, Dargavel called the ARF a monopoly and said it was a threat to the small businessmen throughout the nation because it could possibly discriminate against small business on prices. Gen. Johnson turned the telegram over to the Senate Finance Committee. That group failed to act. However, the issue caught the attention of John J. Cochran, representative from Missouri, who introduced a resolution to investigate the ARF. A new fight was on.

Rep. Cochran became ill soon after his resolution was approved, and the investigation fell to Wright Patman, a congressman from Texas, the next senior member on the Senate Finance Committee. The resolution created a special seven-member committee to investigate the ARF as to its capitalization, its membership, its objectives, the sources of its funds, its financial connections and its officers and agents.

Cochran had been particularly concerned that the new organization might turn out to be a "super lobbying group" and use its considerable wealth to unduly influence members of Congress. Rumors that ARF had pledges for more than $750,000 to use in its lobbying efforts were widely circulated and reprinted in major newspapers. Federation officials downplayed those rumors and said they anticipated that their membership would soon include a number of organizations representing small business. Possible members in this latter group included NARD, the Retail Grocers Association, and the National Hardware Association. Furthermore, ARF prices were to be based on market conditions and would not discriminate solely on the basis of size, ARF said.

Despite ARF's disclaimer, trade association papers added to the concerns of many by reporting that the new group planned to force the smaller, independent retail merchants of America, "engaged in the sale of necessities of everyday life," to contribute an additional $2 million annually to the funds available to this organization in its lobbying activities. Such reporting got Patman's attention. It also got Dargavel's attention. He denounced the ARF for identifying NARD as a "possible member" and sent a telegram to officials at ARF requesting an immediate public retraction. In a follow-up press release, he charged the new retail group with being "a shoddy cloak (for) big and unscrupulous businessmen to cover their real purposes under the guise of representing the small retailers."

He also warned that the ARF had a "diabolically clever scheme of propaganda and wire-pulling intended to promote the growth of great retail monopolies, which if unchecked, will oppress a great number of the workers of the country under conditions approximating economic serfdom." If allowed to succeed, the new method of organizing would leave the "consumer defenseless and bring about the extinction of hundreds of thousands of small businesses throughout the nation."

Patman shared Dargavel's view about the ARF and when the organization moved to incorporate, he decided he needed broader powers to investigate. Returning to his colleagues in the House of Representatives, he gained additional approval to include "the trade practices of individuals, partnerships and corporations engaged in big-scale buying and selling of articles at wholesale and retail." Patman said he now believed the ARF was a group of corporate interests who had "pooled their resources for the purpose of squeezing out the little fellow" through a process of volume buying and price discrimination. Dargavel and members of the executive committee could not have agreed more.

Armed with increased authority, Patman began hearings on June 6. He called the ARF officers to testify. But each denied any motive beyond "gathering statistics on retail distribution not now available to government agencies." Patman was not convinced of their truthfulness, but neither could he break their story. He was to the point of despair when late in the month a staff member, on a tip from Dargavel at NARD, uncovered data of a major consolidation in the grocery business. One firm in particular had received over "$8 million in secret and confidential rebates during 1934, and altogether chain grocery stores did over 80 percent of the cash business in food and grocery sales."

That was the type of price discrimination Patman was looking for and while the data had been compiled from the grocery business, he was convinced it was typical of small business everywhere and he wanted to put a stop to the practice. Dargavel confirmed that independent pharmacists were facing similar proportional losses and he encouraged Congress to act. Patman did not need much encouragement, but Congress adjourned before he could get a bill on the calendar and he was forced to wait until the next session in January 1936 to revisit the matter.

Dargavel and the NARD leadership were disappointed at not getting either a fair trade or price discrimination law passed, but they were encouraged at Patman's progress. When they were not working with the Patman investigation, the NARD leadership devoted time to reworking the association's operating procedures and involving more of the membership in the work.

One criticism of the NARD officers that had developed over the years was that the members of the executive committee tended to ignore resolutions passed by the House of Delegates and to work on their own agenda. President Henry decided to address that. He and the executive committee reviewed each resolution, then assigned it to the appropriate officer or committee. Everyone with any official position was given a direct responsibility for some phase of the association's work.

Henry also established a special "Advisory Committee to the President," composed of the presidents from each state association. He used this group to respond to resolutions and to lobby political leaders in the various districts for specific legislation. Involving more people in the association's activities and the higher volume of paperwork created a shortage of work space in the headquarters office. In fact, Dargavel had been looking for more suitable space for the association's national office since taking over as secretary. When a suite became vacant in the Engineering Building at 205 Wacker Drive, he recommended that space and the executive committee agreed to relocate.

Having so many members with direct involvement in the policy process no doubt contributed to harmony when delegates gathered at Cincinnati, Ohio, for the thirty-seventh convention in 1935. In his presidential address, Henry told the delegates of the leadership's support for the Patman investigation and said they were also committed to getting a fair trade law passed.

He said, too, that he wanted to reestablish the "cornerstone upon which the association was founded — the principle of 33 1/3% margin from the suggested minimum price" on retail products. He pointed out that this was nothing more than the old $2/$4/$8 formula used until World War I disrupted the price structure.

Chairman Ehlers and Secretary Dargavel echoed Henry's sentiments, and the House of Delegates also overwhelmingly endorsed the concept. In another show of unity, the delegates elected Charles Ehlers the new president for 1935-1936 and added Hugh P. Beirne as a new member of the executive committee. Harvey Henry rejoined the committee after completing his term as president. Thomas S. Smith was chosen by his peers to chair the executive committee.

As promised to the House of Delegates, the NARD officer corps resumed their fight against price discrimination and for fair trade in fall 1935. While Congress was out of session during the fall, congressional supporters of the ARF held a series of subcommittee hearings to offset the negative publicity raised by the Patman hearings. But the NARD Executive Committee and its allies recruited from various independent retailers were determined that the corporate interests would not gain the upper hand.

Dargavel organized a number of special "fair trade committees" and kept a steady barrage of editorials, articles, and news releases against price discrimination flowing from headquarters. He also worked through staff attorney Rowland Jones to keep close tabs on supporters in Congress. This publicity did much to neutralize the ARF's counterattack, and when the 75th Session of Congress opened in January 1936, the independent retailers were ready.

As an indication of how popular the price discrimination issue had become in just one year, no less than six new bills on the topic were introduced in the new Congress. Patman reopened hearings in February. In the meantime, Arkansas Senator Joseph T. Robinson, the majority floor leader, introduced a companion to Patman's bill in the Senate. The Senate Judiciary Committee approved Robinson's bill after only two days of hearings and scheduled it for a vote in early April.

Ironically, the quick approval of the Robinson bill caused some trouble for Patman's bill. The ARF, while clearly on the defensive, still had its supporters in Congress and used that organization to good advantage to delay Patman's bill. Since 1936 was also a presidential election year, the realities of party politics began to influence the bill's progress. By March supporters of the proposal were having doubts about whether the bill would get out of committee.

With the Robinson-Patman bill seemingly stalled, Dargavel and the small retailers again sprang into action. Calling for a national "Independent's Day" rally in Washington on March 4, the "independents" flooded the nation with appeals for small businessmen to show their support for the bill. More than 1,700 representatives from thirty-six states showed up in a rousing demonstration. Robinson and Patman both spoke at the gathering. The next day Dargavel led a delegation to meet with President Roosevelt while other independents met with their respective congressmen on Capitol Hill.

The tactic worked. On March 24, the Patman bill was reported out of committee and scheduled for a vote on May 28. Upon hearing of the House's favorable action, Sen. Robinson put his bill on the Senate calendar for April 28. The Robinson bill passed without a dissenting vote after only two days of debate. The House then approved the Patman bill and with quick work in the Conference Committee, the act was ready for the President's signature. He signed the measure into law on June 19.

As finally approved, the Robinson-Patman Anti-Discrimination Act required a seller to extend to all customers, who bought in the same quantities, the same net prices on goods of the same kind and quality. Any differences had to be justified on the basis of selling, transportation, or manufacturing costs. The burden of proof against charges of discrimination was on the accused, and both buyer and seller were liable for prosecution.

(The Robinson-Patman Act in the coming decades became the legal linchpin used to guard against numerous assaults on marketplace "fairness," especially against small businesses such as independent retail pharmacists. The fact that NARD was instrumental, as an organization, in securing its passage led to nationwide recognition of the political clout of the association and its members in Washington, D.C., and elsewhere. The victory became a hallmark in case law as it was tested in the years to come — and NARD's name was attached to it indelibly.)

Dargavel and the members of the executive committee were elated at the victory. Having worked so long for a law, then to see it move through Congress in just a matter of weeks, was particularly satisfying. With that battle behind them, they could now plan for the thirty-eighth convention scheduled for Pittsburgh, Pennsylvania. Congressman Patman was invited to address the NARD House of Delegates. He reiterated a statement made at an earlier press conference — that without NARD the Robinson-Patman bill would not have become law and the association was now a "respected power in the national field."

President Ehlers and Executive Committee Chairman Smith also devoted most of their addresses to the legislative campaign and the implications for the association with Robinson-Patman as law. Both men, along with Secretary Dargavel, reminded the delegates that the association only had achieved one-half of its national legislative package and planned to go after the other half, fair trade, in the next session of Congress. The House of Delegates gave all three men an enthusiastic reception and the old refrain "best convention ever" began to be heard again for the first time in four years. In another show of unity, the group unanimously elected a new slate of officers that included George L. Secord as president. Thomas Smith was reelected chairman of the executive committee.

Within days of the Pittsburgh convention, Dargavel and the executive officers turned their attention to passing a national fair trade bill. They already had a good start. In the last session of Congress, Maryland Senator Millard E. Tydings introduced the National Fair Trade Enabling Act that incorporated key provisions favored by NARD.

Senator Tydings To Introduce National Fair Trade Enabling Act

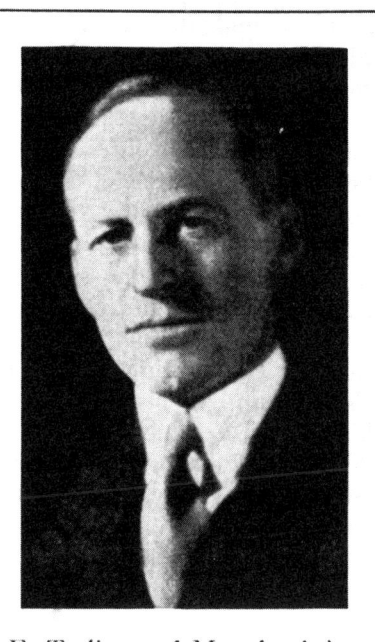

On October 21, Senator Millard E. Tydings of Maryland, in a meeting at Washington, agreed to introduce and sponsor in the coming session of Congress, legislation to remove all doubt as to the legality of the state Fair Trade Acts, particularly in regard to contracts in interstate commerce. The bill will also be introduced in the Lower House by a Representative soon to be selected. This important and highly encouraging meeting was attended by Chairman Swain and Dr. E. F. Kelly of the N. A. R. D. Fair Trade Committee, Herbert Levy, Baltimore, counsel for the Committee; Thomas S. Smith, Wilmington, Chairman of the N. A. R. D. Executive Committee and Rowland Jones, Jr., N. A. R. D. Washington Representative.

From the NARD Journal, November 7, 1935

ion tending to show that price-cutting by retail dealers is not only injurious to the good-will and business of the producer and distributor of identified goods but injurious to the general public as well." The court also ruled that "Fair Trade Acts are not price fixing statutes." Having the court's opinion on free trade before Congress reconvened in January 1937 was a major asset for the movement. Dargavel and attorney Rowland Jones lobbied the Congress in Washington and kept various state leaders informed. Tydings reintroduced his bill in the Senate during the opening days of the new session, and Arkansas Representative John Miller presented a similar bill to the lower house. The bills moved through their respective committees with few changes; Dargavel and Jones were confident both would receive a "do pass" vote by committee members. However, on April 26, the White House released a statement by President Roosevelt asking that further consideration on the Tydings-Miller bill be delayed.

The president's response came as a shock to NARD leaders. In the association's own response to the president, Secretary Dargavel began a series of strongly worded editorials in the *Journal* spelling out what was at stake for independent pharmacists and urging store owners to contact their state's congressional delegation and ask them to support the bill. Jones sent out press releases to the leaders of the state associations asking them to write President Roosevelt. This tactic had worked well in promoting the Robinson-Patman Act, and Jones was hoping for similar results.

Pharmacists responded to NARD's requests. From the various states came a barrage of letters, phone calls, mass rallies, and personal visits to key congressional representatives. Secretary Dargavel wrote that he "was indeed gratified at the spontaneous and enthusiastic support" the membership had given. Dargavel wrote his own "open letter to the President" and asked that he give the small business and trade association representatives time to hear their side of the issue. Tydings and Miller also asked for an audience with the president.

President Roosevelt maintained his reservations about the bill, despite the widespread demonstration of support. Seeing the legislative year slipping away, Sen. Tydings decided to use a parliamentary ploy to move the bill forward. In early July, he attached the bill as a rider to a District of Columbia tax bill. NARD members focused their persuasive powers on that proposal and assisted Tydings in getting a "do pass" on his amendment. The value of this maneuver was that the entire bill would have to be defeated — something the president and most of Congress did not want to do. Tydings was now quite confident that his measure would pass the Senate.

At this point in the political game, Rep. Patman re-emerged to support his "old friends" at NARD. He made a visit to President Roosevelt to present

CHAPTER FIVE — THE FOURTH DECADE: 1929 – 1938

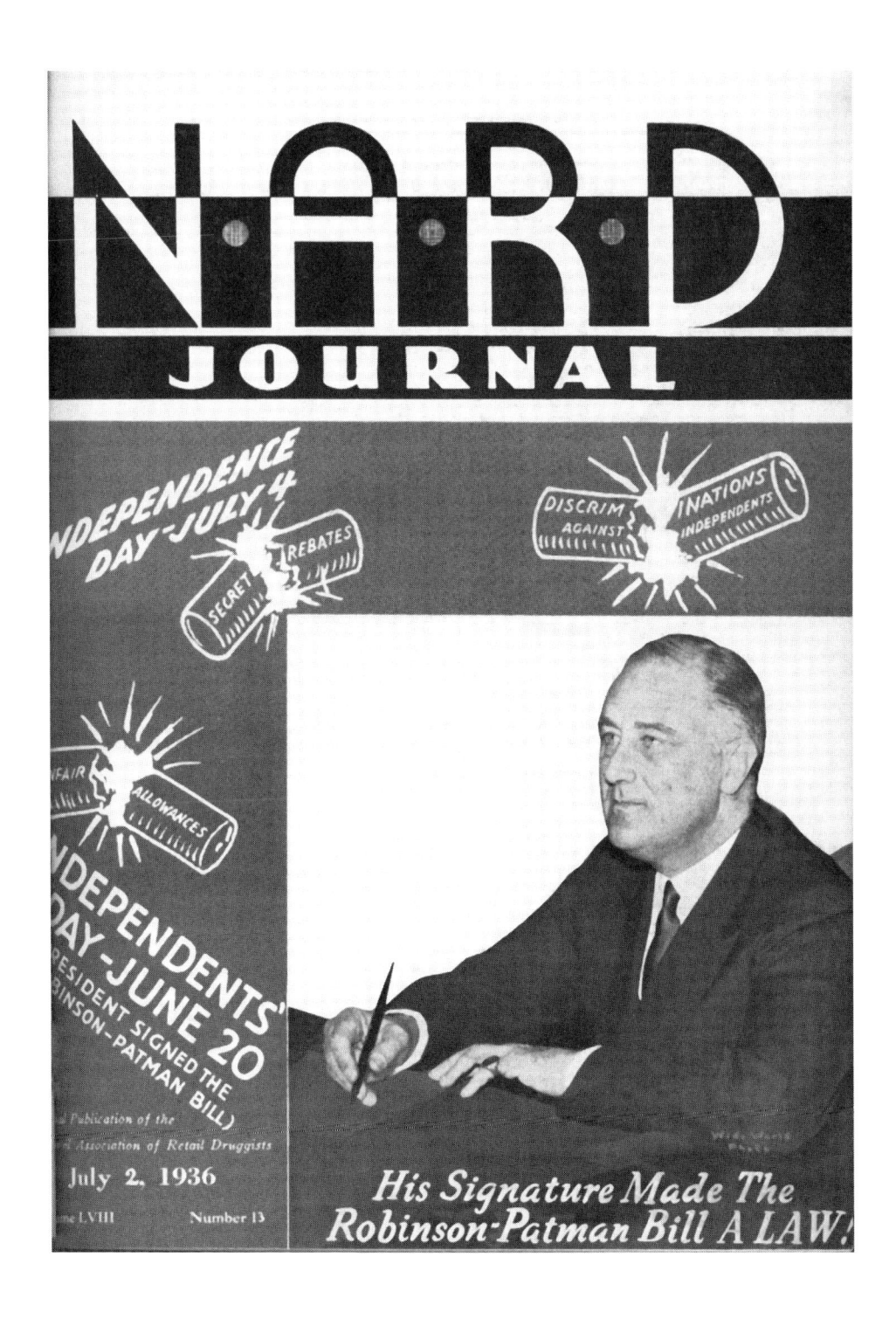

a case for the bill. Given the Tydings maneuver, the personal contact by Patman, and the effective lobbying by NARD and other small retail organizations, the president withdrew his objections — provided the Justice Department was satisfied with the bill. Attorney General Cummings reviewed the bill and made a few minor additions to the text (none of which Tydings or Miller found objectionable). The bill passed Congress on August 4. President Roosevelt signed the Tydings-Miller Fair Trade Enabling Bill into law on August 17 — a second historic victory for NARD in as many years.

NARD's work on the fair trade bill was the talk of the business world. In its August 28, 1937 issue, *Business Week* magazine, in recounting the fight on Tydings-Miller bill, said, "More importantly, it set up the National Associa-

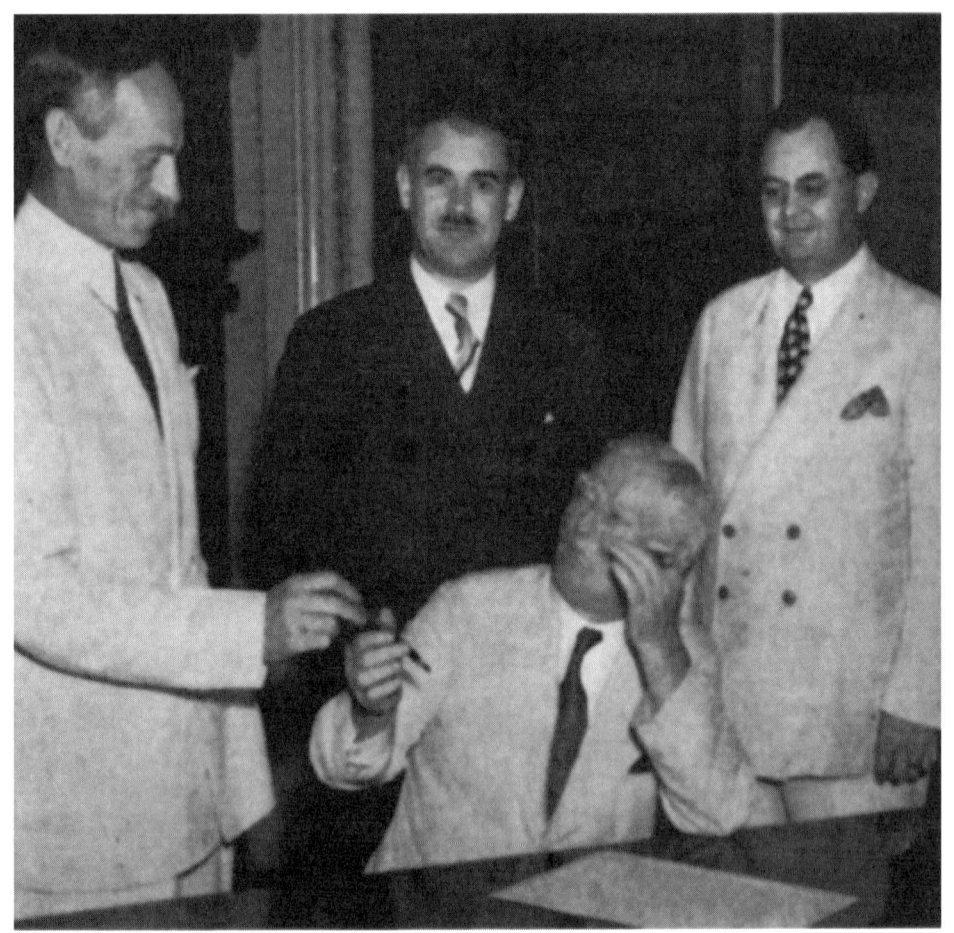

Vice President John Garner hands pen to Senator Tydings (left) after having signed the Enabling Act, with NARD attorney, Rowland Jones, Jr., and Rep. Wright Patman (right) in attendance.

tion of Retail Druggists as a power which in three short years was to roll up a record of accomplishment unmatched by any other pressure group in the country's history. Having won the resale price maintenance fight in the face of the most overwhelming obstacles, the (NARD) is entitled to take rank as the nation's most powerful trade association today." Strong language by an important voice and the mood among NARD members was near euphoric.

Enthusiasm at the thirty-ninth convention in St. Louis was diminished only by the serious illness of President George Louis Secord. He had been hospitalized several times during the past summer and was unable to attend the meeting. Delegates still basked in the association's success, and the old tone of militancy had been replaced by one of enthusiastic confidence. Dargavel felt compelled to tell the delegates that "there is no armistice," but even he took some time to relax.

Delegates unanimously chose Thomas S. Smith as the new president and Hugh P. Beirne was elected chairman by the executive committee. But the prolonged campaign for the Robinson-Patman and Tydings-Miller bills had taken a physical toll. Executive committee members were particularly concerned about Dargavel's health. At times during the Tydings-Miller fight, he appeared near the point of physical exhaustion. Following the St. Louis meeting, members of the executive committee insisted that he take a vacation — his first in six years.

The secretary did not stay away from the association or its affairs for long. He was particularly eager to link the national fair trade law with various state laws. While most states had used the California bill as a model, local political considerations also caused each to be distinct. Identifying those differences and harmonizing those differences from state to state was both sensitive and legally challenging. Dargavel was particularly concerned that too much coordination might result in antitrust charges being filed against NARD.

Agents from the Federal Trade Commission (FTC) visited the headquarters office in December 1937. Their visit was apparently prompted by a letter sent by New York Representative Emanuel Cellar to FTC Chairman W. A. Ayers, charging that the Tydings-Miller bill had been "railroaded through Congress without proper public consideration." Cellar asked the commission to investigate NARD for a possible conspiracy to restrain trade. Ayers responded to the congressman that "you no doubt will be interested to know that the same (NARD) are already under investigation by the commission."

Dargavel assured the membership that NARD had done no wrong and welcomed the investigation to prove it. He blamed the investigation on the "same old enemies" and said, "we have guarded ourselves with sound legal advice as we have gone along and have made no move without having considered all possible effects." He also took the opportunity to remind members that NARD was the target of an investigation because of its standing among the trade associations. As he noted "were the N.A.R.D. still weak, or had it not accomplished something of great benefit to the small independent business man, no mention of N.A.R.D. could be found." The secretary's confidence was confirmed when the FTC found nothing to substantiate Rep. Cellar's charges.

The association's leadership devoted the balance of the year to consolidating the gains made in the two previous record-setting years. The executive committee voted to return to Chicago for its fortieth convention under the theme "The Year of Victory." There were still a number of details to work out in coordinating Tydings-Miller with the thirty-eight separate state fair trade laws, but they were problems leaders of NARD welcomed.

The most significant thing about NARD in the 1930s was the paradox of its poverty and prosperity. Beginning the decade in the grips of a national depression with leadership more inclined to hold onto its past, the organization made a dramatic change in its focus. With almost totally new leadership and an attitude of change and risk-taking, the association became the acknowledged leader among the nation's retail organizations in just five years. NARD became (seemingly overnight) a force to be reckoned with among other national organizations representing a constituency on Capitol Hill.

In the annals of association activity, the achievements of NARD in this decade rewrote the chapters on how to lobby forcefully and effectively. Because of this effectiveness, NARD also experienced a dramatic turnaround in its financial resources and membership. While the decade is recorded as the period of "the Great Depression," most NARD members overcame economic adversity by creating a tide of success and "Great Expectations" for more victories to come.

Chapter Six

The Fifth Decade: 1939 – 1948

Emerging Marketplace Challenges Reshape Association Priorities

As the "turbulent thirties" gave way to the "uncertain forties," few in the National Association of Retail Druggists regretted the passing. For many in NARD, it was a time of turmoil, heartaches, and headaches. But the 1930s, despite their shadows, had patches of sunshine that also saw the association gain some of the greatest victories in its history. During that ten years, the pharmacists of the nation touched the depths of depression in terms of their own business fortunes, but then emerged from these vicissitudes to achieve a more stable financial base on which to grow by 1939.

Based on these improved conditions, NARD entered its fifth decade with excitement and anticipation. Being the acknowledged leader among the trade associations not only helped morale, but also made it easier to recruit members and collect dues and special contributions for the association's "political war-chest." The satisfaction over passing the Robinson-Patman and Tydings-Miller bills still lingered, but NARD leaders knew the high-energy campaigns had taken time away from other association programs and it was now time to place more emphasis in those areas.

Earlier in the thirties, Executive Secretary John Dargavel had articulated a three-point action plan for the association. One focused on the much-discussed national legislative program, a second promoted NARD-state association relations, and a third, the area of "store improvement and operations," was designed to help local store owners compete more effectively in the marketplace.

Since 1934, relations with the state associations and their executive secretaries had improved greatly by enlisting the state executives in the political campaign for price maintenance and fair trade. Former President Harvey Henry also established a President's Advisory Council, comprised of the state association presidents that reinforced the relationship. Beginning with the 1937 convention, Editor George Bender published photos of the state secretaries in the *Journal*. The next year he published pictures of the state presidents, which became an annual feature in the *Journal's* convention edition. While there were still areas of the nation that felt disconnected to the association, those "pockets" were rapidly passing away and a bond of fraternalism began to take hold again.

Building a "democratic organization" was an essential element in Dargavel's management style. He knew that if NARD was to be a viable organization, it must have strong, broad-based support from community pharmacists. But gaining their loyalty would not occur until they were convinced the association knew and was concerned about their interests. As a store owner and former officer of the American Pharmaceutical Association (APhA), he had first-hand knowledge about both the merchandising and professional sides of the retail business and pharmacy profession. He also recognized that the membership was divided between these two phases of store operations. But for Dargavel, it was not a choice of one over the other. Both had to be improved if neighborhood pharmacists were to compete with the chain and the pine board stores.

As Dargavel saw it, the purpose for making legislative strategy a priority was to "give us the opportunity to begin from a more nearly equal basis to that of any of our competitors — but from there on, it will be up to us to make our own way." To make that way he enlisted Editor Bender, the executive committee, and various committee chairmen to promote the local store. The *Journal* was redesigned and enlarged in number of pages — increasing from approximately 40 pages to more than 100 pages an issue and adding new departments featuring both the professional and merchandising aspects of the local drugstore.

One example of professional promotion was a feature article on "Prescription Pricing" written by former President George Secord. Secord was a physician as well as a pharmacist. He developed a "prescription price schedule" in 1930 to assist pharmacists in his home town of Chicago, Illinois, during the depths of the Depression. He revised the list in 1932 and continued publishing it for local usage. Dargavel asked the executive committee to endorse the plan for the membership, which they did, and Bender began publishing the list in the *Journal* as a "suggested guide." Dargavel emphasized, "we must merchandise; we must build up our professional prestige; we must learn to educate our salespeople; to display merchandise, and to sell it. That is the salvation of the retail druggists."

The NARD leadership endorsed one legislative initiative in 1939 — a "Federal Chain Store Tax" offered by their old friend, Rep. Wright Patman. Patman introduced the bill in January but found the reception difficult. NARD officials worked actively for the bill, including joining an alliance known as the Freedom of Opportunity Foundation to help with the lobbying. This organization was assembled to aid Patman in passing the bill and served as a fact-finding body as well as providing a means of intercommunication with other like-minded trade associations supporting the bill. However, NARD soon became preoccupied by various threats to overturn the Tydings-Miller bill and could not give full attention to Patman's new bill.

Against this backdrop of promotional efforts for local store improvements and a more limited political agenda, the forty-first convention convened in St. Paul, Minnesota, in 1939. President John T. Witty told the delegates that "one of our chief activities of the year has been to maintain an adequate defense of the gains of former years." He mentioned the new Patman bill and urged members to support it, but he devoted most of his speech to the merchandising side of pharmacy. Executive Committee Chairman John P. Jelinek told members about efforts to protect the gains made under the fair trade laws and the committee's response to the various resolutions passed at the fortieth convention.

Secretary Dargavel called attention to the new publicity department created at headquarters. The new department, headed by former Minnesota Governor Theodore Christianson, was charged with the responsibility of promoting all phases of the local store. According to Dargavel, "a proper public attitude is indeed important to the drug business, and we believe that through the dissemination of more information, appreciation of the services of the druggist may be increased and public opinion will be more favorable to the profession of pharmacy."

Perhaps one reason the secretary felt a need for better public relations was, as he told the delegates, that "we have had representatives of different governmental bodies making investigations in our office almost continuously since February 1938; first one department than another." Dargavel reserved most of his time to talk about the fair trade situation and the opposition allied against it. He encouraged delegates to be patient and give the plan an opportunity to work. He also said the future was uncertain and for that reason, the membership must stick together as never before since the association's inception.

In other actions, Dargavel told delegates of the favorable decision the association had received requiring physician prescriptions to be sent by first class mail. NARD had opposed the practice altogether, but losing on that ground the association then had argued that since the prescription included "directions written by the physician," the prescription constituted first class mail. He also said NARD was bothered by two potentially harmful actions of the Roosevelt administration. One was the Federal Fair Labors Standards Act, passed in the last Congress, to establish minimum wages and standard hours in the workplace. The bill's original provisions did not extend to pharmacy, and Dargavel assured his colleagues that the association would "resist to the utmost any attempt to bring the retail druggist under the provision on any federal law."

The other object of Dargavel's concern had to do with the Justice Department's charging the American Medical Association (AMA) with being a monopoly in possible violation of the Sherman and Clayton Antitrust Acts. While not anxious to get into AMA's fight, the secretary was concerned that the conflict might lead to federal officials imposing regulations that would "socialize medicine." If that should happened, he warned the membership, "medicine...pharmacy and dentistry will feel the withering influence immediately," and all would suffer.

The wide-ranging topics covered in the leadership's reports were reassuring to delegates attending the forty-first convention in 1939. Before adjourning, the House of Delegates elected Albert C. Fritz of Indianapolis, Indiana the new president. Immediately following adjournment, the new executive committee held its traditional organization meeting and chose George H. Frates of San Francisco, California, as chairman.

The theme for the new year continued to center around fair trade and efforts of the chain drugstores and the corporate retailers to erode it. Dargavel and the executive committee adopted a strategy of showing the contrast be-

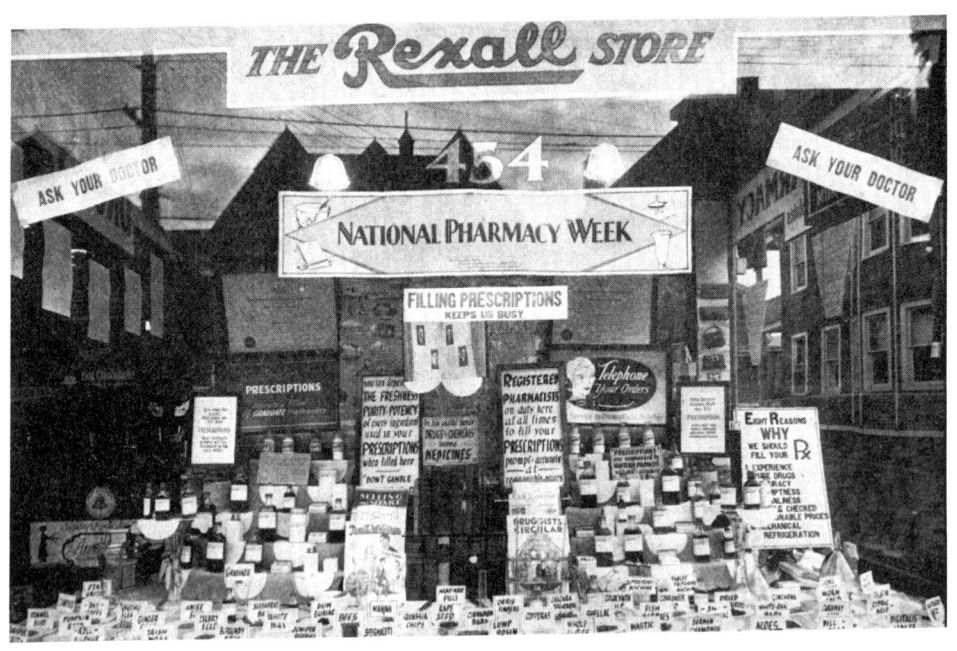

Typical storefront display of the late 1930s

tween community pharmacy and the chain "super-stores" that used the cloak of a health care profession to extend its store hours into the evening and stay open seven days a week. Dargavel called these stores "department stores masquerading as a drug store...their identity is hard to determine because they carry so many identical and overlapping lines."

But he also said that therein lay the opportunity for the neighborhood pharmacists, because in these super-stores, there is "no air of professional service, nothing to create confidence, nothing to appeal to one's senses except glitter and price." For the pharmacist who was "professional-minded, who wanted to retain an air of professional service in his store," here was an opportunity to demonstrate the difference between his store and the impersonal chain store.

Ironically, the association's emphasis on the professional side of pharmacy may have contributed to a division in the ranks. In May, a small group of community pharmacists met in Richmond, Virginia, and organized the "college of professional pharmacists." That in itself was not a problem for NARD. However, when the society drafted bylaws that excluded from membership any store that had "an ice cream, or cigarette sign in the window or that sold food," Dargavel and the executive committee objected. In a pointed editorial in the *Journal,* the secretary wrote that for pharmacy "to try to break up into smaller units, each claiming to be the true representatives of the 'better class' in the profession, is not serving the profession advantageously."

In partial response to the new group, the executive committee created a new professional relations department in the central office. The new office was designed to develop a closer working relationship with those interested in the professional side of pharmacy. Dargavel recruited Edward Spease, former dean of Western Reserve University, to head the office, which gave it immediate credibility with the "college" group. The secretary now had a former state governor and dean of a leading school of pharmacy, not to mention a skilled editor and a stable office staff, working with him. This was quite a change in headquarters personnel in less than ten years.

With 1940 a presidential election year, NARD leaders worried about fair trade as a political issue. That neither Democratic nor Republican party chose to defend fair trade in their respective platforms gave even more cause for concern. Dargavel told the executive committee to get prepared for a new round of lobbying in the next Congress.

Delegates to the forty-second convention met in New York City, New York, in 1940. A key factor in holding the meeting in New York was an attempt to increase association membership in the the largest retail market in the nation. That it was also the home of Representative Emanuel Cellar, viewed by NARD officials as the champion for the corporate retail interest, also had symbolic meaning. President Fritz emphasized the importance of NARD membership in his address to the delegates. He noted the importance of "building from the ground up" and said, "remember, we are all dependent upon one another and the building of any one of the three (associations) is automatically reflected in the strength of the others." He too was bothered by the "college of professional pharmacists" movement and warned the delegates, "as soon as the drug industry of this country starts a movement for the classification of drug stores as good, bad, or otherwise, just so soon is organized pharmacy on the road to disintegration."

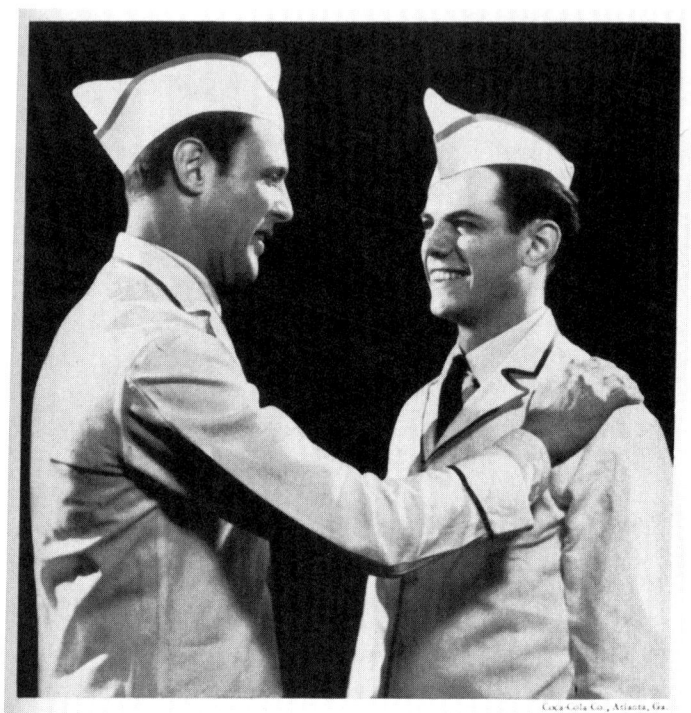

"A fountain that's run right will make money in any man's store"

"*Let me tell you why:*— The fountain attracts more people from the sidewalk into a store than any other department.

"It sends many people to other departments to make purchases.

"It brings customers back again and again—repeat sales which multiply profits and establish habits of buying in the store.

"Ask the Coca-Cola Service Man about it—he can give you the real facts."

Both Executive Committee Chairman Frates and Secretary Dargavel emphasized the importance of fair trade to the neighborhood pharmacist. Pointing to a survey conducted the previous year by the Druggists' Research Bureau, Frates told delegates that here was scientific proof that the "consuming public is paying less for standard, nationally advertised products than before the enactment of these laws."

Frates was also concerned that manufacturers were finding ways to circumvent both Robinson-Patman and Tydings-Miller — particularly the hospitals. Evidence showed, he said, that "the prices quoted hospitals for identical pharmaceutical and specialties are in many instances less than one-half the net price of the retailer. Furthermore, many of the hospitals dispense to outpatients, thus placing the retailer in an impossible competitive position."

Delegates at the forty-second convention were increasingly concerned about the expanding war in Europe and its implications for them. Dargavel acknowledged this anxiety, but also used it as an opportunity to rally support for the association. He reminded the delegates about how the causes for the war developed and noted that "we can now see that the chief reason for the downfall of the conquered nations was complacency — failure to realize danger in time.... Are not the small retailers of the United States making the same mistake? May it not lead to the same tragic consequences?

Before leaving the nation's largest city, delegates amended the constitution to add two more vice presidents, making five total, and created a new "Committee on Reports" charged with reviewing each report presented at the convention and identifying actions needing executive committee attention. They also elected Samuel Watkins to be president. George Frates became the new chairman of the executive committee.

The fall elections returned Franklin D. Roosevelt to the White House. While NARD had been careful not to endorse a candidate, it was an open secret that Dargavel and the leadership were ambivalent toward the president. While agreeing with administration positions on most things, the association's major disagreement on fair trade was significant. Dargavel warned the new executive committee that 1941 would be a political year and to anticipate efforts to amend or repeal the Tydings-Miller bill.

The anticipated attack was not long in coming. Soon after the new Congress convened in January, Representative Hampton Fulmer from South Carolina's Second District introduced a bill to "repeal the Tydings-Miller bill in its entirety." Fulmer based his bill on recommendations from the Temporary National Economic Committee organized by Assistant U.S. Attorney General Truman Arnold. In a series of hearings held throughout 1940, Arnold had become convinced that the fair trade agreements "were in restraint of trade," and repeal rather than amendment was the proper legal solution to the whole issue. NARD's Washington representative Rowland Jones, Jr. alerted Dargavel about the impending bill and said that "if we are to stem and defeat this latest attack by predatory price-cutting and loss-leader selling, we must organize to a man. The seriousness of the picture now presented will admit no slackers in our ranks if we are to succeed." The executive committee quickly set in motion a plan to block the Fulmer bill.

Alerting key people in the state pharmacy associations, so well cultivated in each state over the past five years, the plan went into action. Using direct mail, telegrams, telephones, and editorial pages of the *Journal*, the NARD leadership called upon its members and friends to let members of Congress know of pharmacy's opposition to the Fulmer bill. In urging the membership to take the matter seriously, Dargavel said, "we can take nothing for granted in this fight. The opposition bars no holds and is capable of using all possible methods to destroy Fair Trade."

NARD's all-out effort in opposition to the Fulmer bill kept it bottled up in the House Judiciary Committee throughout the first session of Congress. That pressure, coupled with the growing influence of the war in Europe, kept the principles of fair trade in place at least for the moment.

Legislation in response to the war gradually crowded out most controversial bills. The House Ways and Means Committee began reviewing various revenue-producing measures and in April, President Roosevelt issued an executive order to control prices. The action was prompted because a rapid increase in defense spending had stimulated rising inflation, which in turn threatened the nation's economic recovery. Ironically, this order did more to protect the fair trade issue than all of NARD's lobbying to date. Stability in manufacturing prices had been the fundamental issue in NARD's campaign for fairness, and the president's action reinforced that notion. While the president's action in this instance was welcomed, Secretary Dargavel reminded the membership again that there was "no armistice" in the fight to save fair trade.

It was unfortunate that the store operations section of NARD had to take a back seat to the legislative program. The economy was well on its way to full recovery and had been since 1939. Consumers had more money to spend, and new developments in technology offered neighborhood pharmacists the opportunity to significantly improve store operations. Air conditioning became more cost-effective through improved production, and the advent of fluorescent lighting allowed a wide range of creative designs. The NARD leadership actively promoted new features as they became available. The *Journal* ran regular articles written by experts from industry explaining various products and services and how they could add to store profits. The magazine

CHAPTER SIX — THE FIFTH DECADE: 1939 – 1948   117

also added a special section on the soda fountain and printed anniversary dates for holidays and special events to promote merchandising.

But it was the war in Europe that captured everyone's attention. Even though the United States was officially neutral and public opinion still strongly opposed U.S. involvement, the war dominated domestic issues in this country. By the time Dargavel issued the invitation for the annual convention, Congress was deep into hearings on a new tax bill to fund the mounting costs of defense spending. While quite willing to be a part of the effort, Dargavel

Tin Tube Salvage Poster For Drug Stores

The War Production Board has given final approval to this poster and counter card design, and they will be in the hands of the nation's drug stores about the middle of February. Each druggist will receive one mounted on heavy card, for attaching to collection box; another on poster paper for window use. See Page 189 for complete story.

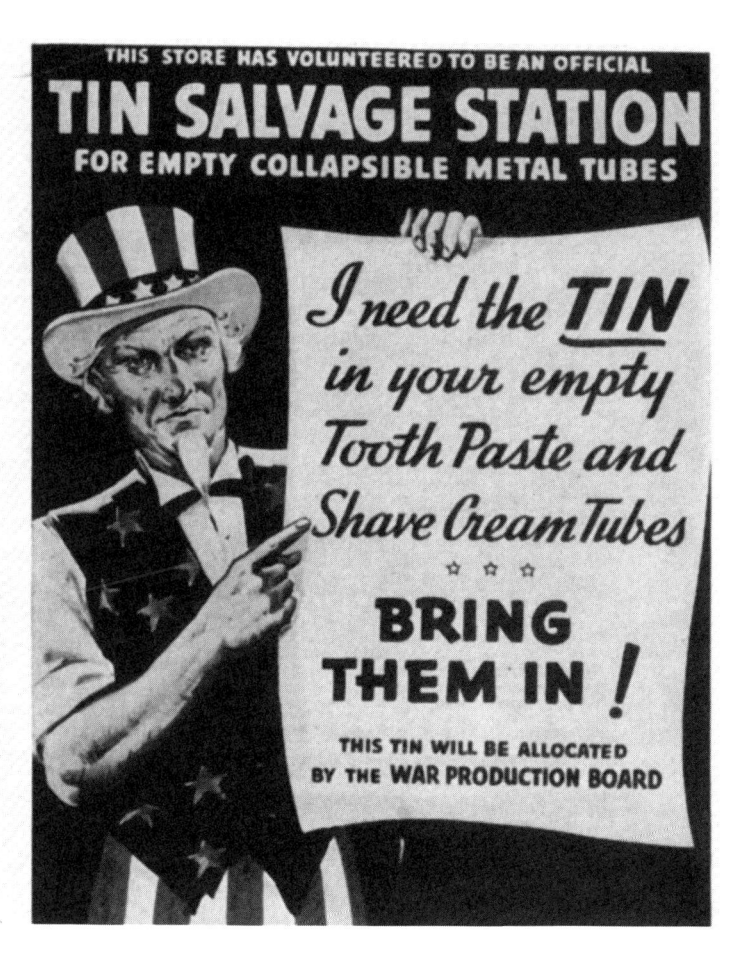

NARD members made their contributions to the war effort.

urged Congress not to place the full tax burden on the small businessman to the exclusion of consumers and manufacturers.

During the interim, as the Ways and Means Committee debated various proposals, NARD joined with the Post Office Department and other trade organizations to participate in "Retailers-for Defense" Week scheduled September 15-20, 1940. The plan was for the postal officials to print a special Defense Savings Stamp that would then be sold in normal retail outlets. This plan was well suited for neighborhood pharmacists, most of whom had long provided limited postal services in their stores. These stamps were then exchanged for Defense Savings Bonds. Stamp purchases had the advantage of raising revenue for a specific purpose, but had a limited impact on inflation. President Watkins headed NARD's promotional efforts, and pharmacists throughout the nation participated in the program.

By the time delegates came together in 1941 in Cleveland, Ohio, the war clouds had grown even darker. Not only did the war in Europe continue to go badly for America's traditional allies, but also the relationship between the United States and Japan had deteriorated to the breaking point. The troubled international situation, the attempt to repeal the Tydings-Miller law, and uncertainty about the meaning of the "college of professional pharmacists" movement brought a more subdued mood to the delegates compared to conventions in the immediate past. President Watkins recognized the atmosphere and reminded members that for the past few years the association had been "in a position of a fast horse which makes a mile in two minutes...but wins out only by a head against another horse running almost equally fast."

Delegates no doubt understood their president's point, but it was still difficult to poise for another race with no assurance of the outcome. Watkins anticipated their response and continued, saying that "it is interesting in that connection to note that our horse seems to be the only one that has not actually lost ground. In every other field of retailing the independent gradually has been losing the race with his corporate competitors; in the drug field only has he been able to hold his share of the business." Watkins attributed this to NARD's sense of organization and its concentration on informing its members of the issues.

Expanding the horse race metaphor, Watkins cautioned that there was a new horse in the field, which he described in terms of an alliance between the drug manufacturers and the hospitals. To the president this was an "unholy alliance" that went to the core of pharmacy as a profession and robbed the pharmacist of his distinctiveness. Pharmacists were being denied "their only reason for existence as...the great pharmaceutical houses place their ready-made preparations in hospitals and in the hands of physicians who dispense them directly to patients." Being "short circuited" was bad enough for the pharmacists, but the "greater tragedy is to the patient (who) in many cases no longer gets the specific and personal medication to which he is entitled." Watkins struck a responsive chord with the delegates with his comments. Executive Committee Chairman Frates built on the president's remarks by explaining in detail how the committee functioned, its defense of fair trade, and its opposition to the Fulmer attempt to repeal the Tydings-Miller law. Secretary Dargavel assured the delegates that NARD had "gained ground" on the fair trade fight and that the association was opposed to the new federal tax bill as currently proposed. He said NARD hoped to amend the bill to prevent it from placing too much burden on the neighborhood pharmacists for collection and bookkeeping.

Dargavel also reported that the association now had almost 28,000 members, out of an estimated 60,000 independent pharmacists. He also released a report showing NARD's annual net earnings as follows:

Year	Amount	Year	Amount
1917	$ 1,749.92	1929	(11,478.79)
1918	8,201.12	1930	(10,749.00)
1919	21,968.19	1931	(9,675.00)
1920	20,499.52	1932	(28,494.29)
1921	17,188.08	1933	(19,407.15)
1922	23,441.76	1934	25,925.19
1923	25,727.23	1935	23,721.99
1924	22,758.79	1936	40,691.24
1925	12,606.47	1937	45,452.82
1926	16,376.05	1938	43,855.02
1927	12,004.10	1939	36,004.19
1928	5,996.26	1940	35,384.86
		1941	26,933.46

Delegates were impressed with the association's financial strength and it served as a fitting closure for the convention. Before adjourning, the delegates elected Hugh P. Beirne as president. Frates was reelected chairman of the executive committee.

No one could have predicted the cataclysmic events that happened hardly sixty days after the conventioneers left Cleveland. Just two weeks before the attack on Pearl Harbor, Hawaii, the executive committee held its traditional November meeting. Among the items of business, the committee selected Los Angeles as the site for the forty-fourth convention.

But life changed dramatically for America's pharmacists after December 7, 1941. Among the casualties was the Los Angeles Convention. The decision of the War Relocation Authority to detain and then confine some 120,000 Japanese-Americans raised questions about national and personal security. Coupled with the logistics and expense of travel, NARD leaders reconsidered their decision and selected Chicago, Illinois, as the new convention site.

Secretary Dargavel addressed the membership through an editorial in the *Journal*. He noted that "whatever may have been our individual thoughts up to December 7, it is certain that today we are all of one mind. We are in the war and our opponents are powerful. They are dangers to be reckoned with. They threaten our way of living. There is but one thing to do and that is, to fight and to win."

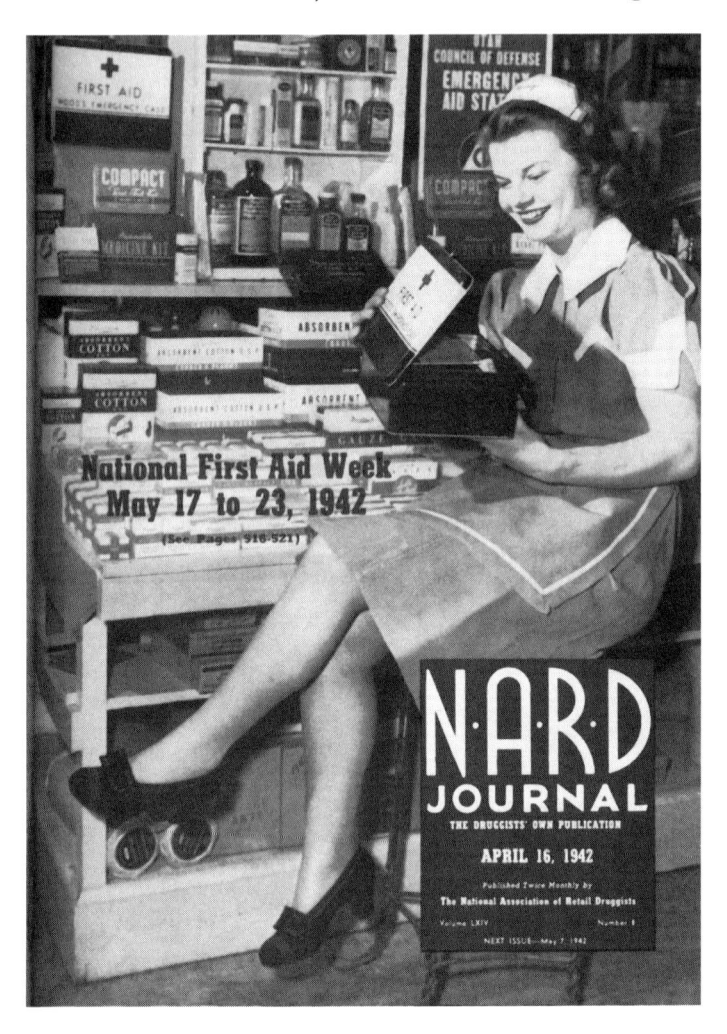

He was referring to Japan and German and their allies. However, even the casual reader of the secretary's comments could recognize the similar language he used against NARD's opponents in the trade wars.

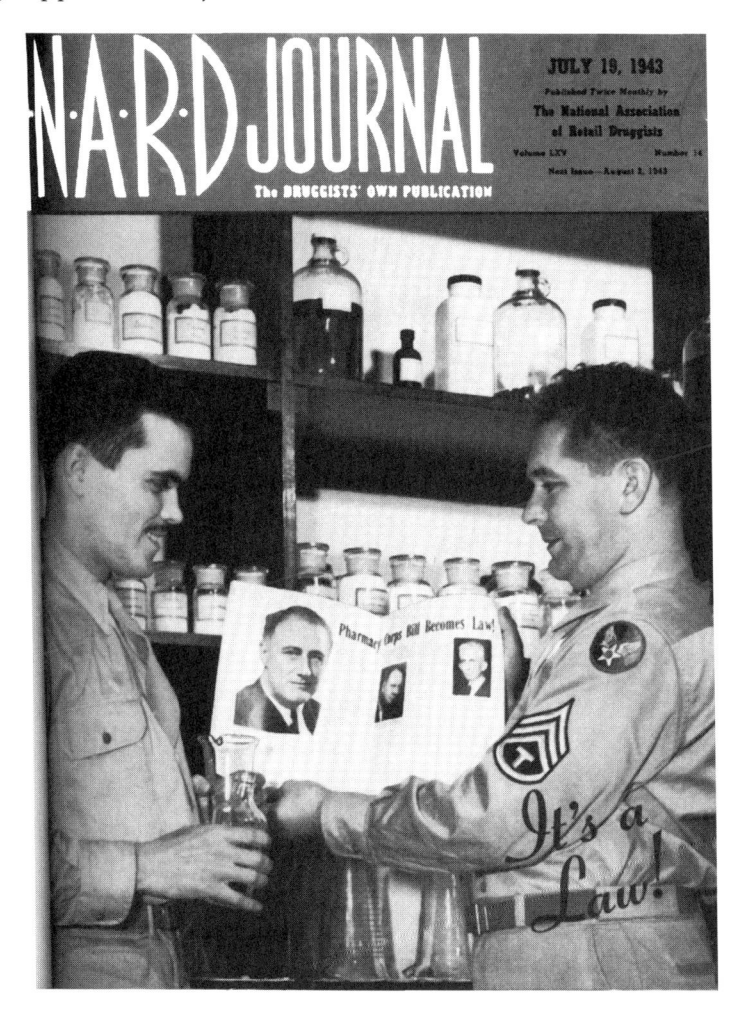

As the nation rapidly mobilized for total war, the executive committee quickly outlined four plans for cooperating with the national defense effort. As a first step, the committee pledged to call on its nationwide network of pharmacists to make their "drug stores civilian defense centers" for their local communities. In a second program, President Bierne appointed a special committee to coordinate local pharmacists' efforts in making surveys and supplying information to the Office of Price Administration for drug procurement and allocation. In a third initiative, NARD contributed to the war effort by establishing a consumer information bureau on drugs and health supplies to keep consumers informed on price trends and market conditions affecting supplies. Finally, the executive committee voted to extend the annual First Aid Week to a full year program. The executive committee also actively pursued a bill to create a "Pharmacy Corps" in the military. Having been thwarted in efforts to establish a corps in World War I, NARD leaders had tried from time to time to get such a bill through Congress in the 1930s. However, the Surgeon General opposed a separate pharmacy corps and the measure lost its way in the fights over price maintenance and fair trade.

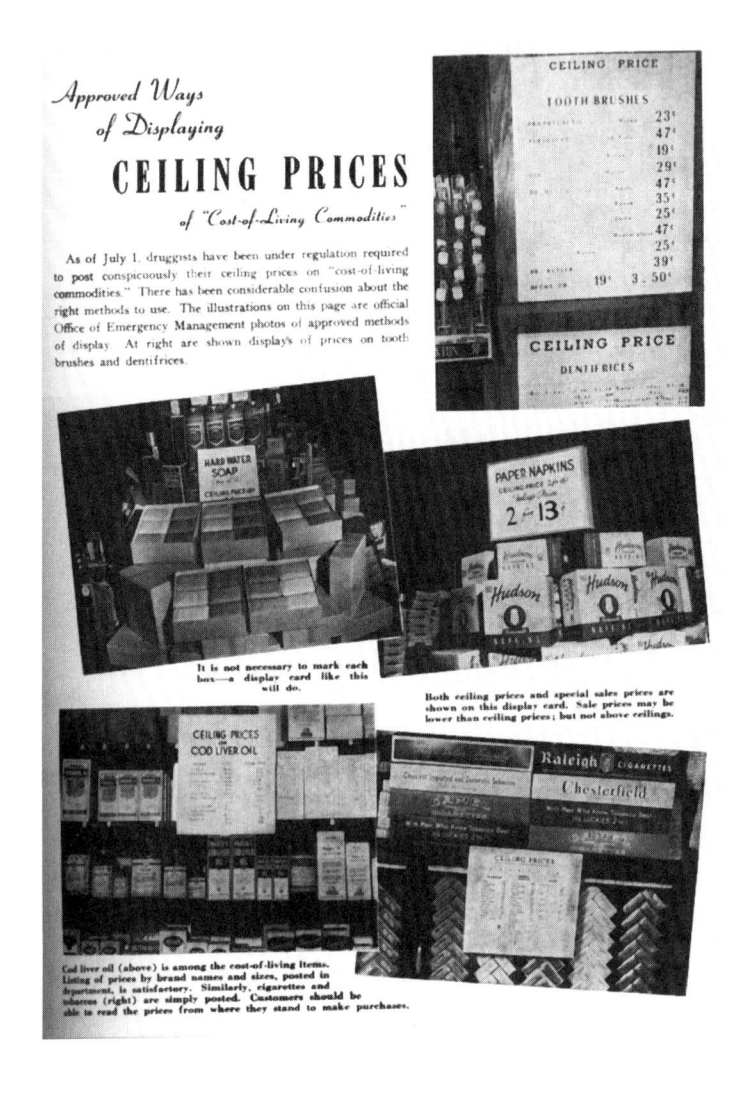

When Congress convened for its regular session in January 1942, the executive committee asked fellow pharmacists Washington Senator Robert Reynolds and North Carolina Representative Carl Durham to introduce a new pharmacy corps bill. While the bill was not a high priority with the administration or the congressional leadership, NARD leaders enlisted support from APhA and the American Legion and finally obtained passage of the Reynolds-Durham bill in July 1943.

Durham, as author of the original bill, was able to keep the corps a part of the "Regular Army," making it a permanent part of the military service. Ironically, although the bill passed unanimously in congressional committee, Army officials resisted implementing the program. The military's action and the continued opposition by the Office of the Surgeon General became a source of significant disappointment for NARD.

Delegates came to Chicago for the forty-fourth convention in 1942. The shortage of workers, the difficulties of travel, and the uncertainty of family members in military service caused many delegates to stay home. Still, others came in "surprising numbers," according to Secretary Dargavel, and the meeting was devoted to exploring NARD's role in the war. The entire opening morning session was devoted to a briefing on the war situation provided by representatives from the Roosevelt administration.

President Bierne reminded the delegates to expect the federal government to become more deeply involved in their affairs. He noted that federal officials "were deeply concerned with two problems — that of conservation of power and fuel; and the fact that we are selling goods at retail far more rapidly than we are able to replace them." But he also noted that druggists could respond to both of these concerns by adopting "earlier closing hours," an issue Bierne had long supported.

J. Otto Kohl from Cincinnati, Ohio, was elected president and George H. Frates was re-elected for his third term as chairman of the executive committee. After the forty-fourth convention, NARD did not hold another convention until 1947. Military needs for rail transportation made civilian travel unpredictable if not impossible. By 1943 the shortage of essential supplies and the need to conserve food and fuel further discouraged a large gathering. Under these circumstances, the association's business was kept to a minimum and carried out by the executive committee. The annual meeting was called a "convention-in-print" and full reports by the officers and various committees were reported through the *Journal*. Kohl and the other officers elected by the forty-fourth convention in 1942 remained in office until 1947.

As the war progressed, pharmacists gradually adjusted to the pervasive influence of federal control on domestic life. The Office of Price Administration became a familiar name as administrators set ceilings on prices, determined cost-of-living commodities, and established a point system for rationing essential food and supplies. To coordinate pharmacy's activities in the war effort, NARD and APhA held joint executive committee meetings beginning in 1943. While the two groups had had representatives meeting on an annual basis since 1927, the joint executive committee meetings were the first time the two groups coordinated policy. The NARD leaders also voted to endorse a bill sponsored by Wright Patman that made it legal for two or more small retailers to enter into an agreement and "bargain" with manufacturers when purchasing merchandise.

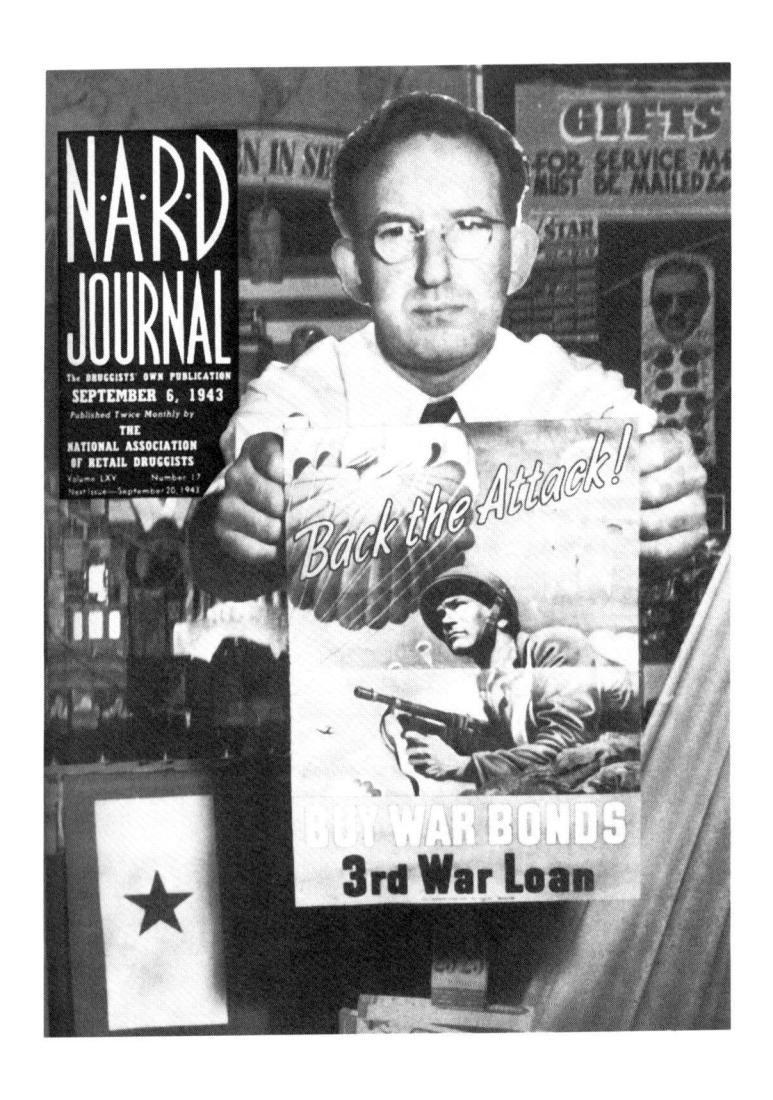

War-time conditions also brought some personnel changes at NARD. Theodore Christianson replaced George Bender as editor of the *Journal*. George Frates replaced Rowland Jones Jr. as the Washington representative in 1943. Beginning in 1944 the executive committee began to alternate its annual November meetings between Chicago and Washington D. C. Because approximately 10,000 pharmacists were called to active duty during the war, dues payments to the association diminished, although NARD continued to make a profit in its other enterprises.

Members of the executive committee began talking about the transition to a peace-time economy as early as 1944. However, they were not prepared for the abrupt end of World War II in August 1945. The rapid demobilization, both in the military and on the home front, led to a period of rapid inflation and a resurgence in competition.

The "supermarket grocery store," a "one-stop market," became the first major challenge for NARD and community pharmacists in the immediate postwar period. In 1945, there were approximately 10,000 supermarkets doing business, and approximately one-half of them sold drug and cosmetic products. But by the end of 1946, there were over 13,000 supermarkets, and seventy percent were selling drugs and cosmetics. Such a rapid change and in such volume was a serious problem for NARD. The NARD Executive Committee discussed how to respond and made plans to resume the annual convention in 1946 and present the issue before delegates. However, military personnel returned from Europe and Asia in such numbers that the convention hotels in every major city were filled to capacity and NARD could not find space to hold a convention.

The association was finally able to get back on track in 1947 with a convention, the forty-ninth, that met in Chicago. President Kohl finally got an opportunity to address the delegates. The "super store" was very much on everyone's mind, but there were no ready answers. Kohl reminded delegates of their protection under the fair trade laws, but then also said that "the fight cannot be won entirely on legislation. It will require education as well. There is a definite obligation of pharmacy to see that the public is protected by laws that confine the dispensing of drugs and chemicals to those qualified to perform that service." This observation was all the more true because of the increasingly common use of complex drug therapy — chemotherapy and antibiotics — in treating or ameliorating the effects of disease.

Delegates at the forty-ninth convention elected John B. Tripeny of Casper, Wyoming, as the new president. He had the honor of serving the association during its golden anniversary. Anticipating a record turnout, the executive committee voted to return to New York City for the special event. More than 3,000 delegates registered for the event. There may have been conventions more memorable for their enthusiasm, or lack thereof, but in a very real sense the "controlled mood" was reflective of an organization that had matured and was confident in its purpose.

Secretary Dargavel spent most of his address to the delegates reflecting on the changes to the association and independent pharmacy over the past fifty years. As he saw it, "the first half-century has proved the necessity of fighting as an army, not as single scouts or individual snipers. There must be a 'grand strategy' in this war to preserve the independent businessman against absorption in a 'capitalistic collectivism' which is moving to take over the economy of the United States."

With those words, the association's leader for the past fifteen years sounded the battle cry for the next half-century. Many of the same problems that had beset pharmacists in 1898 were still around for the first fifty years. Dargavel was to live and lead into the next half-century and wrestle with many of the same problems as his predecessors. The fact that he successfully bridged the half-century mark meant that NARD and its membership were equally up to the task of survival and were, despite many significant challenges, up to the task of building a strong and viable profession that would endure.

Chapter Seven

The Sixth Decade: 1949 – 1958

More NARD Victories in Repelling Assaults on Fair Trade

The post-World War II period found the American public and the nation's pharmacists on the threshold of a vast economic expansion, ending the long drought of the Great Depression. The euphoria associated with the roaring American industrial machine, unleashed from the fetters of wartime materials production, found its way into the retail sector where the public's disposable income and rising standard of living were spurred by enormous leaps in electronics technology and a growing array of consumer goods. The nation's pharmacists also prospered and to some degree the battles of the past over key issues affecting their livelihood on the local level were largely forgotten — except for the vigilance of NARD.

Secretary John Dargavel and the executive committee anticipated another move to repeal the Tydings-Miller Act and perhaps the Robinson-Patman Act as well. The war had brought a momentary truce in the battle over fair trade and price maintenance. With Congress reserving its legislative calendar for matters of war-time emergency in the early 1940s, the battle between NARD and its retail foes was temporarily suspended. However, the aggressive merchandising campaign launched by the supermarket chains immediately after the war was a signal that the truce on fair trade and price maintenance was over.

To prepare for a new round of competition, Dargavel and the executive committee recommitted to the three-pronged strategy that had worked so well before the war. That plan involved the association organizing its personnel and resources to stay actively involved in the legislative game, maintaining a close working relationship with state and affiliated associations, and equipping the community pharmacists to compete in the marketplace.

To finance its ambitious program, association leaders relied primarily on revenues produced by the *Journal* and the annual convention, particularly the "Drug Show." Since it was first introduced in 1907 as an exhibit, the display of merchandise and programs by the manufacturers and distributors in the pharmaceutical industry had become so large that it dominated the space needs of the convention. The executive committee's decision when selecting convention sites was largely determined by space considerations for the drug show.

The accessibility of exhibit space and the opportunity to work more closely with state and local associations prompted the executive committee to select New York City as the site for the fifty-first convention in 1949. The meeting came on the heels of President Harry Truman's announcing his ambitious "Fair Deal" legislative package, which included a national health insurance program. This concept had been talked about from time to time since World War I, and in the 1930s various bills to establish a national health insurnce program for all Americans had been introduced in Congress. None of those bills had made it out of committee. NARD leaders were strongly opposed to any type of national insurance program and had spoken out against it on several occasions, saying such a plan would result in "socialized medicine."

Seeing that federal officials had health coverage under consideration again sparked another reaction from NARD. President Edgar S. Bellis devoted much of his address to the 1949 convention delegates to the issue. He noted that the association was on record as being "in opposition to every program that in (its) operation will deprive medicine and the allied medical groups of the freedom of enterprise they now enjoy." Bellis continued that NARD recognized the need for health care for all Americans, but he believed that was best accomplished "through traditional democratic procedures.... The evidence is clear that compulsory government sickness insurance would be injurious to the profession of pharmacy and to the drug store per se."

Executive Committee Chairman Frank W. Moudry emphasized store modernization as a way of improving store performance so that independents could compete more effectively with the chain stores and supermarkets. He noted that there were too many untidy and dirty pharmacies and said, "it is ridiculous to expect the public to regard the profession with respect when it sees some pharmacies that resemble dives more than they do pharmaceutical health stations."

Moudry also cautioned pharmacists about the competition coming from food stores and supermarkets. Based on information the NARD leadership had collected, he said, these businesses "will grow rather than diminish." To compete in this new market, Moudry urged pharmacists to become better educated on market trends, the rules of merchandising, and business promotion. For example, he pointed out that 40 percent of all health appliances were sold in outlets other than drugstores; only 25 percent of insecticides and repellents and 2 percent of school supplies were sold through pharmacies. At one time, drugstores had dominated in each of these areas. Moudry said it was time for pharmacists to reclaim those markets. But to do so, he said, "it is compulsory for us to go after customers with intelligence and determination."

Dargavel emphasized the issue of discounts in his report to the convention. He noted that the volume of store sales the past year was the highest in history, but profits were down. He believed that was due primarily to an inadequate discount system. "The N.A.R.D. has carried on a determined campaign to persuade the manufacturers to widen the margins and a sizeable number of them have responded," he said, but "many more have continued to ignore the plight of the druggists. They talk about management efficiency and otherwise dodge the issue." He described pharmacists as being on the edge of a financial whirlpool and said, "the issue of discounts must be pushed to a satisfactory conclusion before it is too late to overcome the downswing of business."

What particularly angered Dargavel was evidence that the manufacturers' "own records tell us they have made enormous and outrageous net profits since 1943." In view of that fact, the manufacturers could easily give pharmacists a bigger discount, but, according to the secretary, "they don't seem to give a hoot."

Other matters taken up at the convention included announcing the winner of the NARD Thesis Contest. The executive committee initiated this contest on an experimental basis in an attempt to create more interest among pharmacy students in the retail side of the profession. The first contest was held in 1948 with the association offering $1,000 in prize money. The response far exceeded expectations, and the executive committee voted to establish "The N.A.R.D. Fund for the Betterment of Retail Pharmacy" and make the contest an annual event.

The NARD leadership became increasingly focused on the need to educate both the membership and the general public about the problems facing community pharmacists in the post-war period. Dargavel said that "one of the dangerous situations we face is the ignorance of the public relative to the necessity of small business." If consumers did not understand the principles of the independent retail trade, "they may be influenced to support legislation (that will) open wide the doors of cutthroat competition."

It was the potential "legislation," which rumor said would be introduced in the next Congress, that bothered Dargavel. He was pleased to see a united House of Delegates, which readily endorsed the nominating committee slate of officers. The committee recommended Executive Committee Chairman Frank W. Moudry of St. Paul, Minnesota, as president, and Charles R. Steward of Pasadena, California, as chair of the executive committee.

The leadership prepared to do battle in a new year, and they did not have long to wait. At their November meeting, the executive committee learned that Senate Bill 1008, a measure designed to undermine the Robinson-Patman Act, would be introduced in the new Congress. Without waiting for Congress to convene, Chairman Steward and his colleagues used the pages of the *Journal* to urge pharmacists to contact their senators and representatives and ask them to vote against the proposal.

But unlike the 1930s when much of the corporate world was reeling from the impact of the Depression, the forces of consolidation and monopoly had regained momentum and money. Senate Bill 1008 passed the House quickly; Dargavel and former NARD President George Frates, now representing the association in Washington, managed to stall, but not stop, the bill in the Senate. So powerful was the coalition supporting the bill, political insiders in Washington told Dargavel the battle was over.

However, the secretary was never one to give in before exhausting every possible alternative. He assured those pundits that the fight was not over until the President made his decision. Telegraphing each member of the executive committee and the state executives, he pleaded with them to send "an avalanche of letters to President Truman."

The hard work of the 1930s in developing a strong working relationship with the state associations paid off. The President told reporters he was deluged with "piles of telegrams and letters" urging him to veto the measure. And, despite NARD's failure to endorse his national health insurance program, he was impressed with the response from the "little men." To the surprise of the establishment, he vetoed the bill. Rep. Wright Patman called it "one of the greatest victories of the N.A.R.D."

Not resting on their laurels, the NARD leadership began work on a long-term plan to improve the public image of the fair trade issue. Knowing that their opponents were well financed and that they could not match them on money, members of the executive committee used a strategy of educating the public about the merits of their case. To do this, the executive committee enlisted support from the Bureau of Education on Fair Trade.

Created in 1949, the bureau was funded by NARD, which committed a $30,000 annual contribution, the National Association of Chain Drug Stores (NACDS), a $10,000 contribution, while the wholesalers and manufacturers contributed $40,000 each — a total budget of $120,000. Its purpose was to "enlighten the public on the values that come from fair trade." While the NARD leadership worked to keep the membership involved in the issue, the bureau appealed to the consuming public to support the principles of fair trade and tell political leaders of their support.

CHAPTER SEVEN — THE SIXTH DECADE: 1949 – 1958

In addition to a legislative strategy, the executive committee also discussed plans to help store owners merchandise their products. The idea the committee found most appealing was a "packaged business promotion program," preassembled and designed to assist community pharmacists with promotional materials throughout the year. Included in the package were layouts and installation instructions for specific window and interior displays, mats for newspaper advertising, lessons for educating sales people about particular merchandise, and materials for mail solicitation.

At its November meeting, the executive committee voted to honor an earlier agreement and hold the next convention in Long Beach, California, in 1950. The 1941 executive committee had also chosen this California city, but had been forced to cancel its plans due to World War II. Ironically, by the time delegates arrived for their fifty-second convention, war was again a national preoccupation. Soldiers of the North Korean army invaded South Korea

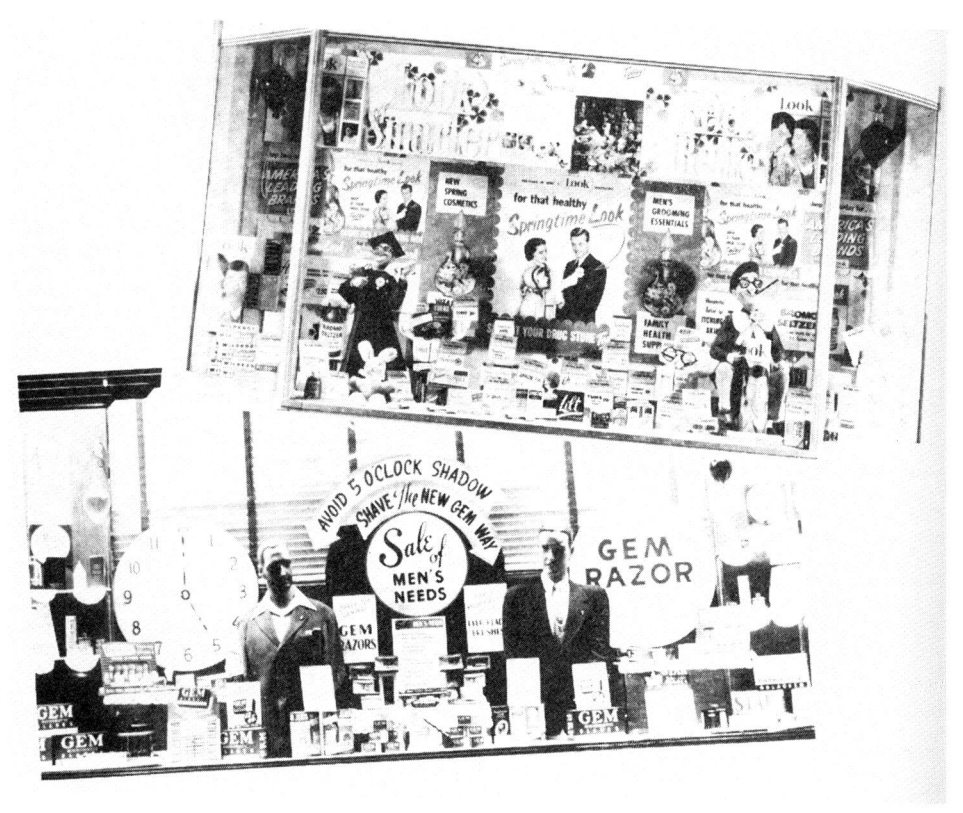

A storefront of the 1950s, designed by pharmacist L.J. (Larry) Carriveau, who won many national prizes for his displays

in October and the United Nations enlisted the support of the United States to repel the attack.

Dargavel was particularly bothered by these developments. The aggressive nature of the North Korean army, coupled with the recent revolution in China and the strong ideological statements coming from the Soviet Union, raised concern about the reality of international communism. The secretary devoted as much of his address to the House of Delegates to the issue of national security and defense of the "ideals of democracy." He told his listeners that "it is folly to minimize the gravity of the situation. Our way of life faces destruction. It must be defended or it will be crushed under the iron heels of Communism. The first line of defense is our own soil...and it runs through your community wherever it may be located."

Then skillfully manipulating his audience's emotions, Dargavel turned the issue from democracy versus communism, "our way of life versus theirs," to retail pharmacy versus the consolidated power of monopoly. "One of the primary elements of national strength is small business," he said. "Small business provides numerous and necessary sources of initiative and to the nation it contributes essential vitality, stability, and progressive flexibility. Anything which hurts small business as such is detrimental to the nation."

Dargavel had not named the opposition, nor had he even mentioned his own association. He did not need to do so. New *Journal* Editor P.J. Sletterdahl reported that the delegates "jumped to their feet...gave Executive Secretary Dargavel an impressive ovation and somebody in the audience called him the MacArthur of the Druggists."

President Frank W. Moudry complemented the secretary's speech by pointing out the mounting threats to community pharmacy. "Three harsh facts stare at me," he said. "One is that less than a fourth of the independent drug stores now in operation can exist alone on prescriptions and sales of drug items. Another is that over 75 percent of the merchandise we must sell to survive is outside the possibilities of restrictive legislation. The third is that the competition of the food outlets and the supermarkets is unavoidable." To counter these circumstances, the president called for "a convention for pharmacy legislation to draft a standard pharmacy act."

Executive Committee Chairman Charles R. Seward echoed President Moudry's theme by pointing out the problem of "duplicated medicinal specialties." He said the NARD leadership had worked hard "to bring about a reduction in the flow of identical prescription products," but so far had not been successful. He predicted the practice would go on "until (lack) of profits hurt the manufacturers."

Before adjourning the fifty-second convention, delegates elected Charles F. Gilson of Centerdale, Rhode Island, their new president. Charles Seward was re-elected chairman of the executive committee.

By 1950, a new issue had worked its way onto NARD's list of priorities. The matter had to do with pharmacy education. In the aftermath of World War II, postsecondary educational institutions of all types saw a boom to their student enrollments. Colleges of pharmacy had graduated a record 5,987 students at the beginning of the decade and estimates were for that trend to continue for several more years.

Responding to the bulging student body, many pharmacy programs began revising their curriculum and some added an additional year of training. NARD leaders were not opposed to more education for pharmacy students; however, they were concerned about the type of courses being offered. At its fall meeting, the executive committee discussed the lack of "retail courses" in the degree programs. Committee members agreed that the issue, insofar as community pharmacy was concerned, was not the length of the training but the lack of courses "covering the commercial aspects of pharmacy." As a result of the discussion on the pharmacy school curriculum, the executive committee voted to request that colleges of pharmacy "include needed practicable courses on business techniques," as well as providing "refresher courses which contain the latest information on pharmaceutical developments."

While pharmacy education was a recent concern, fair trade was long term and continued to dominate NARD. Much of 1951 was again given over to this issue. In May the association and its small business allies received a major setback when the U.S. Supreme Court ruled a section of the Tydings-Miller Act unconstitutional. In a six-to-three vote the court took exception to Section I-A, the so-called non-signer clause of Tydings-Miller (National Fair Trade Law). Language for that portion of the law had been drafted by Edward S. Rogers, a leader in the California Free Trade movement, for a law in that state. Other states had followed that language, as did Senator Tydings when drafting the national law.

Section I-A prohibited "willingly and knowingly advertising, offering for sale, or selling any commodity at less than the price stipulated in any contract entered into pursuant to the provision of Section I of this act, whether the person so advertising, offering for sale or selling is or is not a party to such contract, is unfair competition and is actionable at the suit of any person damaged thereby." The court ruled that the application of that clause "in interstate commerce" was unconstitutional.

While the case did not apply to the forty-four state laws in existence at that time, it was nevertheless a major blow to the national legislation. Fair trade was the talk of the fifty-third convention as delegates gathered at Minneapolis in 1951. General confusion prevailed over what, if anything, could be done, and the membership was in need of strong reassurance from the

NARD leadership. President Charles F. Gilson acknowledged the gravity of the moment and said "public relations now more than ever is compulsory for the druggist." But he said pharmacists must also share some of the blame if fair trade failed because not enough of them were involved in defending its merits. "Somehow," he said, "they must be aroused to the extent that they will help much more than they have in the past to solve the problems of pharmacy and the drug store."

Executive Committee Chairman Charles Seward emphasized the need for NARD to expand its presence and pointed out that NARD had jointly sponsored programs on national television to emphasize the importance of the neighborhood pharmacy. He said the executive committee was also recommending that dues be raised from $5 to $10 to allow greater expansion in association activities.

Secretary Dargavel cautioned the delegates to be patient in their reaction to the Supreme Court's rulings. He assured them NARD was preparing a response, but he said two events were necessary to bring any change in the circumstances.

First, an amendment to the Tydings-Miller bill must be worded in clear and understandable language. But more important than laws, he said, "experience has taught us that it is a serious mistake to have a bill introduced before strong support has been built, (and) it is evident that we lack the militant forces needed to achieve enactment of an amendment. Too many druggists still depend on others to fight for the things that involve the welfare of every independent drug store and the profession of pharmacy in general."

Only after he had raised the militancy issue did the secretary tell the delegates that the leadership had a new bill. It would be introduced in the next session of Congress and promised to provide more protection for fair trade. "You can count on N.A.R.D.," he said, "in the crisis that jeopardizes the survival of fair trade."

Delegates were reassured by the overall convention program, the confidence exhibited by the leadership, and just the opportunity to renew friendships and compare news. The central office staff had also arranged a drawing for door prizes at each business session and that proved to be highly popular with the attendees. They approved the dues increase without debate and elected Elbert W. Gibbs of Birmingham, Alabama, as their new president. Once again, Charles Seward was reelected chairman of the executive committee.

Less than two weeks after the Minneapolis convention, Dargavel was able to report a major legislative victory on prescription labeling. While not a free trade item, the labeling issue had been bothersome due to a ruling by the

Food and Drug Administration (FDA). The FDA ruled that prescriptions were canceled after the initial filling and refills required the same recording as the original order. Moreover, the FDA ruled that the pharmacists had legal liability for all wording on the prescription label if they transferred contents from the manufacturer's original container.

Those rulings and a growing practice by physicians to place prescription orders by telephone without a written record cascaded into a major problem. Not only did the aforementioned rulings require extra paperwork and bookkeeping time, but also the responsibility for certifying the label from the manufacturer was all but impossible. Typically, a pharmacist placed a bulk or multiple count order with the manufacturer, then repackaged the contents in individual dosages or prescriptions.

In an attempt to provide some relief from these regulations, Rep. Carl T. Durham, a pharmacist from North Carolina, and Sen. Hubert Humphrey, a pharmacist from Minnesota, introduced companion legislation in the first session of the 82nd Congress. Among other things, the Durham-Humphrey bill legalized refills except for restricted drugs, allowed oral (telephoned)

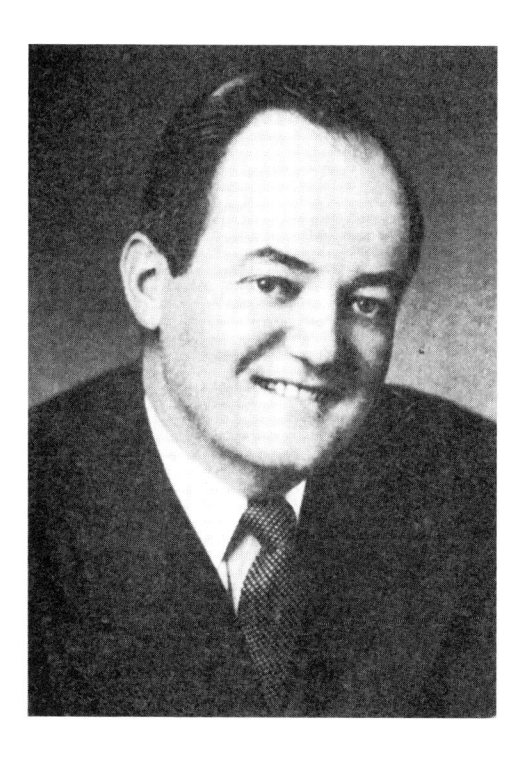

Sen. Hubert H. Humphrey

prescriptions with only a written notation by the pharmacist, established a uniform legend, required manufacturers to affix that legend on all controlled medicinals but prohibited similar labels on non-prescription items, and allowed the pharmacists to reproduce the manufacturer's label and place the exact language on individual orders.

When Durham began to hold hearings on the bill in March, an array of interests lined up to oppose the bill — including the American Pharmaceutical Association (APhA), the American Pharmaceutical Manufacturers Association (PMA), the Proprietary Association (PA), and even the wholesale grocers lobby (the National Association of Retail Grocers). Over the course of the spring and summer, debate on the issue became increasingly polarized. Dargavel was charged by the opposition with introducing the bill for his personal political ambitions and for having a vendetta against the manufacturers for their refusal to correct medicament duplications.

Through innuendo, a news leak suggested that members of "the executive committee of N.A.R.D. were 'pinks'." (The derogatory term, "pinks," was coined by Senator Joseph McCarthy of Wisconsin, head of the Select Senate Investigation Committee, who unleashed a reign of terror on American institutions of all stripes, believing that Communist sympathizers had infiltrated them. Anyone who questioned and possibly threatened American establishments was often referred to as a "pink.")

Despite the allegations and standing alone among the drug trade industries, the NARD leadership refused to yield. Dargavel, who was never one to pull punches, wrote a scathing editorial in the *Journal* in which he referred to the opposition as "misguided and weasel." He reserved harsh judgment on the actions of APhA, which he said "has somehow been deluded to spearhead a plan of legal action that on the surface appears to be aimed to eliminate intolerable restrictions on prescriptions. However, the concealed intention seems to be to serve the manufacturers of drugs, instead of the druggists. It is important to bear in mind, to avoid confusion, that APhA has a membership with varied interests). Various indications suggest that the APhA has lost sight of the independent drug store owners…. The N.A.R.D. represents only drug store owners. It doesn't have divergent interests. Druggists alone dictate the policies and activities of the organization."

Dargavel appealed through the *Journal* and personal contacts for community pharmacists to write or call members of Congress. Again, the network paid off. The Durham-Humphrey bill passed Congress in mid-October and President Truman signed it into law on October 26.

To indicate the significance of this effort, Editor Sletterdahl noted in the *Journal,* "There were 2,743 bills introduced in the Senate…and 6,872 in the House. The Senate passed 1,059 and the House 1,193 — the majority on national defense." He called it "a great victory for the N.A.R.D." As a footnote to the battle, after Durham-Humphrey became law, APhA issued a press release implying that APhA had contributed to getting the bill passed. Dargavel did not contain his anger and denounced APhA for making such statements. "The truth," he said, "is just the opposite. The A.Ph.A. did all it could to obstruct the passage of the proposed measure in Congress." This dispute created a serious rift between the two associations. Since 1927, the NARD and APhA had a joint committee that met annually to discuss issues of mutual interest. During World War II the executive committees from each group held joint conventions. But now disagreement was too great for joint collaboration.

The exhilaration of passing the Durham-Humphrey bill was surpassed only by an even more important bill in 1952. As Dargavel promised the membership in Minneapolis, NARD had a plan for securing the National Fair Trade Law. But the secretary failed to reveal his strategy for getting the bill passed. That maneuvering came to be a bigger story than the bill.

At one of the many Washington social functions, Dargavel met Rep. John A. McGuire, learned that he owned a small insurance agency in Wallingford, Connecticut, and discovered that he had a strong interest in issues important to small business and in fair trade. Dargavel immediately wanted him as an ally, and McGuire agreed to introduce a bill to revise the court's opinion on Section I-A of Tydings-Miller Act.

In the meantime, the NARD leadership organized a "conference of attorneys" attended by twenty-two lawyers representing the various fair trade associations. Over a period of days this group worked out the language that all agreed would pass constitutional muster. More importantly, the group agreed that the best way to protect fair trade was to amend the Federal Trade Commission charter, rather than the Sherman Act.

The reason for this strategy was to get the most favorable hearing in committee. Rep. Emanuel Cellar, the long-time foe to fair trade from New York, had become chairman of the Senate Judiciary Committee. Any bill to amend the Sherman Act would be routed to his committee. By contrast, an amendment to the Federal Trade Commission charter would be referred to the Committee on Interstate and Foreign Commerce. This committee was chaired by Rep. Robert Crosser of Ohio, a staunch friend of small business.

The text prepared by the attorneys was given to Rep. McGuire and he in turn filed it in the House of Representatives. Introduced in October, and passed eight months later, on July 14, the McGuire bill was a "miracle," according to seasoned observers on Capitol Hill. Not only did the bill, and a controversial one at that, make it through Congress in one session, but also NARD won the fight in a most decisive manner — only 10 negative votes in the House and 16 no votes in the Senate. Rather than a miracle, Dargavel chose to believe the bill passed through "marvelous cooperation (with) more than a million individual contributions from drug store owners in the cities and towns from Maine to California." The secretary would probably admit that a major trade war in New York City helped too. Hardly two weeks after McGuire introduced his bill, Macy's Department Stores in New York City announced a major "sale" in certain merchandise with savings over 50 percent off the regular price.

A huge crowd of shoppers filled the store to overflowing and stretched around the block. Violence broke out between competing shoppers and the police had to be called in to keep order. Other stores followed Macy's lead and over the next few weeks the retail market in Manhattan seemed "out of control." Store owners finally conferred and called an end to the price war, but not before the public, and more particularly political leaders, saw the impact predatory price cutting could have on a community.

How much the publicity over the Macy price war influenced the outcome of the McGuire bill was hard to calculate. But, in any event, it did not hurt the cause of small business. It was still in the memory of delegates who gathered in St. Louis in 1952 for the fifty-fourth convention. Because the Durham-Humphrey Act and the McGuire Act had both passed since the last convention, it was a time of special celebration.

Retiring President Elbert Gibbs credited Secretary Dargavel with the association's legislative success and urged the delegates to help him more by becoming more involved in state and local politics. He pointed to a survey the association had commissioned soon after the Supreme Court nullified the non-signer clause in the National Fair Trade Law. The study revealed that only seven percent of the pharmacists were personally acquainted with their congressman and less than three percent knew their senator on a personal basis. Because "pharmacy is the most regulated profession in America," he said, it was "vital that (pharmacists) have a strong voice in politics."

In other action at the fifty-fourth convention, delegates adopted a resolution authorizing the John A. Dargavel Memorial Foundation. The move was spearheaded by former President John Goode and called upon the association president to appoint a committee to develop "an appropriate memorial." Delegates also elected Alexander C. Mayerson of Chicago as the new president.

Fortunately for the NARD leadership, 1953 was a relatively calm year with respect to legislation. Not having to manage or defeat a major bill gave the executive committee time to focus on ways to assist local store owners and to expand NARD's image as more than a powerful political lobbying group.

From a public relations standpoint, the opportunity to promote community pharmacy could not have come at a better time. On November 12, 1952, the Attorney General for the state of New York filed a lawsuit against thirteen Long Island physicians and druggists, charging them with antitrust violations.

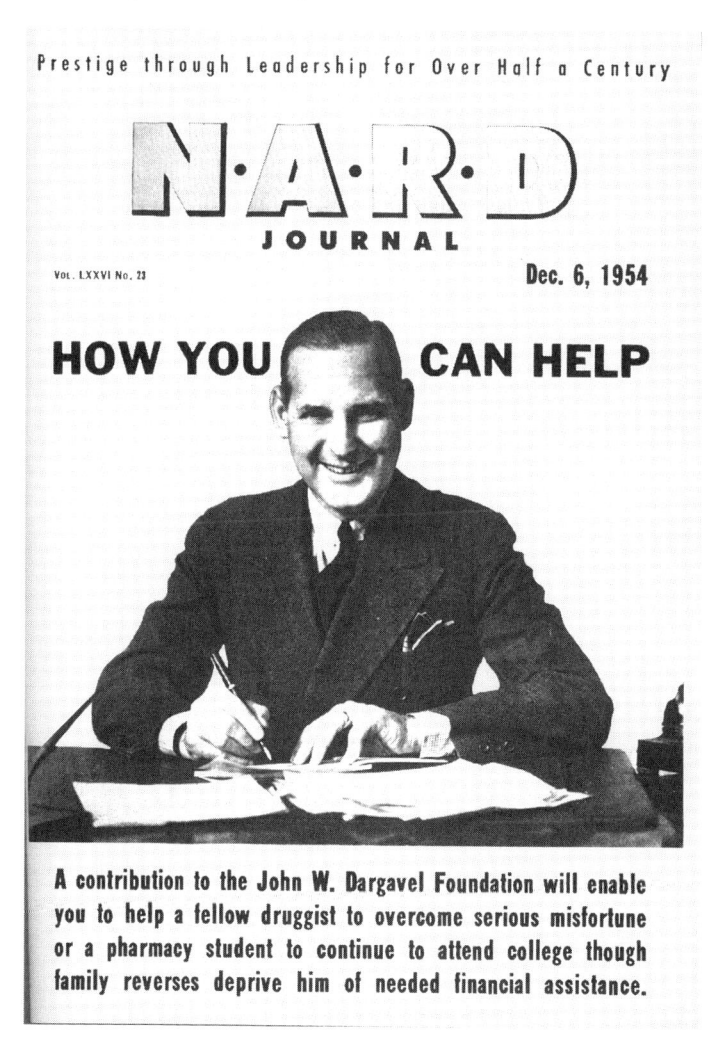

According to the attorney general, neighborhood druggists conspired with local physicians and a local pharmaceutical manufacturer in a prescription racket. Pharmacists bought products produced by physician-owned manufacturers. Physicians then wrote prescriptions in favor of those items and sent patients to the pharmacy having the item in stock. At the end of the year, the physicians and pharmacists split the dividends on the sales. While only thirteen individuals were initially indicted, evidence pointed to several hundred, perhaps over 1,000 being involved.

The suit received "sensational" coverage in local newspapers and became a national scandal. While it did not directly involve NARD, it was a blow to the credibility of the neighborhood pharmacist. Ironically, the executive committee had made physician-owned clinics that dispensed prescriptions an agenda item almost every year since World War II. The association strongly opposed physician dispensing but found only limited political support in the Congress. Beyond pointing out the problem, NARD had no means to force physicians to comply with the law.

The problem posed by the supermarket was equally difficult to solve. According to market surveys done in 1953 for the National Association of Retail Grocers, food stores had found a lucrative market in health and beauty aids and planned to expand their inventories in those areas even more. To counter that move, the NARD leadership conducted its own business surveys and hired specialists to write feature articles for the *Journal* about consumer buying habits and strategies for merchandising.

NARD's analysis of trends in the retail world showed that consumers were less interested in personal service and wanted the opportunity for self-selection when choosing products. There was also a growing "specialty" market and interest in personal grooming, particularly among men. To take advantage of these consumer habits, the association suggested that pharmacists remodel their stores both internally and externally to give a "health center" appearance. This new image emphasized pharmacy as the primary function of the store and featured fixtures and displays arranged for the maximum convenience of the customer.

The NARD leadership further recommended that articles be arranged by departments and that the prescription section be placed at the back of the store to allow customers an opportunity to see other merchandise when entering and leaving the store. While recognizing that product demands varied from one region to another, the NARD leadership noted that the current "baby boom" was nationwide and pharmacists who opened a specialty department in this area could expect a significant increase in sales. Four million babies were born in 1952 alone, and market surveys showed that parents spent an average of $78.25 per child per year, plus another $15.25 for their own needs. NARD's message to its membership was that successful pharmacists must recognize the characteristics of the modern customer and adjust their business habits accordingly.

The executive committee chose "survival problems" as the theme for the fifty-fifth convention meeting in Chicago in 1953. In his presidential address, Mayerson reminded delegates that he was the son of a pharmacist and that he had fond memories of his father's store. However, he said, "the traditional position of pharmacy is in jeopardy." He went through a litany of reasons why that was so — physician dispensing, chain stores, undercutting on price maintenance, and fair trade agreements.

However, Mayerson said the public was turning away from "the neighborhood drug store" primarily because of "the charges we make for prescriptions." While he had no trouble explaining to customers how prescriptions were priced, and that they were in fact low in relation to the costs involved, the public had a different perception. He noted that the association must find a way to educate the public on how prescriptions were priced and to demonstrate to customers what a value prescription medicine was in comparison to the costs of other products. To begin that process, Mayerson sug-

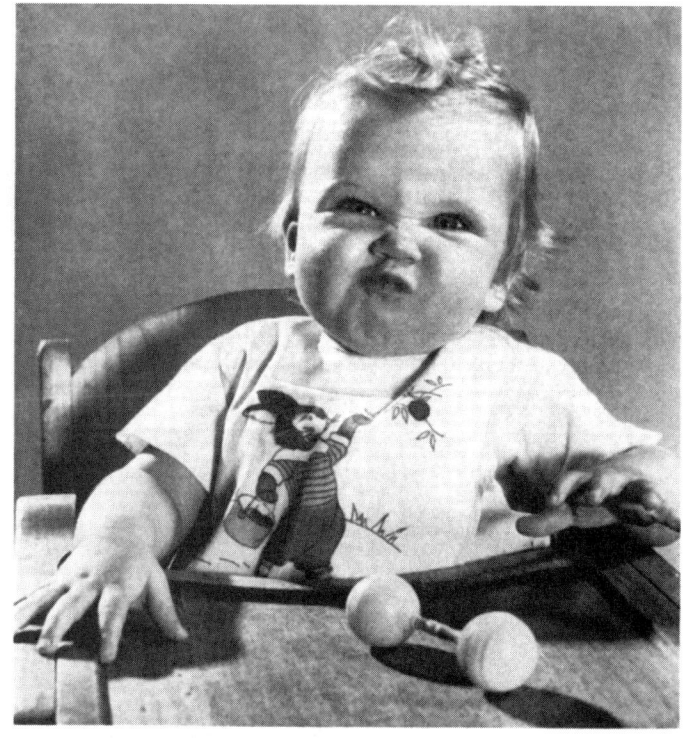

The birth records for 1955 emphasized the importance of the drug store baby department. Tentative estimates tell us that 4,108,000 "bundles from heaven" were born in 1955 (an increase over the year before). One study shows that mothers of the "first baby" are younger today than the mothers of the immediate past generation. Thirty percent are 19 years old or under.

The NARD Journal noted the "baby boom" and merchandising tie-ins to promotional themes, such as National Baby Week.

gested that pharmacists inform customers about the concept of "generic drugs" and encourage them to request physicians to specify A.R.B (Any Reliable Brand) on prescriptions.

Chairman Seward emphasized the problem of "duplication of medicines." He called the large inventory pharmacists were forced to maintain "outrageous" and "intolerable" and illustrated how it contributed to high overhead costs. He also noted that higher fixed costs were seriously threatening the pharmacist's ability to be competitive with the supermarkets. Secretary Dargavel reviewed the leadership's efforts to promote community pharmacy in the past year and told delegates the association had launched a "national public relations program" to coincide with the convention and that the campaign would be continued in the coming year.

In other convention activities, delegates heard a report from former President Frank Moudry on plans for the John W. Dargavel Foundation. Moudry said the foundation established a capital fund of $250,000 to provide loans to pharmacists who lost their stores through natural disasters and to pharmacy students who needed help to complete school. He asked his colleagues to contribute $100,000 to the fund and the foundation would raise the balance.

In one of the last items before the convention, delegates elected Marion V. Hardesty of Louisville, Kentucky, as president. Charles Seward was reelected once again to be chairman of the executive committee.

The new NARD leadership wasted little time implementing the national public relations campaign. Buying space for a major advertisement in the *Saturday Evening Post,* the association promoted the neighborhood pharmacy as a health center "at the corner of life and death." Prominently displaying the NARD emblem (designed in 1950 by Milwaukee pharmacist Larry Carriveau but not profiled until 1953) with the slogan of "Integrity...Safety...Service," the ad graphically promoted the professional side of the local pharmacy and told consumers "there is no more essential merchant in your town than your modern independent pharmacist."

The headquarters office made mats of the ad available to store owners and association leaders to be used in local advertising. The plan was highly successful as favorable reports and requests for mats poured into the Chicago office. When responding to those requests, the staff also included a copy of the emblem and encouraged members to display it on the front door of their stores. Building a national image that transcended, but did not replace, local identities was an important part of the campaign.

Two related parts of the public relations effort were a "consumer relations program that attacked the competition of the food outlets (at their) weakest points" and a "trade relations program center in the *N.A.R.D Journal* to provide closer cooperation between the manufacturers and NARD members." While the public relations campaign was under way, word came of a U.S. Supreme Court decision upholding the principle of fair trade. The case developed when the Schwegmann Brothers Giant Supermarket of New Orleans refused to follow the "fair trade provisions" of the McGuire Act. Eli Lilly & Company filed suit against the supermarket. Lilly won the initial trial and the decision was sustained by the Fifth Circuit Court of Appeals. Schwegmann Brothers then appealed to the Supreme Court. However, the high court refused to hear the appeal and Lilly's suit was upheld.

Dargavel was elated to hear of the decision. He wrote in the *Journal*, "The McGuire Act may now be considered watertight.... From now on there should be much more extensive enforcement.... the manufacturers have an open road on which to drive against the chiselers."

(That assessment proved to be short-lived. A mere three years later, the U. S. Supreme Court ruled in the case of Standard Oil of Indiana vs. Federal Trade Commission that price discrimination was allowable provided the manufacturer acted in "good faith" when establishing prices. NARD's Washington representative, George Frates, had worked hard to build congressional support of a new bill to plug the loophole created by the Standard Oil decision. After weeks of work, Frates persuaded Sen. Estes Kefauver to introduce the Equality of Opportunity Bill designed to correct the "good faith" ruling of the court. However, the oil and gas lobby had more than enough influence to keep the bill tied up in committee throughout the 84th session of Congress.)

The executive committee selected Houston, Texas, for the fifty-sixth convention in 1954, the first time the association had convened its annual meeting in Texas. The local hospitality committee was particularly attentive to the delegates' social interests. President Hardesty used his time before the House of Delegates to talk about "the drug store of tomorrow." He gave an optimistic report and said the future store would be built on five principles: ample floor space, customer convenience, professionalism, business promotion, and community participation.

Hardesty also cautioned his listeners about "laxities found in the state pharmacy acts." He said that failure to pass "corrective legislation" could cause Congress to "vote funds to extend policy activities of the Food and Drug Administration." The reason for this, he said, was because of "the potency of modern drugs."

In an effort to capitalize on the national public relations campaign, the executive committee hosted a meeting for the state and metropolitan secretaries. State presidents and chairs of the state Fair Trade Committees also joined the group. These executives provided an important forum to gain information and promote NARD issues. In other action, delegates elected

Garnet M. Eisele of Hot Springs, Arkansas, as president; Charles Seward was again named chairman of the executive committee.

The highly successful public relations campaign in 1954 was followed by a series of attempts to smear NARD in 1955. At various times in the year, articles appeared in both the trade and commercial press criticizing independent pharmacists for "overpriced prescriptions," for "selling counterfeit merchandise," and for "dispensing substituted medication." Other articles charged store owners with "peddling crime 'comics' and obscene books to youngsters" and for contributing to "juvenile delinquency by providing 'thrill pills' (amphetamines)" to adolescents.

Another major problem developed in March. U.S. Attorney Herbert Brownell, Jr. released a report compiled by a select committee he had appointed to study the antitrust laws. The report called for a repeal of federal fair trade laws and a revision in existing antitrust laws to encourage greater competition. At this point, it was just another study done by a committee. However, to Dargavel and the NARD leadership, it was an opening shot for a new round of anti-fair trade bills.

President Eisele addressed most of these issues in his address to the fifty-seventh convention at Atlantic City, New Jersey in 1955. He said the criticism stemmed from enemies of independent pharmacy and from "the fringe rouges that peddle 'goof balls' and 'thrill pills' and even narcotics...." He insisted

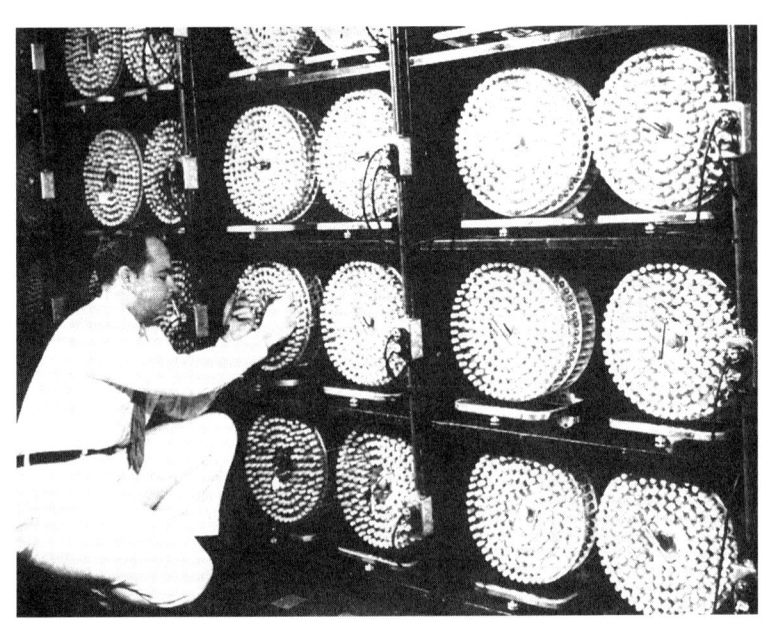

Polio vaccine made its debut in 1954. Roller drums containing hundreds of assay tubes with the Salk vaccine are shown in the incubating rooms above.

that the rogues were a small minority and that it was time for professional pharmacists to stand up and defend the profession. "The stake we have in this deplorable situation," he said, "is prestige." With reference to the Brownell report, he noted that his committee had "labored in a vacuum remote from the economic facts of life."

Secretary Dargavel reported on his trip to England on behalf of the association. He was invited to visit Great Britain by the Proprietary Article Trade Association to speak on behalf of fair trade to various pharmacy associations and to the British Parliament. The secretary told of Britain's commitment to fair trade and reported to his surprise how loyal the pharmacists in that nation were to socialized medicine.

Before leaving Atlantic City, delegates elected John J. McKeighan of Flint, Michigan, as president for 1955-1956. Charles Seward was again chosen to lead the executive committee.

Stung by the highly publicized criticism attacking their professionalism, NARD leaders moved to neutralize as much future negativity as possible. Another bothersome issue was word that the American Medical Association (AMA) had amended its code of ethics to allow physicians to own a pharmacy. The offending amendment read, "It is not unethical for a physician to prescribe or supply drugs, remedies, or appliances as long as there is no exploitation of the patient." Dargavel and others thought such practice was unethical. However, rather than continue the negative publicity that would come with a fight to get the offending words removed, he recommended a meeting to work out the differences.

At its fall meeting in November 1955, the executive committee voted to accept the secretary's recommendation and host a joint meeting with AMA. In an effort to "mend more bridges," the executive committee also invited APhA to join the meeting. Each association agreed to a three-member delegation.

But, despite the best intentions, the representatives of the three groups found it difficult to reach agreement, and the matter was still unsettled when the fifty-eighth convention met in Cincinnati in 1956.

President McKeighan avoided a direct reference to the AMA amendment. However, he said that "a code of ethics which cannot be enforced counts for nothing in the mind of the pharmacists." Following the official policy of conciliation with the AMA and APhA, the McKeighan told the House of Delegates that pharmacy must be known for its integrity and to remember that "it is important for all of us to retain the gentle spirit of the deepest interest in mankind."

The convention was remarkably subdued in comparison to many in the past. There were no major new issues. Even Secretary Dargavel lacked his usually fiery rhetoric. He seemed almost resigned to the current economic playing field as he told the membership that "independent druggists and small retailers in general will have to live with the changes that came with the postwar revolution in distribution."

Charles Seward of Pasadena, California, after serving seven terms as chairman of the executive committee, was elected president for 1956-1957. H.E. Henderson of Seattle, Washington, was selected as the new chairman of the executive committee. Soon after the convention adjourned, rumors circulated in some trade journals that Secretary Dargavel planned to retire. However, at its fall meeting, the executive committee extended the secretary's contract another five years through 1961.

Despite having a new Congress in session, legislative action involving issues of concern to NARD were minimal. The "interprofessional committee" (NARD/AMA/APhA) continued to meet, but still did not resolve the basic "ethical" questions separating the associations.

The fifty-ninth convention returned to Minneapolis in 1957. President Seward voiced hope that the physicians and pharmacists "will eliminate the

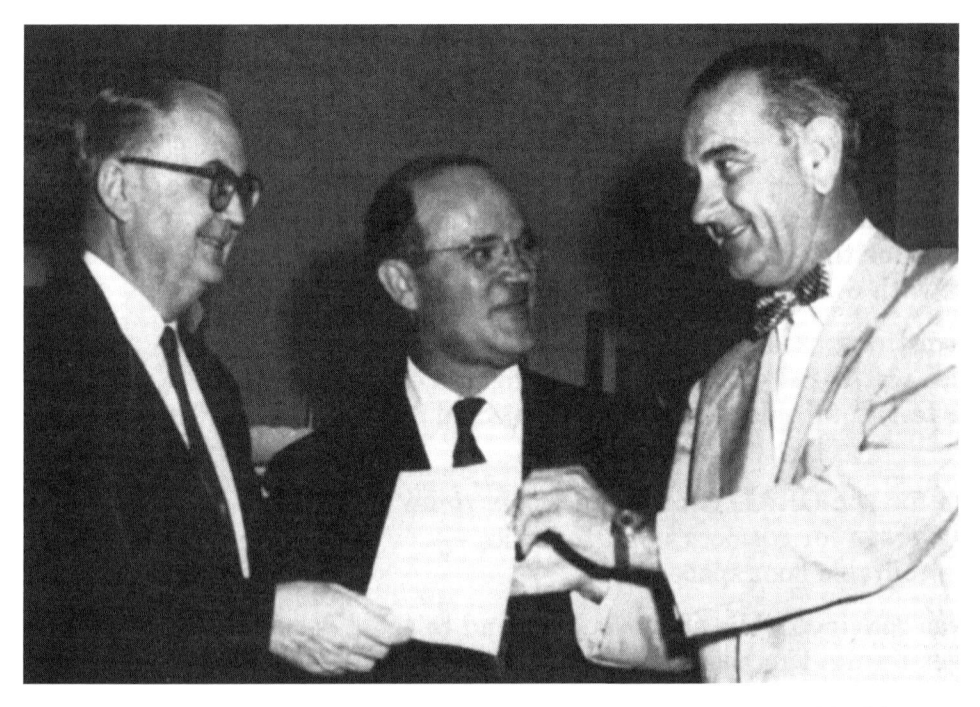

Rep. Wright Patman (left) and Sen. Lyndon Johnson (right), as co-authors of the Johnson-Patman Act in 1958, congratulated Mills B. Lane on the first investment company (Citizens & Southern Bank, Atlanta, Georgia) formed to operate under the act. The act authorized investment of federal funds to support small businesses.

differences that interfere with harmony in inter-professional relations." He also decried the problem of "duplication" and suggested that "a provision be placed in the code of pharmaceutical manufacturers to correct the flow of imitated products."

Chairman H.E. Henderson used his time before the delegates to talk about the need to revive political action. He noted the "forces arrayed against one program or another directed by N.A.R.D." and urged the membership to get ready for a new round of political action.

Secretary Dargavel discussed economic trends and business activities for the past year. He reported that it had been a very average year for most pharmacists. Moreover, he said, "it is obvious that around half of the independent retail pharmacists in 1956 earned too little to save the money needed to finance expansion of facilities necessary to keep up with competition."

While the general business activities may have been flat or nearly so, NARD continued to have major growth in its finances. In 1957, the association passed $1 million in assets and news of that milestone sparked some life in the delegates. Also H.E. Chapman, secretary of the Proprietary Articles Trade Association in England, became the first foreign pharmacy official to address the House of Delegates and he too received a rousing reception.

The delegates elected H.E. Henderson president. Willard Simmons of Texarkana, Texas, was chosen as the new chairman of the executive committee. The NARD leadership entered the last year of their sixth decade much as they had the first year. The "cat and mouse" game with the forces opposed to the principles of fair trade and price maintenance continued to dominate the legislative agenda.

The association received a blow in April 1958 when its president, H.E. (Ned) Henderson, died from a sudden illness. In special session, the executive committee selected Angus H. Taylor of Minneapolis, then 1st Vice President, the new president. When delegates gathered in Philadelphia for the sixtieth convention, they did so under the cloud of Henderson's death and a new round of negative publicity. Nationwide criticism had been directed against prices on prescribed medications. The consensus among the trade paper journalists was that such prices were unjust and that pharmacists were responsible for the high costs of prescription medicines.

President Taylor lamented the "reverses that have struck fair trade" and he said that "the mutilation of anti-trust statutes has resulted in the return of desperation to the independent retailers in the marketplace." He described the situation as "tragic" and said, "you talk (to individual store owners) and they soon make it plain that they wonder how soon (before) they too, will lock the front door for the last time."

The new association president may have been a bit pessimistic as he addressed the House of Delegates for the first time. But such was not the case for "the old war horse," John Dargavel, who was completing his twenty-fifth year as secretary. Over those years, he had developed an understanding of when to be militant and when to be reassuring. This was the time to reassure the delegates. He reviewed the history of the fair trade movement and NARD's role in it. He told his listeners that "a fair trade law has never been repealed."

In a rousing close to his speech, Dargavel said, "I am confident that the N.A.R.D. will continue to march with progress and that it will grow in influence to be even more significant to the independent retail pharmacist than it is today. Of that I am certain."

CHAPTER EIGHT

THE SEVENTH DECADE: 1959 – 1968

NARD Grapples with Seismic Change in the Marketplace

*T*he seventh decade of NARD's history witnessed an upheaval in American society, as well as a seismic shift in pharmacy's relationship with the federal government. The "Great Society," Medicare/Medicaid, and public pharmaceutical benefit programs were all born in the 1960s.

The placid 1950s gave way to the tumultuous '60s. The French Indochina War of the 1950s in Southeast Asia became an American nightmare as the "local" conflagration blew up into a full-scale war midway through the '60s, lasting well into the next decade. The Vietnam conflict became a contentious issue that divided American society as few others had. The civil rights movement also increasingly became a divisive issue as most of the nation's major cities were racked with violent demonstrations against existing social policies.

Much of this discontent began on the nation's college campuses, traditionally one of the most reliable agencies for transmitting national culture. The assassinations of President John F. Kennedy in 1963, as well as Martin Luther King Jr. and Robert Kennedy in 1968, added to the emotional upheaval.

Against this ongoing background of tumult, NARD found itself throughout the decade coping with simultaneous assaults on fair trade, the emergence of a vast federal presence in the marketplace (Medicare/Medicaid), and the passing of a great leader in its history — John Dargavel. The mettle of NARD as an organization for the remainder of the century was forged here in the 1960s.

As the decade opened, the association found itself under attack for allegedly driving up prices on prescription medicines. Moreover, the organization found itself increasingly isolated from other trade associations on the issue of fair trade — the life-blood of small business. While respected and even feared in some circles as the premiere organization when it came to political lobbying, NARD was still a "small voice" in the great wilderness of the retail world. With a peak membership of 36,000 community pharmacists, out of a total of some 60,000 independent stores, it took a supreme effort from the leadership, and even some luck, on every political issue.

Having failed in the 85th Congress to gain any substantive revision in the fair trade laws, the NARD leadership concluded that to be effective, it must have a broader base of support. This was particularly true since community pharmacy had borne the brunt of the criticism about high prescription prices. It would take time to educate the public about the pricing issue. In the meantime, association leaders could not risk having their opponents use the negative publicity to get fair trade laws revised or, worse yet, repealed.

As a first step in this strategy, members of the executive committee moved to build an alliance among groups who shared interests similar to their own. Without shared interests, it was unlikely that NARD could persuade the dry goods, cosmetics, jewelry, and similar groups to work with pharmacy. The executive committee also set a goal of placing a pharmacy representative "on local, county, and state health boards and in the federal health agencies." Having pharmacists directly involved with these groups would allow NARD an opportunity to provide them with direct information about pharmacy issues and a better chance of gaining their support on political issues.

The trend in retail sales was another reason for building alliances. Secretary John Dargavel and the central staff collected volumes of materials on market trends for the executive committee. In analyzing this data, the executive committee identified trends that "ran against independent pharmacy" in the retail field. These trends included hospitals opening their own pharmacies for outpatient care; clinics and group medical practice units dispensing their own prescriptions; and labor unions, as well as state and federal agencies, contracting with specific stores, usually a chain, for their pharmacy needs. Each of these areas was growing rapidly and was projected to continue to do so for the foreseeable future.

The above data also revealed other disturbing information. The American Association of Retired Persons (AARP) was in the process of developing a plan to provide its members with a "national mail order pharmacy." While still in the planning stage, the prospects of the more than 50,000 (and growing) members channeling their pharmacy needs to a single source was a real challenge to NARD. Information from another source indicated the emergence of "giant retail centers" where nonfood merchandise made up more than half the floor space and annual sales exceeded $20 million. According to the survey, these stores offered prices "that (made) the discount houses look like gougers."

Evidence of the mail order potential for organizations and businesses having interstate connections forced the executive committee to change its schedule on new fair trade legislation. Mail order became a sensitive issue because the U.S. Supreme Court ruled in General Electric vs Masters in 1958 that "a sale by mail need not conform (price wise) with the laws of the state into which the goods are shipped." Getting a new bill to amend the original Tydings-Miller Act before the new "mail order pharmacies" became operational was now imperative.

Dargavel and Executive Committee Chairman Willard Simmons contacted George Frates, NARD's Washington representative, to discuss a new bill. Frates had been the association's "man in the Capital" since 1943. Given the association's current public image due to the prescription price issue, as well as the growing opposition to fair trade from diverse and well-funded groups, Frates suggested that the executive committee employ an additional legislative specialist to help him. Simmons and Dargavel agreed, and upon Frates's recommendation, they hired Philip F. Jehle, the chief counsel to the Senate's Small Business Committee. Jehle was thoroughly familiar with the fair trade issue and began work on January 15, 1959.

While recruiting a new member for the legal team, Dargavel also talked with several in Congress about a new bill. Minnesota Senator Hubert Humphrey was quite willing to introduce a bill in the Senate, but the unruly House of Representatives presented more of a problem. Ironically, the representative most interested in fair trade was another Arkansan, Fourth District Congressman Oren Harris. He agreed to sponsor the measure, and the Harris Fair Trade Bill (H.R. 1253) was introduced in the second session of the 86th Congress. Sen. Humphrey was joined by Wisconsin Senator William Proxmire and the two cosponsored a companion bill (S. 1083) in the Senate.

When Rep. Harris opened hearings on his bill, Dargavel counted fourteen different groups lined up to speak against the proposal. The executive secretary sent out his usual call to the NARD membership for a "flood of letters and telegrams" to Congress in support of the bill. But, as he said, "the immediate response amounted to only a trickle." Waiting a couple of weeks, he again appealed for support, but again "the responses were too meager to count for much." Meanwhile, representatives of the American Federation of Labor and Congress of Industrial Organizations (AFL-CIO), the American Farm Bureau, the Grocery Manufacturers of America (formerly the National Retail Grocers Association), the Departments of Agriculture, Commerce, and Justice, and numerous others spoke against the bill.

It was at this point that Jehle's legislative experience became vital. Using his former Capitol Hill contacts, he managed to build some support, and with Harris's strong commitment, the bill was reported out of committee with a "do pass" resolution. However, with presidential elections scheduled in 1960, the Senate bill got caught in the last-minute political maneuvering and did not get scheduled for a vote. Dargavel was forced to tell the House of Delegates at the annual convention that much more work was ahead.

The sixty-first convention returned to St. Louis, Missouri, in 1959. President Taylor joined Dargavel in urging delegates to be more supportive of the Harris bill in specific and fair trade in general. "We are convinced," he said, "that minus the legislation, the small independent retailer is doomed to eventual extinction."

Executive Committee Chairman Simmons reviewed the survey results on trends in the marketplace taken the previous year. He also mentioned that community pharmacists were being unfairly compared to the "mail order houses and peddlers" who sold "nostrums" with limited medicinal value. Because of these promotions, he said, "it is evident that the efforts to enlighten the public on the cost of medication have failed to count for much. Complaints continued unabated." But he said the executive committee would continue to seek a solution to this issue since "the problem of the common attitudes toward the prices charged for prescriptions is too serious to minimize." Before adjourning, the House of Delegates elected Ralph R. Rooke

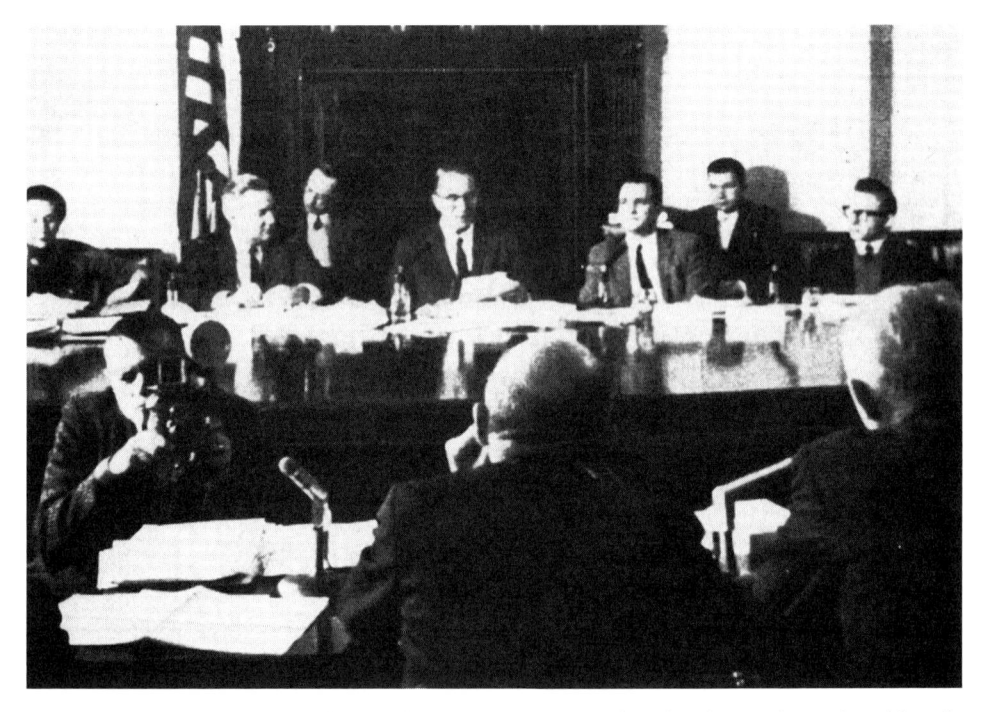

As a one-man subcommittee, Sen. Kefauver (center) carried on his drug price probe with only a few staff members in attendance. The cartoon at the right demonstrated NARD's view of the hearings.

of Richmond, Virginia, as president. Willard Simmons was again chosen chairman of the executive committee.

Within days after returning from the St. Louis convention, Dargavel heard that Tennessee Sen. Estes Kefauver planned to conduct an investigation into "the high costs of drugs." That report was confirmed on December 5, when Sen. Kefauver called a press conference in Washington and said, "our country has the finest drugs and medicines in the world, but prices are so high that such items are becoming unavailable to many people." He continued to talk about "the uniformity of drug prices," which gave indication of "administered prices by which competition is absent and prices may be raised even though demand falls off."

The report caught Dargavel and the NARD leadership by surprise. Sen. Kefauver was thought to be a supporter of small business and had introduced a bill for NARD in 1957 to amend (favorably to NARD) the Robinson-Patman Act. But the publicity about high prescription prices had caught his atten-

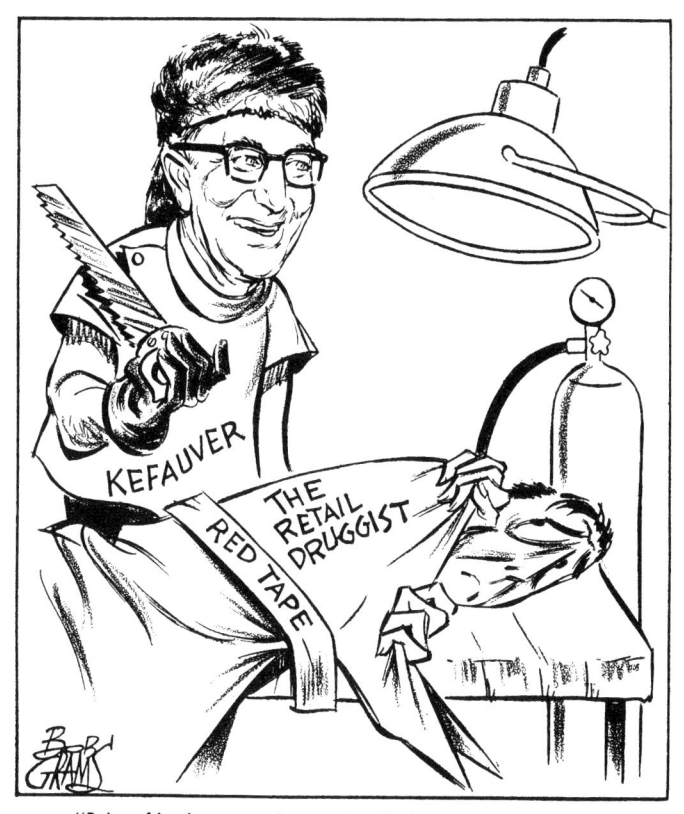

"Relax, friend, my appointment is with the drug manufacturer."

tion, and he said he intended to use his Senate Antitrust and Monopoly Subcommittee to investigate. While most of the attention appeared to be directed toward the manufacturers, Dargavel and his colleagues knew that community pharmacy would also be affected by association with those companies.

In light of the publicity surrounding the "Kefauver probe," the executive committee decided not to push the Harris Fair Trade Bill in the second session of the 86th Congress. Instead, members concentrated on the internal affairs of the association. One of their first decisions was a vote to reestablish the printing operation for the publicity department in the central office. For the past year the association had contracted with a private firm to provide this service. In conjunction with that decision, the executive committee also asked the staff to prepare a brochure highlighting the membership benefits offered by the association.

The list of services NARD offered to its members for one annual fee was impressive. Included was the Washington Office, which monitored legislation and lobbied public officials. The central office in Chicago included the legal department, which provided members with counseling on contracts, leases, claims, and related matters; the publicity department published the *Journal,* the Washington *Newsletter,* and other timely information; the modernization department helped with store layout, fixtures, and trends in merchandising; the public relations department promoted public and interprofessional programs; and the "Bureau of Education on Fair Trade" kept the membership and other trade organizations informed about business practices and efforts to maintain stability in the marketplace. The *N.A.R.D. Almanac,* a promotional give-away to customers that could be personalized with the store's name, was available at a small additional cost to members.

In another action, the executive committee accepted a bid from the Mutual of Omaha Insurance Company to establish a personal insurance program for the membership. Coverage included both major medical and life insurance. This was the first time the association had offered this member service, and it quickly became popular with not only the rank-and-file but also new member recruits as well.

Rep. Harris re-introduced his fair trade bill in the second session of the 86th Congress — even though Dargavel told him NARD could provide only limited support. The bill attracted the same opposition as before, but again made it through committee. This time, however, the bill was referred to the Rules Committee and died. Dargavel tried to rally enough support to bring the bill to a vote, but failed to do so. It was still in committee when delegates gathered for the annual meeting.

The executive committee selected Denver, Colorado, for the sixty-second convention. Delegates gathered there in 1960 in the words of editor Sletterdahl in a rebellious mood. Most of the members who came to the national meeting were well informed on association activities and worked hard to support its programs. It had not been a good year in external relations. Beginning with the Kefauver investigation, and continuing with the battle on the Harris bill, NARD had not won a victory this year — a situation foreign to its experience.

President Rooke highlighted the problems with unfair competition and said, "deception through juggled prices is just as effective today as in bygone years. It seems that honest prices amount to robbery prices in the mind of the public. The predatory merchants never appear to think about integrity or the rules of fairplay." He mentioned specifically the grocery outlets, noting that between 1950 and 1958, they increased their volume in medications, health, and beauty aids by 1,000 percent. During the same time, "drug store sales of the same products went up 65 percent." He concluded by saying those who did not believe that "pharmacy is threatened by grocery outlets are living in a delusion."

Executive Committee Chairman Willard Simmons addressed the issue of monopoly. He noted that with all the business consolidations in the 1950s, fewer than 500 corporations now controlled commodity production and distribution. To make matters worse, neither political party responded to NARD's appeal that a pledge to protect small business and fair trade be included in the party platforms. Instead, he said, "both parties devoted only gestures to the march of monopoly in the distribution of commodities.

Simmons also talked about the difficulty NARD had in trying to develop an interprofessional relationship with the American Medical Association (AMA) and the American Pharmaceutical Association (APhA). Previously, the AMA never participated in the National Pharmacy Committee on Relations with the Health Professions, of which NARD was a charter member. But now, for unspecified reasons, the APhA also pulled out of the alliance. Simmons reported that the NARD would continue with the National Pharmacy Committee, but currently the interprofessional relations aspect of the committee was dead because of "an action of the A.Ph.A. The blame for the demise belongs alone to the A.Ph.A."

Secretary Dargavel sounded despondent as he talked to the House of Delegates. He recounted the glory days when NARD overcame all odds to pass the Robinson-Patman, Tydings-Miller, Humphrey-Durham, and McGuire Acts. But he said the Harris bill failed because the "predatory merchants were aggressive and through unscrupulous propaganda, mobilized extensive opposition to the bill." However, he said a more important reason the bill failed was that "the independent druggists of the country in total failed to provide more than meager support for the bill. Less than a dozen of the state pharmaceutical organizations were active in the front lines of the fight to save fair trade."

If the Harris bill had had the support of the previous bills, Dargavel was confident it would have passed. He asked rhetorically, "Why the letdown? How is it explained? I admit I am baffled in the search for an answer." He also mentioned that while the association had a record year in income, it had also been the most expensive in history and the organization was in need of money. He recommended that dues be increased from $12.50 to $17.50.

Delegates approved the dues increase, but designated $2.50 of the increase to go to the John A. Dargavel Foundation. They also elected Tom C. Sharp of Nashville, Tennessee as president; Simmons was again elected chairman of the executive committee.

A number of issues confronted the executive committee as members gathered in Chicago, Illinois, for its annual November meeting. Chief among them was a bill sponsored by Rhode Island Representative Aime Forand to add health care benefits to Social Security. Senator John F. Kennedy of Massachusetts had cosponsored the bill in the previous session of Congress. Since his election as president of the United States, the odds were good that he would again support the bill. NARD had repeatedly opposed all suggestions of "socialized medicine," and the executive committee served notice that it would oppose the new Forand bill, too.

Other legislative matters included a bill Sen. Kefauver planned to introduce to place price restrictions on the pharmaceutical manufacturers; a new proposal initiated by the Food and Drug Administration (FDA) to open all store prescription files to agents of the FDA; and possibly another attempt to repeal the Tydings-Miller Act. In view of these developments, the executive committee decided to delay a decision on sponsoring a new fair trade bill until they could get a better understanding about whether they could effect passage of it.

Prior to the 87th Congress convening in January 1961, an article about discount drug prices appeared in a pharmacy trade journal. The article was based on a survey that Dargavel conducted or a least had attempted to conduct. When the story was published, his efforts to collect the data collapsed. Dargavel acknowledged that he sent a questionnaire to thirty-seven pharmaceutical manufacturers requesting information on how each priced products. As Dargavel explained, "I kept quiet about the questionnaire in order to avoid publicity that might interfere with the responses…and with the hope that the industry would clean up the prevalent unfair discount policies."

Publicity may have foiled the executive secretary's ability to gather information, but it served as an alert to the Federal Trade Commission (FTC). In short order, the FTC filed suit against the thirty-seven pharmaceutical manufacturers, requesting that they make their pricing policies available. The larger companies receiving the order responded by announcing a "uniform, single-price system" in which all customers paid the same price "irrespective of functional status." However, the "fine print" of the policy also stated that "purchases on a direct-basis...in (sufficient) quantities" received a discount. This loophole for the larger chain stores and hospitals was evident to all, but it did not violate fair trade principles.

To counter the "single-price dodge," the executive committee reconsidered its strategy on legislation. Rather than waiting until they had time to "read Congress's mood," the group decided to sponsor legislation without delay. Rep. Harris and Senators Humphrey and Proxmire were willing to resume the battle on NARD's behalf. The new legislation was called the "Fair

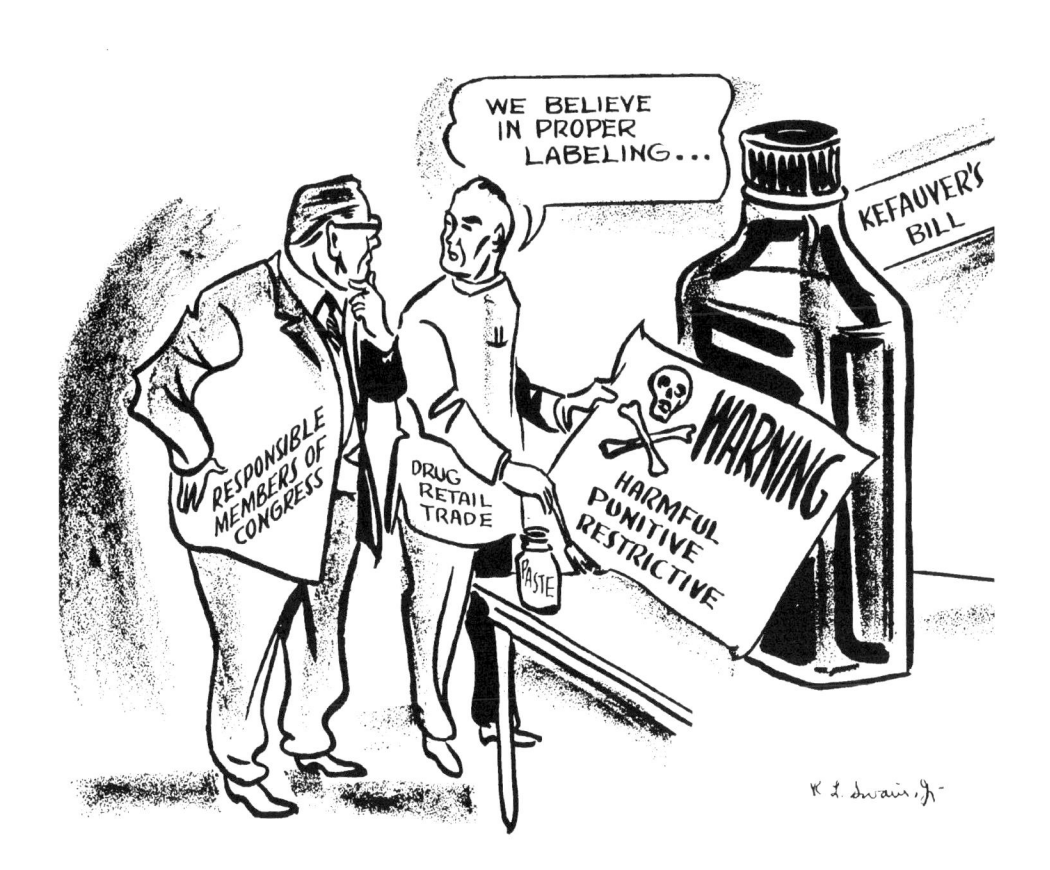

Competitive Practices Bill" and was introduced in both houses of Congress in the opening weeks of the session.

Product pricing proved to be an important issue in the 87th Congress. In addition to the Competitive Practices bill introduced by Rep. Harris, two members of the Indiana delegation, Rep. Ray J. Madden and Sen. Homer E. Capehart, introduced a similar proposal, which they called the Quality Stabilization Bill. While intended as a fair trade bill, this measure excluded language requiring manufacturers to set a minimum price for "brand-name" products, and there was no penalty provision for "resellers" who violated the law. The sponsors' intent was to avoid the antitrust challenges that the Harris-Humphrey bill was expected to draw. But to the NARD leadership, the Quality Stabilization bill was also too soft on enforcement. While not opposing the bill, Dargavel let it be known that NARD preferred legislation reflected in the Fair Competitive Practices Bill.

As before, both bills became bogged down in committee. Dargavel, Simmons, and Jehle worked in vain to get a "do pass" vote. Community pharmacists were apparently not feeling the pressure of economic hard times and not willing to risk their "momentary" prosperity to mount an aggressive political campaign. The NARD leadership's call to action before "the forces of monopoly" took control of the marketplace went largely unheeded. It was not so much that the leaders's message fell on "deaf ears," but more so that the membership did not see the problem with the same urgency.

Another reason the NARD leaders failed to get a vote on the Fair Competitive Practices was that they became distracted by a dispute with APhA. Under new leadership, APhA began an aggressive campaign to become the recognized leader of the profession. As part of that strategy, the association came to the defense of the Northern California Pharmaceutical Association (NCPA) in early 1961, when that organization was charged with violation of antitrust laws. APhA requested support from other pharmacy organizations, and Dargavel volunteered NARD's services.

However, representatives of the two groups strongly disagreed on how to prepare a defense in the case. APhA took the position that "pharmacy is excluded from antitrust legislative restrictions" and hired an attorney with limited antitrust experience to defend the California group. NARD strongly objected both to the interpretation of the law and to the lawyer retained to prepare the defense. When APhA refused to yield on either point, NARD withdrew from the case. In subsequent district court action, the California association was found guilty of violating the Sherman Antitrust Act and fined for its actions.

APhA announced its intent to appeal the decision and sent a letter soliciting financial support to the various organizations in the pharmacy profession. The letter was sharply critical of NARD for failing to actively support the Northern California association and noted that APhA was the only association "fighting for the cause of pharmacy." The solicitation letter said that if the lower court's opinion was allowed to stand, then "the future of pharmacy will be jeopardized." It also included an application for membership in APhA. Clearly, the association was seeking to take over the leadership role for pharmacy and increase its membership at the same time.

The California case and the Fair Competitive Practice Bill were still unresolved when delegates gathered in Miami Beach, Florida, for the sixty-third convention in 1961. President Sharp told the delegates that "it is evident that various difficulties which the drug store owners must contend with cannot be eradicated. So we must insist that the rules be enforced and, where necessary, amended." He also counseled, "it is unwise to become frightened and intimidated by the problems on a rampage in the retail drug field. The gloom and doom 'hucksters' care nothing about the solutions of problems in pharmacy."

Simmons addressed NARD's inability to pass major pieces of legislation in the last two sessions of Congress. He said, "we must fight with more anger than we have displayed in the recent past as we tried to bring about the enactment of legislation necessary to the collective stability and prosperity of the small retail firms of the country."

Secretary Dargavel explained his role in the pharmaceutical survey and the dispute with APhA. With respect to the survey, he said, "legitimate druggists (expect) nothing more than they are entitled to receive from pharmaceutical manufacturers...the same prices granted to the hospitals, clinics, physicians, and every other customer." As far as APhA was concerned, Dargavel asked the delegates rhetorically, "why throw money away on the case (Northern California) since the defense is based on false claims? Furthermore, why should money be provided by N.A.R.D. to help finance the propaganda of the A.Ph.A.?"

The House of Delegates chose Bert C. Corgan of Denver to be president. Executive Committee members chose Frank Lobraico of Indianapolis, Indiana, to be their chairman. Delegates also agreed with the executive committee's recommendation that "enactment of the Fair Competitive Practices Act" should be the primary legislative objective for the coming year.

But plans for NARD's sixty-third year were abruptly interrupted by the sudden death of Executive Secretary Dargavel. Arriving in Chicago from the Miami Beach convention, he suffered "a coronary occlusion" at 10:00 p.m. on October 9. He was sixty-seven years old. The shock reverberated throughout the pharmacy world and left NARD members in a collective state of shock. As the driving force for the organization over the past twenty-eight years,

Dargavel's name had become synonymous with NARD. Almost half his life and nearly half the association's history had been intricately intertwined. Tributes to Dargavel poured into NARD headquarters from throughout the nation.

As tragic as the circumstances were, members of the executive committee realized that they must quickly choose a new executive secretary. After first considering the possibility of promoting one of the current staff, the committee decided instead to turn to a former chairman of the group, Willard Simmons. After considering the offer for a couple of days, he accepted, and the association began a new era under its fifth executive secretary and general manager.

Simmons, born in Myrtis, Louisiana, received his training in pharmacy at the Little Rock College of Pharmacy in 1924 and was licensed to practice in both Arkansas and Texas in 1925. He worked in his father's pharmacy in Bloomburg, Texas, for several years, then the two formed a partnership and bought a store in Texarkana. He became active in NARD soon after World War II and beginning in 1950, served as an officer, member, and chairman of the executive committee. He had just opened his second pharmacy in Texarkana when the executive committee called. Simmons was also active in

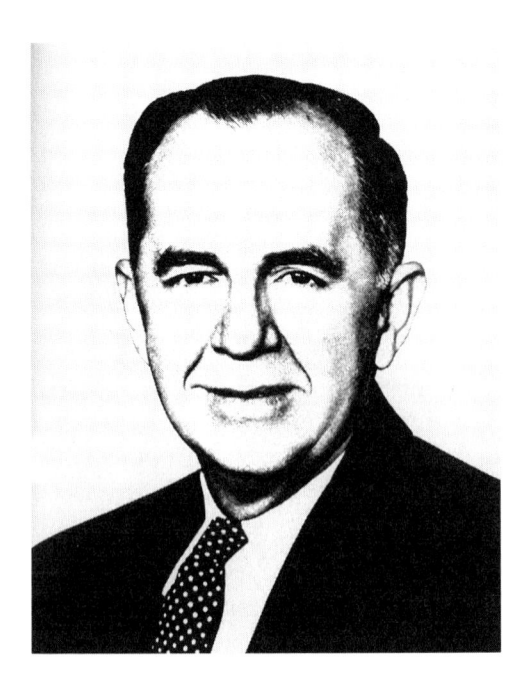

Willard B. Simmons, NARD Executive Secretary, 1961 – 1976

Texas politics, having worked as an "advance man" for Lyndon B. Johnson's first run for political office.

As was the case twenty-eight years earlier, albeit under different circumstances, productive activity was again the prescription for overcoming tragedy in the association. The legislative agenda was crowded, and new leadership offered an opportunity to remind the membership about the association's continuing mission. Respected as a "thinker in depth," being a student of history, and having been intricately involved in association policy for a decade, Simmons stressed continuity rather than change as he assumed his leadership responsibilities.

With the U.S. Congress scheduled to reconvene in just over two months, NARD leaders focused their attention on finding the best strategy to protect fair trade. In meeting with legislative leaders, it became apparent that if the fair trade interests continued to divide their support between two bills, the Harris Fair Trade Bill and the Quality Stabilization Bill, they would lose both.

In view of that prospect, Simmons, in his first major executive decision, recommended that NARD switch its support to the Quality Stabilization Bill and rally the votes needed to get it passed. The Fair Trade Bill was scrapped. Sen. Humphrey, who had become majority whip of the Senate, and Rep. Harris, who had become chairman of the Interstate Commerce Committee, agreed to introduce the revised Quality Stabilization Bill.

As a new leader, Simmons also initiated contact with APhA and AMA to discuss common interests. Both organizations indicated a willingness to reopen a dialogue and meetings were held in November 1961 and June 1962. At the latter meeting, representatives from the AMA's Judicial Council submitted a "joint code of cooperation." While not entirely to NARD's liking, the document at least provided the basis for more substantive discussion.

But when talk turned to specific language in the code, the AMA representatives decided they did not have time to prepare a new report for their House of Delegates before their next annual meeting. Simmons said he did not doubt "their sincere desire...for eliminating the causes of antagonistic attitudes...between pharmacists and physicians," but still there was no joint agreement and he admitted the groups would have to meet again.

While the three groups were together, NARD and APhA representatives were reminded that their associations had held joint meetings for years before being discontinued soon after World War II. From those discussions, the two groups agreed to "explore" the possibilities of resuming the "joint conference."

Simmons also had an early opportunity to focus on NARD's relationship with the state associations. In early December, the Veterans Administration (VA) announced that it was canceling the so-called "hometown pharmacy program," which administered prescriptions through contracts with the state associations. This arrangement had been developed soon after World War II and had forty-seven of the state pharmacy associations participating. But according to officials at the Justice Department, these contracts were in violation of federal antitrust laws and had to be discontinued. The VA said the program would end September 30, 1962.

The new executive secretary called Jehle in the Washington office and, together with Jehle's new associate, Joseph Cohen, the three planned a response to the Justice Department ruling. All agreed that personal contact with the antitrust division at Justice would be an important first step. However, officials there refused to discuss the matter. Simmons then called upon APhA and the state pharmaceutical association secretaries for support, and a delegation from the three entities scheduled a June meeting in Washington with VA officials. Simmons told the VA he was confident the contract could be revised, but the states needed more time to rework the language. However, the VA representatives refused to extend the deadline.

Failing to make progress through negotiation, Jehle called Rep. Patman and informed him of the situation. Patman arranged another conference with the VA for August. At this meeting, VA officials still refused to make any commitments on a revised contract, but did agree to extend the program until December 31. While the "hometown pharmacy program" had not been saved, Simmons at least convinced state leaders that their partnership with NARD was still strong and in good hands.

Simmons also got an early opportunity to work directly with store owners. The issue involved a new bill on Medicare. This concept had been around since the 1920s, became the topic of debate in the New Deal days of the 1930s, and was even introduced as a bill in the Truman administration. Since 1950, some type of compulsory health insurance program for the elderly had been introduced in each session of Congress. NARD had routinely joined with AMA and other health care providers to oppose what they considered a form of "socialized medicine."

By the 1960s, proponents of Medicare had become quite sophisticated in their efforts to gain public support. The 87th Congress saw Medicare coupled with Social Security. This made it a particularly difficult bill to argue against on its merits. However, as Jehle, Cohen, and the executive committee reviewed its provisions, they were convinced the cost estimates "left more to the imagination than reliable actuarial estimates" and that it was fundamentally unsound. The executive committee voted to oppose the bill.

To explain NARD's position, Secretary Simmons mailed out over 40,000 posters, highlighting the bill's provisions and explaining why it was not a good proposal for the members. He also provided pharmacists with a prepared text for speeches and a compilation of data to illustrate the bill's weakness. The issue gave Simmons and NARD an excellent opportunity to make contact with community pharmacists and work on building a network of common interests. Moreover, since AMA was so adamantly opposed to the legislation, NARD had the luxury of watching the physicians block the bill while not expending the association's own political capital in the fight.

An issue involving public relations became another opportunity for Simmons to stamp his brand of leadership on the association. The case involved the FDA, which had long sought to examine prescription records of community pharmacists unannounced and indiscriminately. Since 1950, the agency had tried repeatedly to achieve its objective. Each time, Dargavel and his colleagues had been able to amend the bill to forbid indiscriminate searches and allow agents to inspect prescription lists only upon presenting evidence of wrong doing by the pharmacists.

In August 1962, drug agents thought they had a case of wrongdoing. On a routine inspection of a New York pharmacy, officials found evidence that a controlled drug, thalidomide, had been repackaged from its factory-labeled container and made available in smaller dosages "on drug store shelves."

The *New York Times* covered the story and quoted an FDA agent as saying "historically retail druggists have been the main source of illegal diversion of prescription medications." Simmons immediately challenged the story's veracity and charged that the profession was being tainted by generalizations. However, the agent's statement was entered into testimony before Rep. Harris's House Interstate and Foreign Commerce Committee. Harris's committee was holding hearings on the FDA's perennial bill to broaden its investigatory powers.

Simmons and the executive committee countered the testimony by citing results from the FDA's own files. The agency had taken surveys between 1949 and April 1962. For that period of almost thirteen years, the FDA's records revealed community pharmacists had violated drug enforcement policies just over 1,000 times, an average of 85 violations per year. When that figure was compared to the 55,000 independent pharmacies, and over 40,000 community pharmacists employed in those stores, Simmons said the FDA data was "statistically of no consequence."

As a follow-up, the executive secretary released statements made by FDA Commissioner George Larrick praising community pharmacists for "assisting the F.D.A. in the enforcement of the fedcral drug laws." NARD was again able to block the FDA's efforts to get statutory authority for unrestrained prescription list searches.

By the time the sixty-fourth convention met in New York City, New York, in 1962, the NARD leadership had been able to recover, somewhat, from

Dargavel's death. Still, his spirit filled the House of Delegates as various speakers referred to his actions or events reminded everyone of his presence. President Corgan recalled Dargavel's "fighting spirit" and how he "gave his all" for pharmacy. He called upon the younger members to remember the association's heritage and how difficult it had been to build a legacy. But he noted that the cornerstone of NARD's legacy was built on "the human qualities (of caring) which count large in the operation of a community drug store."

Chairman Lobraico echoed President Corgan's comments about Dargavel. But he also praised Willard Simmons's work and noted the variety of activities the new executive secretary had to deal with in such a short period of time. Lobraico particularly singled out Simmons's work with the thalidomide case. He said situations like this developed primarily because pharmaceutical manufacturers were "still overloading physicians with sample medications when there is no reason to supply them at all." The chairman also warned about the new practice of "dispensing medications by nurses in hospitals and physicians' offices through vending machines."

Executive Secretary Simmons reviewed his first ten months of work and said he hoped to restore pharmacy's reputation for integrity and regain respect from the public. Delegates gave the new executive secretary an enthusiastic reception. Before adjourning, they elected Frank Lobraico as president. The executive committee chose T. Donald Perkins of San Diego, California, to chair their group.

The second year in Executive Secretary Simmons's tenure proved less eventful than the first and gave him an opportunity to work more on internal affairs. One item of interest and identifiable need was more office space for the headquarters staff. The executive committee reviewed the matter at the November 1962 meeting and authorized Simmons to seek new property. The executive secretary found a new site at One East Wacker Drive, just a short distance from the existing offices. The building was still under construction and would not be ready for occupancy for a year.

Simmons also created a new "Department of Merchandising" and employed Donald B. Reynolds, an authority on advertising and buyer habits, to run the department. The new unit was designed to help community pharmacists modernize their stores and provide expert information on market trends and consumer interests.

Continuing with his plan to improve interprofessional relations, the executive secretary drew up an eleven-point "Code of Cooperation" with the AMA. The code was a wide-ranging statement on matters of common interests, but included a section opposing physician-owned pharmacies. Representatives from the physicians' group stopped short of endorsing the code, but did promise to take it under consideration. In the aftermath of discussing the code, the AMA agreed to help form a "Commission on Medicine and Pharmacy" and to cosponsor a "Community Health Week." The latter became an annual event. However, it did not take Simmons long to recognize that AMA's response was only "cosmetic" and ignored the fundamental issue of physician dispensing and competition with pharmacists.

When it became apparent that AMA was not willing to take a stand against physicians owning pharmacies, Simmons broke off discussions. The aggressive efforts of APhA to become the "voice of pharmacy" were also offensive to NARD leaders. The majority of APhA members were not retail pharmacists and, in fact, many spoke contemptuously of "commercial pharmacy." Little progress was made in forming a true alliance.

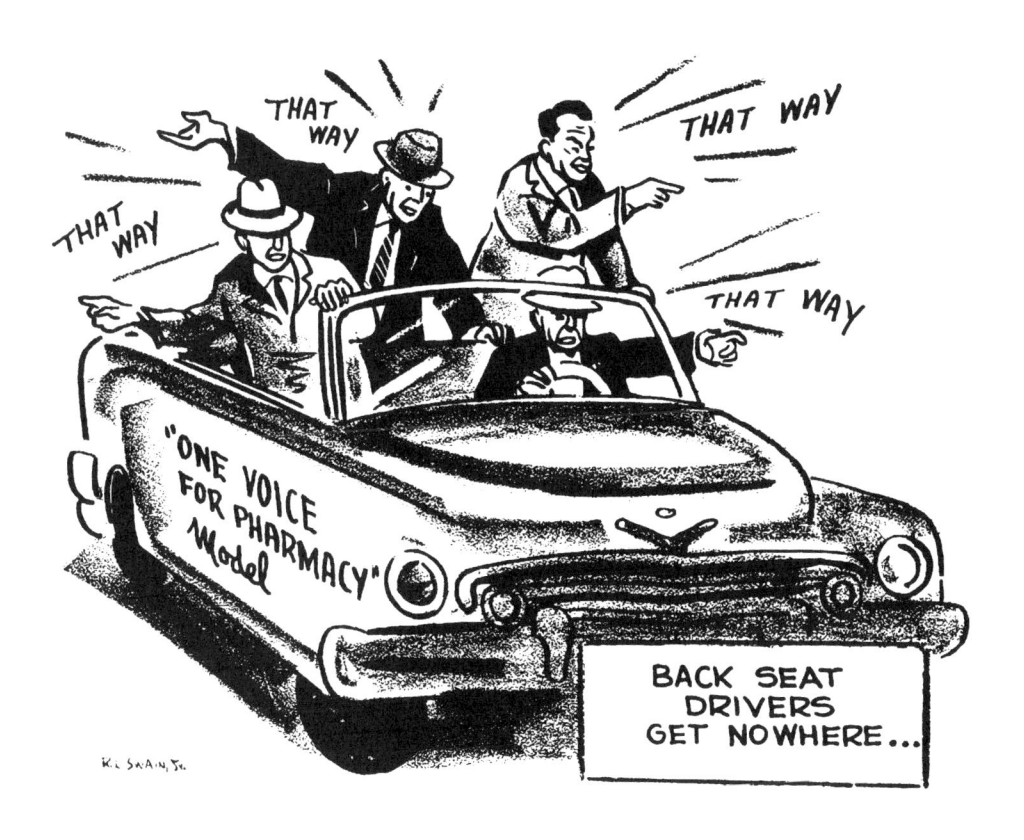

NARD Journal view of "pharmacy unity" in 1962

Still in the vein of improving professional relations, Simmons received executive committee approval to explore a joint marketing project with the Proprietary Association (PA). The eight-month-long project was centered in thirty-three "medium-sized retail drug stores" chosen by A.C. Nielsen in the company's nine survey districts. Simmons said that the project would test several marketing ideas and "the ideas that achieve desired results will be adopted for recommendation to independent pharmacists everywhere."

The sixty-fifth convention returned to Chicago in 1963. President Lobraico devoted most of his time before the House of Delegates to decrying NARD's treatment from AMA and APhA. He criticized the AMA for refusing to revise its code of ethics to prohibit physician-owned pharmacies. He was even more critical of APhA's insistence on being the voice of pharmacy. He believed that their membership was too diverse to ever get a consensus on any controversial topic. In truth, he said, "the A.Ph.A. speaks for nobody in pharmacy."

Executive Committee Chairman T. Donald Perkins said the committee believed the best way to solve the physician-owned pharmacy issue was to take it to the state level. Consequently, the committee hired an attorney to prepare a "model state law" and made the text available to the states upon request.

Simmons reported on the status of the fair trade laws and noted that "it is difficult to keep fighting for legislation after repeated rebuffs from Congress." NARD had still not been able to bring the Quality Stabilization Bill to a vote. However, the measure was still alive in the 87th Congress, and Simmons was confident that it would eventually pass. "I believe," he told the delegates, that "today the majority of congressmen recognize the urgency of legislation to make it possible for independent enterprise to survive."

To assist in the fair trade fight, Secretary Simmons also recommended that the association enlist the support of women. Noting that this group had usually been overlooked, he said that "wives, mothers, daughters, relatives, and employees will allow the association to double its support." He admitted that NARD and most pharmacy groups had a group identified as an "auxiliary," but he said "that designation sounds like a term applied to a machine and the connotation is mechanical." He preferred to call them "Women of Pharmacy" and urged his colleagues to enlist their support. In 1962, eight of the state association secretaries and two of the metropolitan secretaries were women.

Simmons's call for support from women was welcome news to WONARD. Since its founding in 1905, the organization had been primarily a spouses' group and had worked to fund scholarships for pharmacy students and to provide cultural enrichment at NARD's annual convention. But over the years, as an increasing number of women chose pharmacy as a profession, WONARD enlarged its charter and its membership became more than a "wives club." As partners of pharmacy, the organization became an important source of grassroots support for NARD's legislative program. WONARD had also made regular contributions to the John A. Dargavel Foundation.

Delegates at the sixty-fifth convention elected T. Donald Perkins to be president and Leonard J. Dueker of St. Louis, Missouri, was chosen chairman of the executive committee. Barely a month after the convention adjourned, President John F. Kennedy was assassinated in Dallas, Texas. The national mourning that followed that event and the elevation of Lyndon B. Johnson to the presidency reshaped the political agenda.

Most of NARD's political issues knew no changes in 1964, but there proved to be other challenges to the organization and its membership. The most significant new issue to arise was a move by APhA to persuade FDA to adopt a new drug classification system. With growing societal abuse of amphetamines and barbiturates, APhA insisted there should be four classes of controlled drugs. Leaders of that group planned to get the reclassification by amending the Food, Drug and Cosmetic Act and wanted NARD's support. Simmons and his colleagues, while not opposed to reclassification, were more concerned about legal liability, recordkeeping, and the costs of maintaining inventory. They were reluctant to endorse such a proposal until they could see provisions addressing their concerns.

For the sixty-sixth convention, the executive committee voted to return to San Francisco, California, in 1964. President Perkins chose to make "professionalism and store improvement" the theme of his address to the House of Delegates. He pointed out that the "marvelous advancement in medication in the last 25 years caused changes in the practice of pharmacy that could be described as 'revolutionary'." To cope with those changes, Perkins said, "the proprietor of a drug store must never cease to be alert to fluctuations " and understand "the necessity of adventure in business."

Simmons told the delegates about the disappointment of the past summer when, with six members absent, the Senate Commerce Committee voted six to five to table the Quality Stabilization Bill. Fair trade was again denied a vote by the full Congress. Simmons said that he hoped the fall elections would bring the changes necessary to get the bill passed. He also encouraged the delegates to support fellow pharmacist Hubert Humphrey, the vice presidential nominee for the Democratic Party in the upcoming elections.

The executive secretary devoted a portion of his speech to information on "improving store conditions." He urged his listeners to watch for two new features soon to appear in the *NARD Journal*. One section would provide information on "Advertising Ideas"; the other would focus on "Remodeling Rewards" for the local store owner. Articles on these topics would be run on a monthly basis. Before leaving San Francisco, delegates elected Leonard Dueker to be president. Members of the executive committee chose Charles B. Dunnington of Brockton, Massachusetts, as their chairman.

The November presidential election went as most in NARD hoped as Lyndon Johnson and his running mate, Hubert Humphrey, were swept into office by one of the widest voting margins in history. At its fall meeting less than a week later, the NARD executive committee reviewed a list of agenda items that were becoming all too familiar. These included better and closer relations with APhA, pharmacy ownership, drug reclassification, outpatient prescription services by hospitals, and procedures and suggestions for the Congress on Medicine and Pharmacy.

The executive committee also "after detailed discussion" decided to delay a decision on what to do about fair trade legislation until its members could "confer with friends...in Congress" for guidance. As a final decision, NARD decided to hold the 1965 convention in Washington, D.C.

In the new year, the association made little progress on its agenda. APhA continued to seek ways to be the "voice of pharmacy." Its latest strategy was called "affiliation," whereby it would become "a protective umbrella" for all the pharmacy-related organizations. The NARD leadership, while continuing a long-held policy of "working with everyone who promoted the cause of retail pharmacy," refused to work with "anyone who sought to subvert its autonomy." A similar impasse developed on the other issues.

When the new Congress opened in January 1965, it soon became apparent that the Johnson administration was focused on passing a Medicare bill. The outline of the new bill was not unlike the trial balloons of past sessions. However, there was a resolve to get it passed, and NARD had little input into the process. Washington Representative Joseph Cohen (Phil Jehle having left for other employment) worked diligently to get pharmacy costs included in the bill, but without success. The only drugs covered in the bill were those "commonly provided by a physician in his office, and which cannot be self-administered."

(Hindsight is 20-20 when viewing actions in their historic context, but NARD's failure [and certainly that of other pharmacy organizations as well] to have written into the bill prescription drugs as a mandatory provision rather than as an option proved to be an ongoing nettlesome issue for decades to come. As one astute political observer noted years hence, "it is always tougher to get [your issue] in later rather than at the beginning.")

In anticipation of a growing federal involvement in the world of health care, the executive committee made a strategic decision to significantly increase its Washington office. To assist Cohen, the committee hired Earl Kintner, a specialist in antitrust law, as well as J. Baxter Funderburk and Wil-

CHAPTER EIGHT — THE SEVENTH DECADE: 1959 – 1968 169

liam E. Woods — "two experts in government relations and legislative liaison."

When the sixty-seventh convention opened in Washington, D.C., Simmons introduced the new legal team to the delegates. He explained "the greatly enlarged staff" by saying "government, through legislation and regulation at federal, state, and even city levels, has always significantly influenced the ...operation of our drugstores." The new staff was recognition that a new era was emerging in the pharmacy world, and "two-way communication" between government and the association must be "firmly established."

The highlight of the convention was Vice President of the United States Hubert H. Humphrey's address to the House of Delegates. Having been a

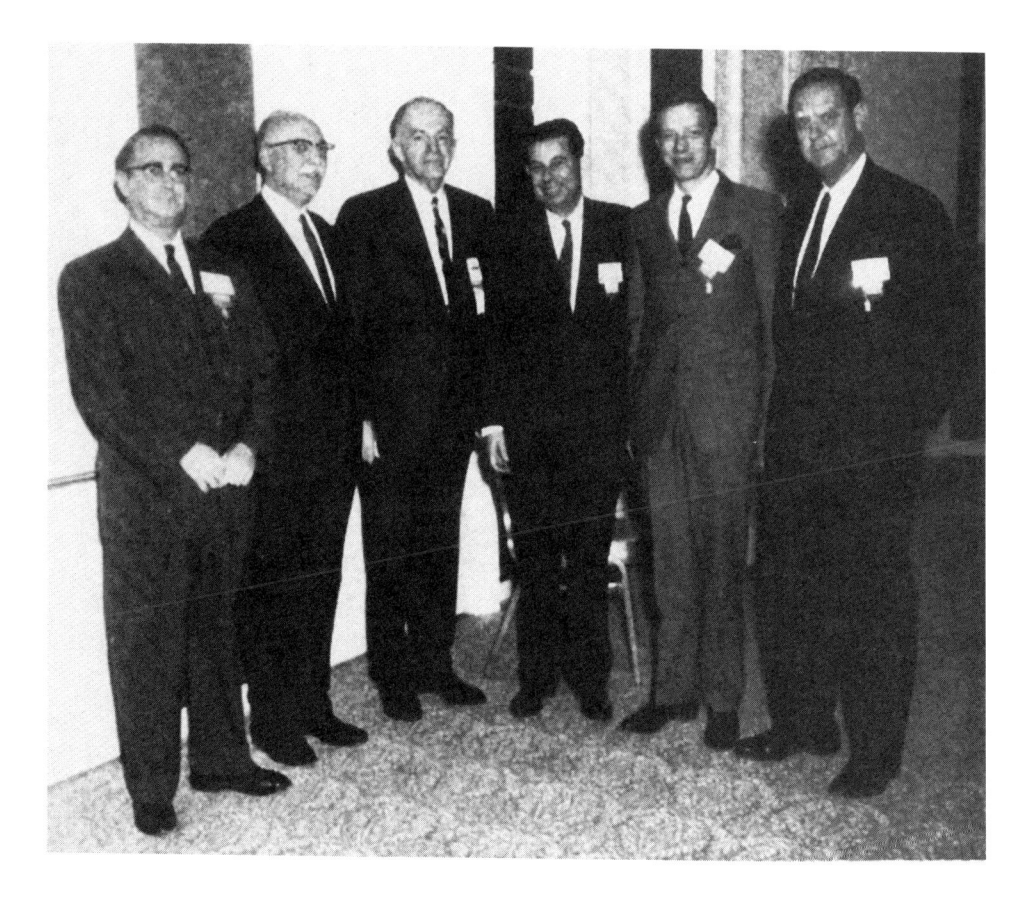

NARD expanded its Washington presence in the 1960s to include (left to right) J. Baxter Funderburk; Joseph Cohen; Simmons who was located in Chicago; Earl Kintner and his associate, Jack Lahr, and William E. Woods.

regular on the convention program for several years, it was a special moment for the community pharmacists to see one of their own in such an exalted position. In other convention action, Executive Secretary Simmons announced the retirement of *Journal* editor Peter Sletterdahl after eighteen years of service. He had suffered a heart attack shortly after the 1964 convention and had never fully recovered. The new editor, Louis E. Kazin, was a native of Bridgeport, Connecticut, and a graduate of the University of Connecticut College of Pharmacy. Delegates elected J.C. Cobb of Tishomingo,

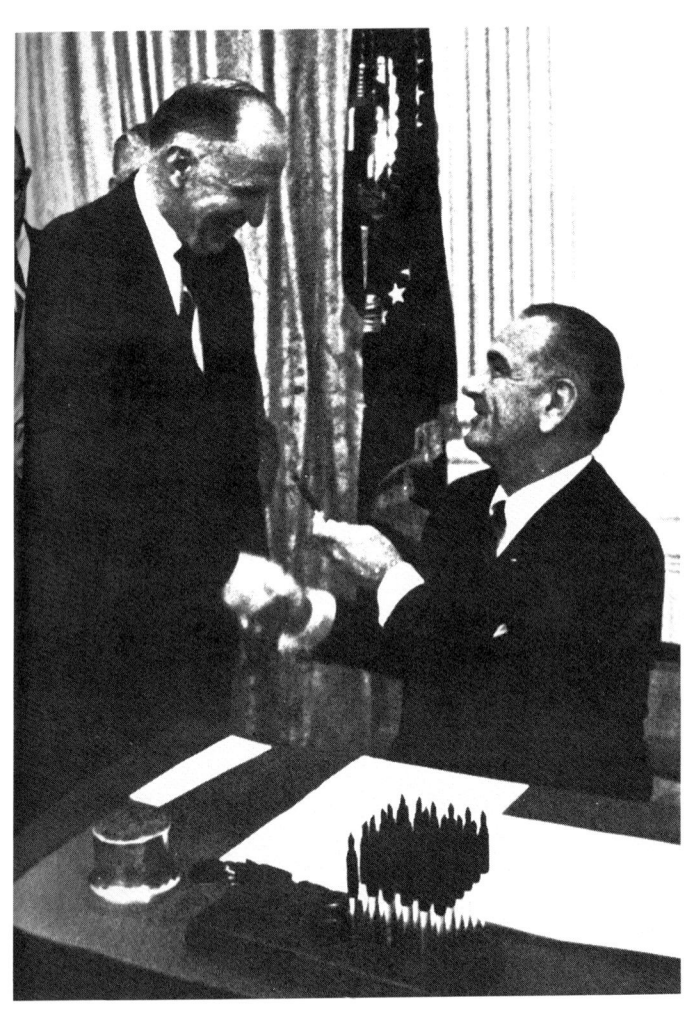

NARD's Willard Simmons attended a bill signing ceremony in the White House with President Lyndon B. Johnson in 1965.

Oklahoma as president; Charles Dunnington was reelected as chairman of the executive committee.

For NARD the most pressing need in the new year was to get clarification on the drug dispensing provisions in the Medicare bill. The law was scheduled to go into effect January 1, 1966. Simmons and the executive committee asked for a meeting with officials from the Department of Health, Education, and Welfare (HEW), as well as Social Security to discuss the matter. In this meeting, Undersecretary of HEW Wilbur J. Cohen explained that no direct payments would be paid to pharmacists. However, pharmacists would be reimbursed based on "the actual cost of the drug, plus administrative expenses in handling the drug." Obviously, the greatest challenge for NARD would be to help its members in defining administrative expenses.

Two other provisions in the Medicare Act, "Extended Care"(Nursing Homes) and the "Supplementary Medical Insurance Program" to cover equipment rentals and home health needs, held more promise. In both cases, payments would be made directly to pharmacists. However, the "supplemental insurance" was not to go into effect until July 1, 1966, and the nursing home phase would not begin until January 1, 1967.

In another year-long activity, NARD contracted with the Ohio State University School of Pharmacy to do a national survey on pharmacists' needs and views of the profession. Among other things, the survey showed that between 1954 and 1964, the percentage of manufacturers' sales of ethical drugs to hospitals and physicians went from 9 percent to 17 percent. The percentage going directly to community pharmacists increased from 29 percent to 31 percent and that percentage sold through wholesalers dropped from 58 percent to 48 percent. In share of the market for toiletries, community pharmacists dropped from 37 percent to 26 percent. Overall, "drugstore sales as a percentage of total sales...declined in 18 of the 27 categories surveyed." Estimates were that independent pharmacists would continue to lose in the overall share of the market.

Another part of the survey dealt with individual opinion. When asked what support pharmacists wanted from NARD, 64 percent said a national public relations campaign to promote a positive image of the independent pharmacist. When asked what the most important national level activity NARD had been involved in, 46 percent indicated the association's efforts to secure "fair trade legislation." Clearly, NARD had work to do to strengthen its membership and make them more competitive in the marketplace.

Simmons thought the new Medicare program might be able to do that. As he and the legal staff analyzed the massive number of regulations implementing the legislation, he noticed that Title 19 applied to state welfare drug programs. Typically, medical care among the various welfare recipients was administered thorough charity hospitals. However, the Medicare program proposed to "pay what the private patient pays," giving welfare recipients an opportunity to select their own physicians and pharmacies. While the guidelines would have to drafted state by state, Simmons believed that would be possible. With approximately 35 million people in the category to receive welfare benefits, he said it would be worth the effort. He noted that as the programs were implemented in the states, "it will not be uncommon to find many independent retail pharmacists receive $10,000 to $20,000 annually in welfare prescriptions.

The role of government and the expanding health care field dominated NARD's agenda throughout 1966. When delegates assembled in St. Louis, Missouri, for their sixty-eighth convention, there were still many questions about the long-term impact of the Medicare program. President Cobb told the delegates that "the growing health consciousness of our people, combined with the government health and welfare programs, have generated a force affecting the lives and habits of all our citizens." Moreover, he said, "the demand for health services and products...outstrips anything we have known before in the United States."

Chairman Dunnington reported that the Medicare program had "occupied a great deal of time and attention on the part of all officers and staff members." Among the issues that the executive committee studied included the "prepaid prescription insurance programs" circulated by various companies and prepared guidelines for the "nursing home phase of the Medicare program." He said that he believed "the nation is beginning to recognize the role of pharmacy in the maintenance of health." However, it was necessary for NARD to "maintain a special relationship with government administrative agencies to assure the professional correctness of decisions that affect pharmacy."

Dunnington was elected president and George Wilharm of Minneapolis, Minnesota, was chosen chairman of the executive committee. Responding to the Ohio State survey, the executive committee voted to implement a national public relations campaign in 1967. The plan was to emphasize the community pharmacists' contribution to public health and do so through "all types of media." A professionally produced film, "Bartlett and Son," featuring an independent pharmacist and the role of a neighborhood pharmacy in the community, became a key component in the campaign.

As part of the public relations campaign, Simmons worked out a cooperative "drug education program" with the Chicago public school system. This was also in response to the Drug Abuse Control Act passed in the 89th Congress, which encouraged pharmacists to assist in educating the public about the problems of drug abuse. To implement the school program,

Simmons arranged a meeting with more than sixty editors of various school newspapers. He provided them with literature depicting "the growing dangers of drug misuse and abuse" and received a commitment from them to help educate their classmates.

In addition to the media campaign, Simmons and representatives from the executive committee held a series of regional meetings in Memphis, Tennessee; Los Angeles, California; and Portland, Oregon. These meetings not only gave the NARD leadership an opportunity to get a better understanding of local needs, but also gave many pharmacists their first contact with NARD.

The sixty-ninth convention was held in Houston, Texas. In his address to the delegates, President Dunnington said pharmacy was in the "midst of a heightened evolutionary period...(and) it is pharmacy's responsibility to continually be on guard against attempts to destroy or impair existing or traditional services while moving to adjust to new demands of a health conscious citizenry."

Chairman Wilharm reviewed more than a dozen bills that had been introduced in the 90th Congress. The Washington office had indeed been busy, and in view of that activity, the publicity campaign, and the extra demands of Medicare, the association required a dues increase. He proposed that dues be raised from $17.50 to $25.00. Wilharm also noted that joint relations with AMA and APhA had disintegrated and in view of that circumstance, NARD would have an even bigger role to play in educating the public about pharmacy.

Simmons told the delegates that as government moved into a new partnership with health and welfare services, "there must be recognition on the part of all those who go to make up this type of union that much can be learned from each other." The executive secretary was also concerned that too much change was coming too quickly without proper regard to tradition and established procedures. He was particularly bothered by the "mandatory requirements for generic drugs." He said that many of these drugs "were of unknown therapeutic equivalence on a cost basis."

Related to the generics issue, the NARD leadership was also concerned about attempts to establish a standard formula for prescription pricing. Simmons said the method "should be the sole responsibility of the individual pharmacist, and furthermore, it should be based on a series of facts which take into consideration elementary cost accounting factors."

Delegates at the sixty-ninth convention elected George W. Wilharm president and the executive committee selected Michael M. Perhach of Binghamton, New York, as chairman. The executive committee chose Boston, Massachusetts, as the site for the seventieth convention in 1968.

As the NARD leadership prepared to close out the last year of the association's seventh decade, it was all but overwhelmed with the variety of programs and needs. After spending the first half of the decade with little variation, the last five years were all but traumatic. The expanding role of the federal government through President Johnson's "Great Society" and the rapid military build-up in Vietnam affected pharmacy in a dramatic way.

The Medicare program increased the number of customers in the store. It also opened a range of new opportunities in home health care, equipment rental, nursing home care, and professional consultant. It also increased paperwork and recordkeeping. The rapid changes and the tremendous increase in the amount of money being spent on health care contributed to a widening chasm in the health care arena.

President Wilharm addressed these divisions in his message to the House of Delegates at seventieth convention. He said, "we cannot close our eyes to the damage being done by the enemies of retail pharmacy. I think that we have already begun to perceive the results of this divisiveness.... These people have indeed created a climate of fear and unreliability through their appeals for professional glory at the expense of a sound economic and profit-making drugstore operation. The president continued, "there is a sincere desire and determination among our people to continue the good record which the community pharmacy has earned in its service to the public."

Chairman Perhach continued the theme outlined by President Wilharm. Noting that NARD objectives were being achieved, he said, we "are willing and ready to cooperate with any organization of benefit to retail pharmacy — but your organization is not going to sacrifice your interest. We will not surrender your best interest for the sake of trying to establish some sort of nebulous relationship called 'One Voice for Pharmacy'."

Even the normally controlled and analytical Executive Secretary Simmons took an aggressive tone in his speech to the House of Delegates. Commenting on how long it had taken to build the association into a society recognized for its "excellence of performance," Simmons said the NARD leadership was "determined that neither self-serving elements within pharmacy, or power-hungry officials outside our profession shall tear down this great structure of pharmacy." He promised the delegates that "the people of these United States shall all have the best pharmaceutical service that they can render, the sick shall have the true medicine they need, at stores of their own choice, in places convenient to them, at prices equitable for substance and service rendered."

This commitment to customer service would be carried into the next decade as NARD faced even greater challenges than it faced here on the beach head of change in the health care delivery system.

Chapter Nine

THE EIGHTH DECADE: 1969 – 1978

NARD Meets the Storm's Center in Washington

*T*he turbulent and troubled 1960s yielded to a decade of crisis in the 1970s. The period had hardly begun before rumors circulated that a break-in at the Democratic Party's campaign headquarters in Washington, D. C. was more than a "two-bit burglary" gone bad. As innuendo gave way to evidence, the "Watergate incident" provoked a crisis in the executive branch of government and forced the first resignation of an American president — Richard M. Nixon.

Another crisis began to take shape even as the U.S. Congress investigated Nixon's role in the Watergate issue. This one involved an oil embargo imposed by the Organization of Petroleum Exporting Countries (OPEC). Shortages in gas and oil products quickly evolved from an inconvenience to a full-blown energy crisis midway through the decade. Double-digit inflation, interest rates, and unemployment, driven by high energy costs, dropped the nation into a serious recession.

For a brief eighteen months Americans were able to put off their concerns about shortages and uncertainties to commemorate 200 years of nationhood. This Bicentennial Celebration was a needed tonic to a people overwhelmed by social and economic upheaval. But, for many in the United States, reflecting upon the nation's history only served as a reminder of how far their generation had drifted from the founding fathers' objectives.

For many of the 30,000 community pharmacists organized as the National Association of Retail Druggists, the 1970s marked the beginning of a prolonged crisis surrounding the reimbursement policies nurtured by the Medicare/Medicaid program. MAC, or Maximum Allowable Costs, and its derivatives under federally funded drug benefit plans were under constant assault during the 1970s and subsequent decades. In addition to this stranglehold on the level of reimbursements, pharmacy billings were being held hostage by long delays in federal payments through the program.

At the beginning of the decade, Medicaid patients represented about 15 percent of a typical pharmacy's business. But almost a third of the pharmacies participating in the program reported delays of more than sixty days in getting paid for Medicaid prescriptions. Some were forced to obtain business loans to compensate for cash flow problems, and all reported spending an inordinate amount of time filling out claims forms associated with the program.

It was in this context that the NARD leadership chose to elevate member concerns in a unique face-to-face dialogue with federal officials of all stripes in its first-ever Conference on National Legislation and Public Affairs held in Washington, D.C., soon to be the association's permanent home. Invitations were sent out in February 1969 for the conference scheduled in April. Officers and administrators in the state associations, pharmacy manufacturers, trade representatives, various political leaders, and executive branch officials working with the new Medicare/Medicaid program were invited to attend.

The scope of new legislation affecting the distribution and control of narcotics and other controlled drugs, discussions of Sen. Phil Hart's bill to

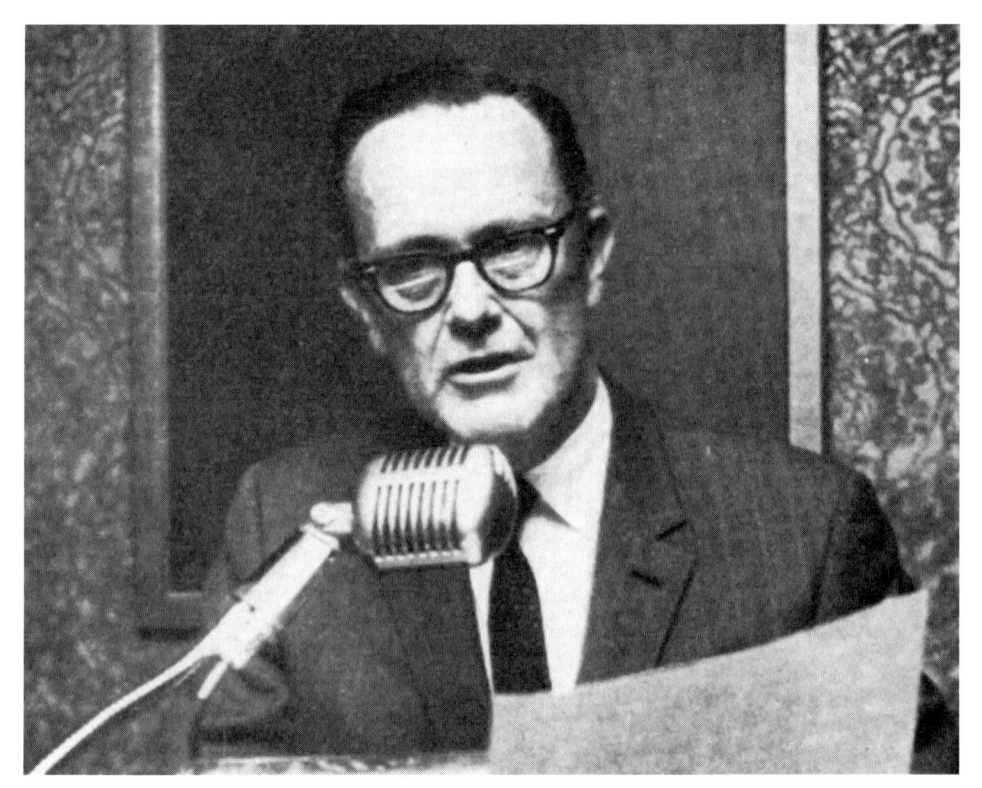

Sen. Philip A. Hart, lead-off speaker at the first NARD Legislative Conference

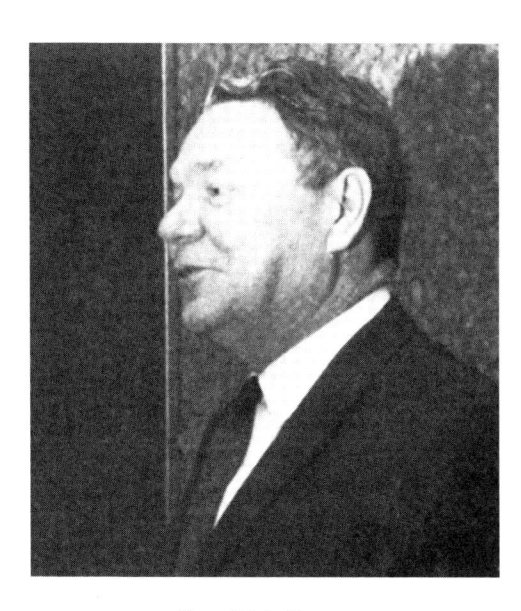

Rep. Hale Boggs

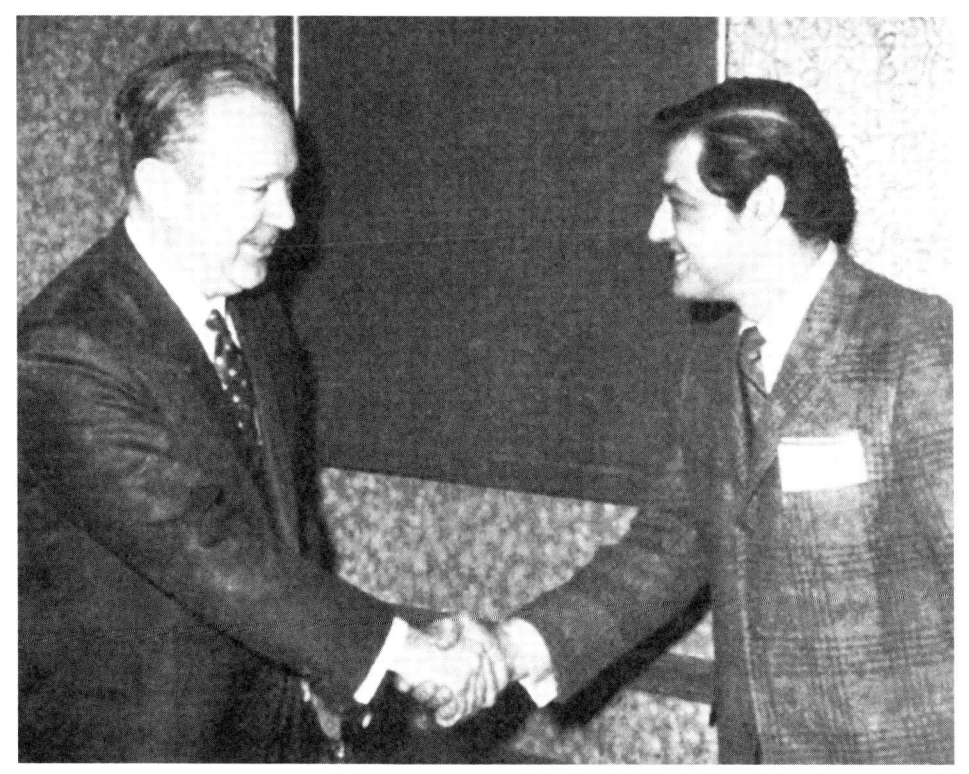

Sen. Russell B. Long (left), greeted by Salvatore D'Angelo, NARD second vice president

prevent physician ownership of a pharmacy, the unveiling of a new type of prepaid prescription program, and further probing into the brand vs generic name controversy dominated the discussions at NARD's first Annual Conference on National Legislation and Public Affairs. In issuing the conference call, Willard B. Simmons, NARD executive secretary, noted that "this session of Congress will be enacting much legislation within the next year affecting pharmacy practice. Pharmacy's voice must be heard at all levels of governmental activity during this next session of Congress."

The roster of invited speakers featured three of the most powerful congressional figures of the decade. The lead-off speaker was Sen. Philip A. Hart, who announced he was again introducing his bill calling for the elimination of physician ownership of pharmacies. The senator indicated that he was "frustrated" over the lack of progress made on this issue, which he said could have been eliminated by the Senate Antitrust and Monopoly Subcommittee when it investigated the anticompetitive effects of "doctor merchants" five years ago. The powerful Michigan legislator reported that the harmful effects of such physician competitive activity were readily ascertained by the Senate subcommittee. "The number of doctor-owned pharmacies and drug repackaging companies today is greater than five years ago," he said.

Rep. Hale Boggs of Louisiana said that one of the "most glaring weaknesses in the Medicare program was the absence of any provision enabling recipients to obtain necessary drugs and pharmaceuticals." Any attempt to provide such drugs without utilizing the services of the nation's retail pharmacists, he said, "would be a mistake."

Sen. Russell B. Long of Louisiana emphasized the fact that pharmacists participating in public programs should be paid the same for prescriptions under such programs as they are by private patients. His new bill, to be introduced shortly, would for all intents and purposes allow a continuation of the "usual and customary" compensation charge favored by NARD.

The conference was highly successful. NARD President Michael Perhach presided over the plenary sessions, and members of the executive committee chaired sessions devoted to specific topics. The meeting gave the association a new presence in Washington, and it gave key leaders the "facts and figures" they needed to lobby their respective congressional delegations.

As a follow-up to the Legislative Conference, the NARD leadership devoted additional attention to its national public relations campaign. That renewed emphasis was needed, in part, because community pharmacy had received a national "black eye" from bad publicity. In January 1969, a national television network produced a program on the high costs of health care. According to the network, a considerable part of that cost was due to the pricing practices of local pharmacists.

Simmons and the executive committee took exception to the reports and asked for a retraction or equal time to present the case for community pharmacy. The network allowed "equal time," and Simmons was able to explain to a national audience that, "according to the government's own figures," the prices for "prescriptions have dropped markedly in comparison with other commodities." The executive secretary was also able to quote from an NARD-University of Oklahoma survey taken the previous year about how frequently neighborhood pharmacists were called upon to provide health care information. Simmons's television appearance was a public relations bonanza for the association. Criticism about excessive drug prices, so severe in the previous decade, became muted, and public confidence in community pharmacy began to rebound. The association received additional positive exposure by being the first national organization to develop a drug abuse education program. Launched the preceding year in 1968 with Chicago area high schools, the program was so successful there, the executive committee voted to fund the costs for extending it throughout the nation.

The drug abuse program brought the association White House recognition. President Richard M. Nixon, during a meeting with NARD officials there,

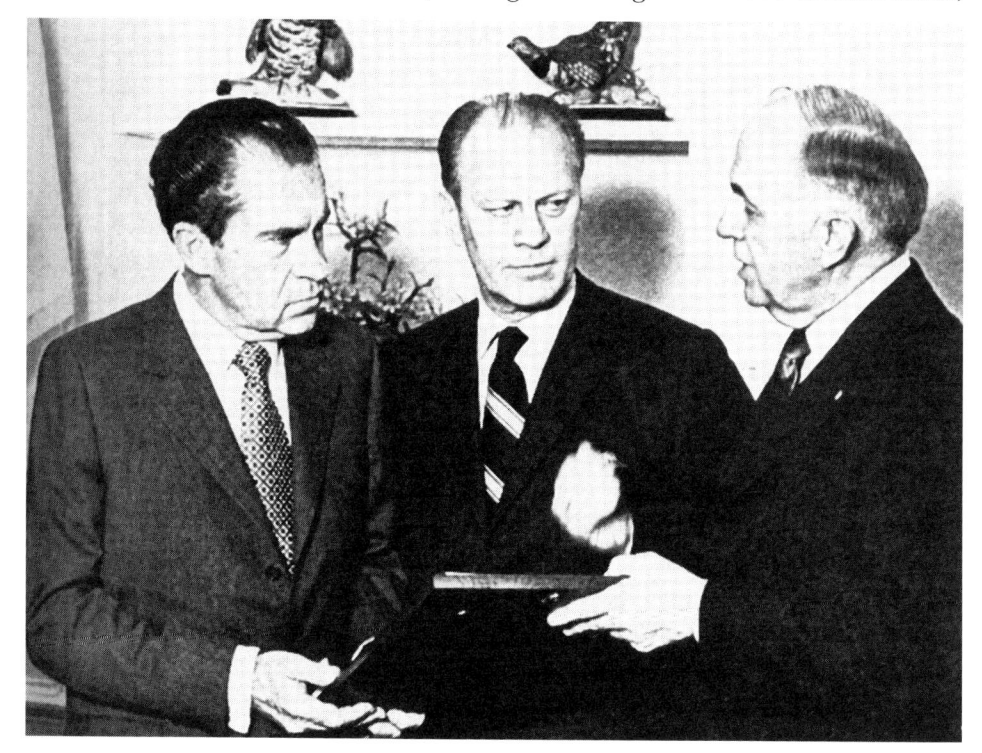

NARD's drug abuse effort was discussed at the White House with (left to right) President Richard M. Nixon, House Minority Leader Gerald R. Ford, and NARD's Willard Simmons.

heartily endorsed the association's comprehensive program of education against drug abuse. Following a report on the program from Simmons, the president said NARD and its members "could do no more important work than to expand and intensify their program against drug abuse, which is now directed to teenagers."

Mr. Nixon said it was highly encouraging to see a professional and business organization undertake such a vital national program entirely in the public interest. The president told the group during the meeting in his office that he believed it was most appropriate that the corner drugstore be the place where young people can go for information and dependable advice concerning proper drug use, as well as regarding misuse of drugs.

In commenting on the White House event, NARD Executive Committee Chairman Nick Avellone said the program "has achieved national recognition and has been received enthusiastically by a large number of civic, educational, labor, church groups, judicial and enforcement agencies." He noted that "may we state with pardonable pride that the NARD pioneered this drug abuse educational effort throughout the country."

The underlying economic pressures of funding both the ever-costly and escalating war in Vietnam and a sputtering economic expansion at home had its influence on American business. The costly Great Society legislation of the mid-1960s proved to be expensive, providing the springboard for government attacks on those segments of the health care system that seemed most vulnerable to federally mandated cost reductions.

Independent retail pharmacists were caught in a squeeze. Drug manufacturers continued to "pass along" to pharmacists the cost of doing business in developing and marketing new drug therapies. The high cost of drugs thus continued to be passed through to consumers, many of whom now were covered under the Medicaid program, where the cost of drug therapies attracted the attention of new governmental entities such as the Health Care Financing Administration (HCFA). The health care landscape had suddenly become very complicated and was to remain so for decades to follow.

The federal intervention into pharmaceutical reimbursement soon created an interlocking web of difficulties for the nation's independent pharmacists. Public relations about the high cost of drugs targeted independents again. At the seventy-first convention in Las Vegas, Nevada, in 1969, President Perhach told the delegates that "the public is still confused about some of retail pharmacy's procedures and objectives and in a few instances, the governmental agencies concerned don't understand our position and are openly hostile." To help correct the problem, he encouraged the leadership in the coming year to "improve its communication with the public and the areas of government that are most concerned with the consumer's welfare."

Third-party reimbursements was also another problem. Executive Committee Chairman Nick Avellone termed it "the number one concern of pharmacy today." Executive Secretary Simmons reported that "there is a confusing array of third-party payment plans developing around the country (and they have) occupied a great deal of our attention." He said, "NARD maintains that the usual and customary charges method is still the fairest and most equitable way of compensating for third-party payment prescriptions."

Beyond payment, Simmons was also concerned about community pharmacy facing a continuing intrusion from federal agencies. He was particularly bothered by the Office of Economic Opportunity's practice of allowing its "Neighborhood Health Centers" to dispense medications. By law, these centers were to "consult with local pharmacists before dispensing. However, in reality that seldom happened. Simmons said, "We are confronted with the spectacle of a tax-supported agency (government) adopting practices which can destroy those tax paying neighborhood drugstores that provide useful services and employment for residents of the area."

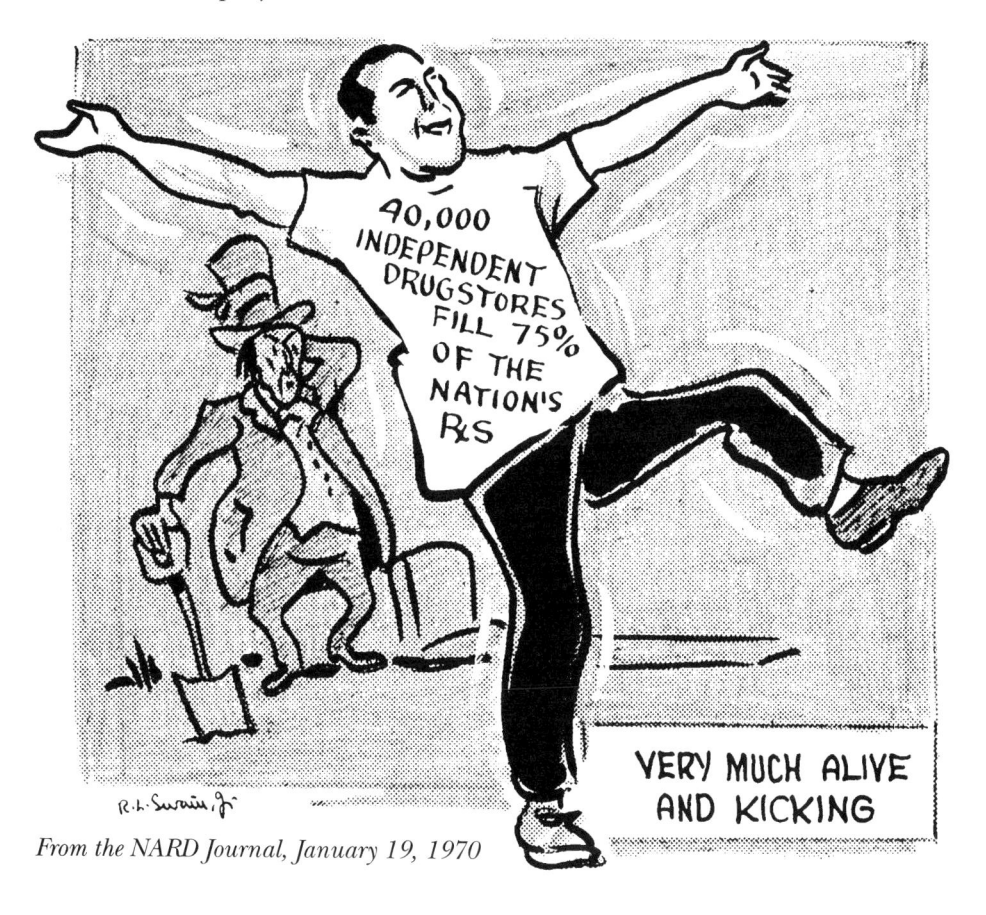

From the NARD Journal, January 19, 1970

The House of Delegates voted to support the executive committee's recommendation to make the NARD Legislative Conference an annual event. The delegates also endorsed the executive committee's recommendation that "usual and customary" be the standard for computing prescription reimbursement — an important position that was to be offered time and again as pharmaceutical reimbursement continued to be subjected to federal assaults.

Before adjourning, the delegates elected Chris Haleston of Portland, Oregon, as president. Nick Avellone was reelected chairman of the executive committee.

Much of the work for the new year focused on the method for calculating the costs of prescriptions. As health care costs continued to escalate at a rapid pace, Simmons and the executive committee recognized their members would lose public confidence unless the association could be more definitive in defining their costs. To assist in that effort NARD joined with the National Association of Chain Drug Stores (NACDS) and hired R.A. Gosselin & Associates to make a comprehensive statistical study of variability in prescription charges and operating characteristics among the nation's pharmacists.

The Gosselin study was detailed and took a year to complete. But from the data assembled, NARD leaders were confident they had reliable information. The report documented that "variations in prescriptions from one pharmacy to another are due to identifiable and quantifiable characteristics of pharmacy operations and given demographic factors." With this information, Simmons hoped to alleviate any public criticism and to give the association legal team data to make a case for professional fees in third-party plans. One immediate result of the survey was agreement between NARD and NACDS to develop a standard drug claim form to use in third-party payment.

In other matters, the executive committee voted to oppose efforts to abolish "anti-substitution laws," as well as plans to "eliminate brand-name prescribing." Most states had adopted such laws in previous years, and federal reimbursement officials and other providers saw an opportunity to cut drug prices. Executive Secretary Simmons reviewed these issues with the executive committee, but in their collective judgment, "nothing has altered circumstances enough so that the public would be less vulnerable to the obvious dangers of free substitution and elimination of prescription brands." Free substitution, in the executive committee's judgment, "would expose pharmacists to serious liability risks against which they could not protect themselves."

By 1972, NARD was in another period of transition. The Medicare program had been joined by Medicaid, which had then a full five years of experience. The detail of its multiple initiatives was overwhelming to almost everyone in the front lines of health care delivery. Medicaid's complexity forced almost all other legislative issues to the background at both the local and national levels. The time required to comply with the regulations, not to mention the procedural constraints limiting independent store owner decisions, sapped the energy of community pharmacists. NARD's central office also absorbed substantial financial costs of its own in responding to the many changes and helping members understand the changing reimbursement provisions.

The changes in retail pharmacy were reflected in the annual Lilly Digest for 1972. According to that report, "average" sales rose only 2.2 percent for the year. This increase was due solely to gains made in prescription revenue, which was 6.5 percent. Other sales declined by 1.2 percent. Moreover, prescriptions represented 46.6 percent of total store sales — then an all-time high. Also an important gauge to the overall health of the profession, net profit was only 3.6 percent of sales — an all-time low.

The stress of the mounting red tape spawned by the new federal programs began to take its toll on NARD. Policy decisions were harder to develop and less enthusiastically endorsed within the executive committee. Regions of the nation were affected differently by the Medicare/Medicaid programs and that was reflected in the attitude of community pharmacists. Forging consensus became more difficult than ever. Ironically, this internal pressure began to mount just as the profession turned the corner on its poor public image.

For a time Simmons and his colleagues tried to focus attention on the professional side of community pharmacy. Those familiar with the NARD story recognized this as a proven strategy. At the seventy-fourth convention in Chicago, Illinois, in 1972, the officer corps worked hard to remind delegates about their heritage and the importance of taking pride in the profession.

President E. Crawford Meyer sounded the pride theme in his address to the House of Delegates. Referring to the multiple players in the health care field, particularly the "bureaucrats," he said that "we don't deny their right to be there, but it certainly is not justified in terms of their health care knowledge or special expertise they possess in the treatment of the sick. They participate for economic and political reasons. We participate for sound health care reasons." As he pointed out, "the public is rightly concerned with skyrocketing costs of health care — particularly medical and hospital costs...we have held the line on price. No other division in the health care professions has done so well."

Executive Committee Chairman William Wickwire supported that view. He told the delegates that consumers were not only concerned about costs, but also apprehensive about personal care. "Nowhere," he said, "is resistance to regimentation more acute than in relation to individual health. When their own health — or the health of their loved ones — is involved, people do not want to be reduced to the status of cold, unfeeling numbers. They want to know that there is a friend down at the corner — a professional, well-trained, well-seasoned, and well-experienced (community pharmacist) who will give them the counsel and guidance and understanding they need to get through the problems and perils of individual illness." He urged his colleagues to continue to follow this route rather than "becoming employees of large-scale operations (chain drugstores), which promise income and security without so much involvement in the lives of people served."

To top off the convention theme, Executive Secretary Simmons reminded the delegates that "the people have not turned against us.... On the contrary, those in our profession who work most closely with the people know it is exactly the opposite. On every tongue there is a cry for restoration of the personalized and unregimented care our forefathers knew." Simmons noted, "If we are going to be the trusted consultants of the lay consumer on matters of health care, we face the challenge of continuously educating the public whom we serve."

That theme resonated with the more than 4,000 delegates in attendance. George Benson of Seattle, Washington, was elected president for 1972-1973. William Wickwire continued to serve as chairman of the executive committee.

Benson set two goals for the year. First, he planned to have legislation introduced that would allow pharmacists to supply medicine "for the patient at home, under Medicare." He also wanted to continue efforts to pass a bill that would "enable retail pharmacists to meet with third-party providers and administrators and negotiate the just terms under which we shall be reimbursed for our services."

The new president saw his bill introduced in the House of Representatives, and the NARD team worked hard to resolve the third-party payment issue — but without notable success. Members of the House and eventually all of Congress became more and more distracted by the developing "Watergate Scandal," which threatened to bring down a sitting president, and the "Energy Crisis," which ushered in a period of high inflation and interest rates that threatened the American economy. The latter was touched off by a five-month oil embargo, which lasted through the fall and winter of 1973-1974.

For NARD and its members, neither the issues nor the rhetoric changed during the year. Convention delegates assembled in Portland, Oregon, in 1973 for the association's seventy-fifth "Diamond Jubilee Anniversary." Notwithstanding the turmoil surrounding the Nixon administration, Gerald R.

Ford, then House Speaker, was the designated keynote speaker for NARD's convention.

A week prior to the convention, Vice President Spiro Agnew resigned amid scandal, and Ford was appointed to take his office. Simmons called Vice President Ford to give him the opportunity of withdrawing his convention engagement under these circumstances, but Ford's response was, "I've made a promise and I'll be there." In the words of NARD's Benson, that commitment "really set the tone for the convention. Mr. Ford, even as a politician, was true to his word."

At the convention, President Benson expressed his concern about the Veterans Administration's (VA) recent action to administer its own prescriptions through mail order. As Benson noted, "how tragic it will be for society and for pharmacy to see the mails filled with stimulants, depressants, and other potential drugs of abuse, accessible for illicit diversion."

Delegates elected Harold J. Shinnick of Chicago president and William Wickwire continued as chairman of the executive committee. Former NARD President Benson left association office to seek a seat on the Seattle, Washington, City Council. In December 1973, Benson won a seat on the council, which he held for 20 years, while his pharmacist wife, Evelyn, managed their drugstore for the entire period. As Benson wryly notes, "the saying around our house was that 'Evelyn runs the store and George runs the city.'"

While most of the nation continued to focus on Watergate and the energy crisis, community pharmacists became more concerned about crime. Federal enforcement of the Controlled Substances Act of 1970 reflected a growing national concern about crime involving illegal drugs and created the Bureau of Narcotics and Dangerous Drugs with a wide-ranging authority. While pharmacies were the most common target for drug robberies and burglaries, it was unclear how community pharmacy might be affected by the new law. The NARD leadership originally took a "wait and see" attitude with respect to the new bureau, but the association membership believed that the act placed community pharmacies — by virtue of their profession — in harm's way.

The membership got its way, and the NARD leadership began to prosecute on Capitol Hill over many years the reality that pharmacies had become "outposts" in efforts to control drug misuse. Because pharmacists were so vulnerable to robberies and burglaries, NARD sought legislation to make an attempt to obtain a controlled substance from a pharmacy a federal offense. However, officials in the Department of Justice opposed such legislation and the bill struggled for many years.

An "incident" in 1974 added to the strained relations with the American Medical Association (AMA). The controversy became categorized as a dispute over "patient consultation," but in reality it was a problem in labeling. Manufacturers of certain over the counter (OTC) medications accepted a recommendation from a team of "outside consultants" to change the OTC product label. The new wording advised the public that they may obtain more information about the product by "consulting a pharmacist or physician." Historically, the labels had only mentioned the physician. The AMA became upset over the possible implications of pharmacists advising patients and filed a complaint with the Food and Drug Administration (FDA). The FDA ordered a return to the original wording.

NARD held its seventy-sixth convention in Las Vegas, Nevada, in 1974. The VA's entry into the "prescription by mail" business had begun to make an impact by the time the delegates assembled. President Shinnick reported that "our drug distribution system is in chaos" and "the day has long since passed when any of us can look up the price of a product in the Blue Book." (The Blue Book was a standard drug pricing reference at the time.)

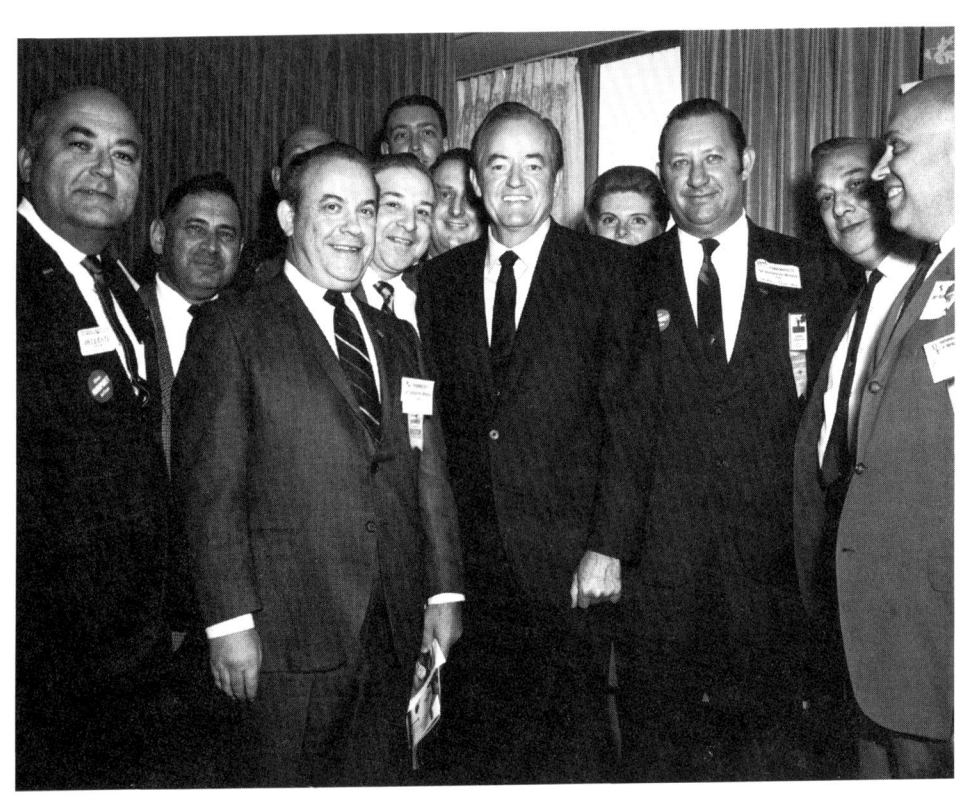

Senator, then Vice President Hubert H. Humphrey (center) was a frequent speaker at NARD's Annual Legislative Conferences and Conventions during the 1960s and 1970s.

Shinnick said it was time for NARD to revive the fight against discriminatory pricing and cited the VA's program as a case in point. He reported that "we can see more and more prescription medication being funneled through government hospital facilities." Shinnick deplored this practice. He said, "All NARD wants is that each independent pharmacist be given an equal opportunity to compete on equal terms and conditions with the hospital, the government, and the discounter. We ask no special favors, no special discounts for ourselves, just an opportunity to buy on equal terms and equal prices." This argument was to become the core premise of the decades-long fight over discriminatory pricing.

Throughout the 1974 convention, the growing federal intervention into health care was a resonant theme. The association's leaders attempted to decipher and explain these developments to the membership, but they were without a full understanding of what course NARD should charter.

Chairman Wickwire alerted the delegates to be prepared for a "National Health Insurance" plan that was being discussed in Congress. While it was still too early to know what form, if any, the proposal would take, it was another indication of "big government" intruding into health care. Wickwire was also able to report a bit of a thaw in relations with APhA. Representatives from NARD and APhA had held several meetings over the past year and had formed a Committee on Pharmacy Economic Security (COPES) to "study the third-party prescription" issue.

Simmons seemed to have lost some of his enthusiasm for the cause. As in 1973, his address to the House of Delegates lacked the fire and drama of his earlier presentations. He devoted almost half of his speech to the "crisis in the Presidency," Richard Nixon's resignation, the new role for Gerald Ford, and to reviewing the association's financial situation. With respect to issues, he said, "The reality is there. The literature is there. The words are there. But when we move out into the realm of relations and interactions with others in the health care community, there comes back the old and unaccountable attitude that somehow, pharmacy's place is at the second table." Finding a way to move from that position was the NARD leadership's biggest challenge.

E. Boyd Garrett, of Nashville, Tennessee, was elected president and Sam A. McConnell, Jr. of Williams, Arizona, was chosen chairman of the executive committee. For much of the year NARD leaders were locked into intense negotiations with officials in the Department of Health, Education, and Welfare (HEW) over pricing policy in the Medicaid program. HEW officials wanted to establish a schedule of Maximum Allowable Costs (MAC) that it would pay for Medicaid prescriptions. These government officials wanted to base MAC on the Office of Veterans Affairs's prices. Garrett, McConnell, and NARD staff pointed out that the VA could buy from the manufacturers at a

75 percent discount below what community pharmacists paid. Rather than setting maximum costs, NARD argued that HEW should follow the guidelines established by the Robinson-Patman Act, set minimum prices, and allow market forces to determine the price to consumers.

Through a series of meetings and four draft documents, NARD argued its case, but without success. In August 1975, HEW published the MAC regulations and said they would go into effect January 1, 1976.

Losing the MAC debate was disheartening to NARD leaders. Knowing that non-elected officials were in position to arbitrarily decide what pharmacists should charge for their services without regard to market forces or professional judgment was difficult to accept. Equally disturbing, the MAC debate revived talk about repealing the Robinson-Patman Act. Even though opponents had been able to find many loopholes and federal officials were extremely lax in enforcing its provisions, the act still stood as a symbol for small business. If allowed to function as its sponsors intended, NARD officials were convinced the Robinson-Patman protective umbrella would continue to be beneficial to all concerned.

Another issue, prescription price advertising, also illustrated the philosophical differences between NARD and others in the health care industry. Members of the executive committee thought the concept was wrong professionally. Advertising would not only confuse the public about the nature of prescription medicine, but it would also minimize the professional services provided by the pharmacists. It was wrong from a business standpoint, too, in NARD's view, because the advertising costs would be added to the price, thereby negating the original argument that competition lowered prices. With persistent effort, NARD's Washington representative, William E. Woods, was able to keep bills to allow prescription advertising confined to a committee.

Given the costs of responding to so many political issues, McConnell and the executive committee decided it was time to convert its fledgling political action committee, the concept of which was announced a year earlier, into a formally registered entity. Kenneth G. Mehrle of Cape Girardeau, Missouri, guided the effort to form the National Association of Pharmacists Political Action Committee (NAPPAC), with the help of NARD legal counsel Sidney Waller. NAPPAC was eligible to receive tax deductible contributions of up to $100 per person and could use that money to financially support political candidates — which NARD as an association could not do. NAPPAC, pharmacy's first political action committee (PAC), eventually became a powerhouse among association PACs.

The events of 1975 found NARD continuing a lonely battle against price discrimination. President Garrett noted in speeches to the membership during his travels that "customers in our independent pharmacies have to pay extra for prescription drugs to cover the discounts that manufacturers give to the government, the hospital pharmacies, and to the discounters and corporate chains." He noted that association leaders had tried to involve the APhA and the Proprietary Manufacturers Association in the fight, but without much success. He also used his various forums to sound a warning that "should discriminatory pricing continue to help eliminate community pharmacies, the drug manufacturers will find themselves in a difficult position."

During the seventy-seventh convention in Miami Beach, Florida, in 1975, Chairman McConnell reported that the executive committee "devoted more time to developments in Washington than to any other subject." This focus had become expensive, and the executive committee had worked with Executive Secretary Simmons to "develop more precise information about the association...so that we can continuously keep expenditures in line with income."

McConnell was also concerned that resolutions and motions from the floor during the House of Delegates business meeting might sometimes cause the association to take ill-advised actions. This was particularly true given the complexity of current issues. "Would it be advisable," he asked "for the NARD executive committee to present to the delegates — for vote — position papers on some of the more important or controversial issues?" While many delegates saw the logic of the chairman's question, a majority did not want to give up their individual input from the floor.

As part of the "spontaneous" action, delegates approved a resolution asking the executive committee to immediately begin research on the possibility of filing an antitrust law suit against third-party prescription plans." Delegates also agreed to increase their annual dues to $45, created an ad hoc committee to draft "Community Pharmacy Standards" and heard a report from the Committee on Form and Organization on the issue of a name change for the association.

They also approved a resolution commending the work of *NARD Journal* editor Louis E. Kazin who was leaving that position and extended greetings to Richard W. Lay, the new editor. (The hiring of Lay marked the first time in the association's history that a nonpharmacist had been awarded the position of *Journal* editor. Other Journal editors who followed in Kazin's footsteps were hired as communications professionals who not only learned the issues of the profession, but also were equipped to effectively articulate association points of view.). As a final action, delegates elected William D. Wickwire of Los Altos, California, president. Sam McConnell, Jr. continued as chairman of the executive committee.

During the coming year, the nation was wrapped up in its Bicentennial Celebration. For community pharmacy, it was anything but a celebration.

The profession watched the MAC regulations being implemented. The squeeze between what HEW officials determined to be the pharmacists' "estimated acquisition costs" (EAC) for prescription drugs and the maximum allowable costs (MAC) the agency would pay as reimbursement was hardly a festive occasion.

The new pricing structure for Medicaid prescriptions was difficult enough for pharmacists to swallow, but it positively choked them in downtime and exorbitant paperwork requirements. For example, Michael Bongiovanni, president of E.R. Squibb & Sons, conducted a study on the new regulations and how they might affect his company. He reported that it would "take 130 million man-hours" to fill out the required government forms, and he estimated the paperwork "added $750 million to the cost of prescriptions." The NARD leadership was not satisfied with the new guidelines, but having lost the debate on MACs in the past year, they felt there was little now they could do.

In addition to the EAC/MAC bind, pharmacists and the nation were stuck in "stagflation," as inflation, interest rates, and unemployment continued to rise near double-digit numbers. The depressed economy began to take its toll on advertising revenue in the *Journal,* and at the spring executive com-

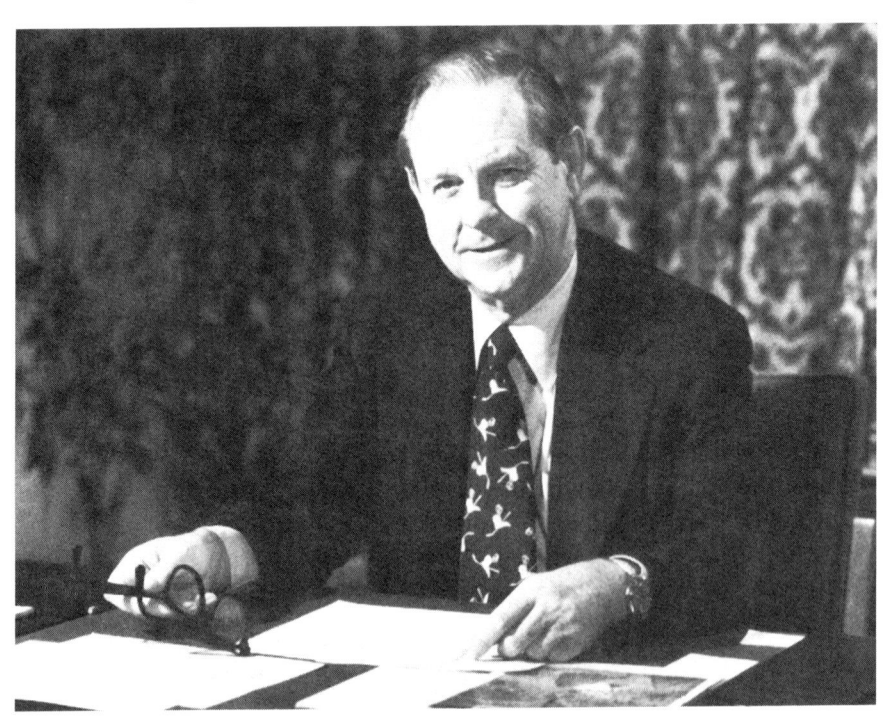

William E. Woods, NARD Executive Vice President, 1977 – 1984

mittee meeting, Executive Secretary Simmons reported that sales on rental space for the annual drug show at the fall convention were behind schedule. Some members of the executive committee were concerned about the association's long-term financial status. While it was not a crisis for the association to maintain two offices as operational costs were increasing and revenues were not keeping pace with inflation, the overall situation was nevertheless viewed as serious.

Under these conditions, it was difficult to justify separate offices. But which office should be closed? There was much to be said for the central offices remaining in Chicago, Illinois. However, the growing federal presence in health care and impact of those programs on community pharmacy made a strong case for moving the association to Washington, D.C.. In addition, the argument that the nation's capital was the proper site for a national organization had been part of an ongoing dialogue within NARD since the 1920s.

Given these circumstances, the executive committee decided in August to close the Chicago office and move the association's corporate offices to Washington. Simmons, having invested sixteen years in Chicago, decided not to move with the office. The executive committee, after rewriting Simmons's contract to officially end at the end of December 1976, then hired Woods as the new General Manager effective January 1, 1977. Simmons remained as association secretary.

The executive committee's action was not generally known until delegates began to assemble in San Francisco, California, for the seventy-eighth convention in 1976. Simmons told the delegates about the changes as he finished his sixteenth report to the House of Delegates. He said, "As some of you know, I made a significant decision in 1961 when I became your Executive Secretary and General Manager to move to Chicago. I uprooted my family, sold my drug stores, left my many friends and familiar surroundings in Texas to settle in Chicago. I cannot at this time in my life proceed to make another drastic change of this nature." He pledged his support to the association and to Woods as the new Executive Secretary.

Simmons's announcement was only one of several emotional issues. The Committee on Form and Organization reported a survey of the membership supported another name for the association. The proposed new name, subject to voter approval at the next convention, would be the "National Association of Independent Pharmacists." (A decision regarding a change in name was ultimately postponed until the late 1980s at which time the House of Delegates approved "NARD" as the official name of the association, later to become the National Community Pharmacists Association [NCPA] in 1996.)

The delegates also heard a motion for NARD to merge with the APhA — this coming from the floor after APhA President Bill Apple addressed the audience and strongly urged the merger. The motion was overwhelmingly defeated. In a different kind of emotional moment, Executive Secretary Simmons announced that Rep. Wright Patman had died earlier in the year and asked to approve a resolution honoring him for his "tireless and dedicated efforts in behalf of his community pharmacists and pharmacy owners of the nation."

Before leaving San Francisco, delegates elected Salvatore (Sal) D'Angelo of New Orleans as president. Neil Pruitt of Toccoa, Georgia, was elected chairman of the executive committee.

The change in leadership, while a surprise to many, was not like the shock of John Dargavel's death. The transition was made quietly and with little fanfare. Woods, a graduate of the University of Texas College of Pharmacy and a lawyer, brought a new perspective to the office. Having been Washington representative and Associate General Counsel for the past twelve years, he was familiar with most aspects of the association.

Woods thought it was important to build a Washington office, not just relocate the Chicago staff. In his first report to the membership in early January 1977, he said he was "in the process of defining and developing our new emphasis. We will be rebuilding our staff in an organizational structure designed to meet the needs of the membership.... We will not continue programs or activities just because we have always done them." Over the next six months he revamped every department. He made a major push to attract new members, redesigned the *Journal,* reworked the convention program, and increased the lobbying efforts. He also relocated the John A. Dargavel Foundation and NAPPAC to the Washington office.

By the time the association's seventy-ninth convention convened in Washington, D.C., in 1977, the transition to the "new look NARD" had been largely completed. President D'Angelo reported to the delegates that he had traveled over 73,000 miles in the past year and felt he had "gotten a good feel for the issues independent pharmacists were most concerned about." He called these the "gut issues" — the restraints placed on pharmacists by the MCA/EAC rulings under Medicaid, the VA's mail order program, and the inability to gain acceptance for "usual and customary" reimbursement on professional fees. D'Angelo encouraged his colleagues to stand firm because "NARD never has and never will support the fixed fee concept. With fixed fees we solve a problem today with a two-bit crumb and then we have the same problem tomorrow."

Executive Committee Chairman Pruitt explained the committee's efforts to ensure a smooth transition in relocating the general offices and working with a new administrative officer. In the life of associations either of these major changes would require a period of adjustment; having both in the same year doubled the readjustment.

To assist in making the changes, the executive committee brought in a management consultant team to review the office set-up and recommend organizational realignments. Prutt said the committee was presently at work on a "five-year comprehensive statement of operating policy" and delegates would see more results from that planning in the future. Part of this planning was redefining the job description of the General Manager and the role that position played in the association. After some discussion, the committee agreed to keep the secretary's position free from administrative responsibilities and change the manager's title to Executive Vice President.

Delegates approved the executive committee's recommendations and elected Sam A. McConnell, Jr., a veteran of the executive committee, to be president. Neil Pruitt was re-elected chairman of the executive committee.

The NARD leadership spent the last year of the association's eighth decade in "self-analysis" and "introspection." All "activities, relationships, and services" were evaluated and a decision made on what to eliminate and what to continue. One activity, that of the "field men," or "organization men" as they were known in the earliest days of the association, was terminated. The executive committee also worked hard to cultivate a closer relationship with the state associations and to give special recognition to each state's incoming president each year.

The executive committee also hosted a meeting for the association's corporate members, the first meeting of this type for NARD. In view of the new title and job description for the organization's chief administrator, the committee proposed amendments to the constitution to add secretary to the treasurer's position and to make necessary editorial corrections wherever the word secretary was used inappropriately or was unnecessary.

By the time delegates came together in New Orleans, Louisiana, for the eightieth convention in 1978, their mood was upbeat, and there was a degree of optimism in the hotel corridors. President McConnell had made increased membership his major theme for the year and was pleased to report a healthy increase. He was also proud to announce a new organization — the Joint Commission of Pharmacy Practitioners (JCPP) — that NARD had been instrumental in developing. This, yet another attempt at interprofessional cooperation, was an outgrowth of Past President D'Angelo's unsuccessful efforts to revive the Committee on Pharmacy Economic Security (COPES). McConnell was hopeful that this new start, which represented more than 90 percent of the practicing pharmacists in the nation, would be an asset to NARD's efforts to lobby Congress and the various federal agencies.

Chairman Pruitt reviewed the events that had transpired over the past eighteen months with the move to Washington. The accomplishments were remarkable. The central office staff had increased from five to thirty full-time members. Office space had increased 30 percent, and the executive committee was recommending a historic $2 million budget for 1978-1979. It had taken the association 59 years to reach its first $1 million budget in 1957, the second million came in less than 21 years. Pruitt admitted that in the previous year the association had a $20,000 deficit; however, he was confident that the new growth the committee anticipated would more than recover the loss.

Pruitt also cautioned the delegates to be on guard for economic panaceas being offered by various sources. "Ten years ago," he said, "we predicted that a fixed fee determined unilaterally by a government agency would reduce pharmacy services to the lowest common denominator and, in many areas, it has. A brief point today, however, is to warn you of an even more ominous cloud on the horizon. The fancy bureaucratic title is a 'uniform accounting system.' Please don't confuse this high sounding title with what retail pharmacy really needs, which is a system to determine the costs of filling prescriptions."

Executive Vice President Woods reviewed the challenges of building an office staff and getting settled in at the association's new headquarters at 1750 K Street, N.W. He also called attention to the programs on personnel management the association had developed in the past year through a contract with Roche Laboratories. As he concluded his report to the House of Delegates, he noted, "I am determinedly dedicated to one personal goal of honoring our commitment to give you a total program that recognizes public affairs and member services as what you are paying for. I am equally determined that our programs will be of high quality and up to date."

Delegates to the eightieth convention elected Kenneth J. Mehrle president. Neil Pruitt continued as chairman of the executive committee.

The decade of crisis saw NARD weather a mild crisis of its own. Changing its executive leadership and relocating its corporate offices are major events in the life of any association. But to one battling for its economic life against mounting governmental constraints on one hand and a growing concentration of wealth on the other, it was little short of miraculous. Lacking the legislative success of some of the previous years, the eighth decade, nevertheless, saw NARD finish the period bruised, but not defeated, and in an aggressive mood for action.

CHAPTER TEN

THE NINTH DECADE: 1979 – 1988

NARD Wins Battles in the Legislative Trenches

*I*f the 1970s were times of crisis, the 1980s were days of "revolution." The Cable News Network (CNN) went on air June 1, 1980 followed by Music Television (MTV) in 1981, precursors of a revolution in communications and technology. The "Reagan Revolution" fundamentally changed the American economy for the first time in fifty years. In foreign affairs, peaceful revolutions in Eastern Europe brought an end to a forty-year reign of communist rule.

Revolutions of different types also occurred. Acquired immune deficiency syndrome (AIDS), first identified in 1981, brought dramatic life-style changes to many Americans. The Economic Recovery and Tax Act of 1981, which cut personal income taxes by twenty-five percent over a three-year period, was followed by a sharp two-year recession. A "deregulation" revolution beginning with energy policies in the late 1970s become full-blown by the mid-1980s, and contributed to a record number of corporate consolidations. Record tax cuts were followed by record deficits in the federal budget, as well as in the nation's savings and loans institutions. Then there was a record collapse of the stock market in 1987.

For NARD, the challenge was to craft a strategy that responded to these rapid changes while anticipating the future. Eighty years of experience had convinced many association members that stability was the best response to many, if not most, of the "revolutionary" changes, and NARD leaders worked hard to provide consistency for the membership. That said, the association's leaders were also mindful of new developments. New marketing and merchandising services were launched, and a wide array of emerging niche marketing opportunities were exploited in the pages of the *Journal* and elsewhere.

This blending of tradition with change was reflected in the area of member services. Mindful of its responsibility to provide members with the tools "to stay competitive in today's market," the association began to offer a number of new services early in the decade. One of these, a "Merchandising Alert" column began appearing regularly in the *Journal* in January 1979. This monthly feature informed community pharmacists about "new pricing, promotion, and sales information" for the top-selling "front end" items in the store. Categorized by region, this service gave each NARD member definite guidelines on how to better merchandise the various departments in a typical pharmacy.

Another service provided members with a variety of media programs. For example, with "Bookstore by Mail," NARD members were able to order books and audio cassettes on various subjects pertinent to their business and professional development. Another series featured a videocassette demonstration on "product placement," "selective buying," and "understanding accounting records." The NARD/Roche "Guide to Good Pharmacy Management" continued to be a force in promoting store management and customer care.

Executive Vice President William Woods and the executive committee also gave considerable attention to store modernization. Many neighborhood pharmacies had been built or remodeled in the 1950s and had had only minor alterations since that time. By contracting with companies specializing in pharmacy design, the association was able to furnish members with expert consultation on refurbishing their stores. For a fee, these same companies offered comprehensive assistance in supervising store design from layout to installation and leasing.

The association also focused more attention on customer relations. In addition to promoting better communication with customers, the NARD leadership produced special publications on the emerging niche markets of "nursing home care" and "home health care." The Health Supports and Appliances (HSA) program, organized in the late 1970s to provide orthotic and prosthetic appliances, continued to grow in importance and numbers. By 1980, that niche included some 3,500 pharmacists in 1,500 NARD-certified pharmacy facilities. The growing enrollments in long-term care facilities led the executive committee to ask Executive Committee member H. Joseph Schutte to design a handbook detailing government regulations and special services pharmacists could offer patients in nursing homes.

Maintaining liaison with other pharmacy groups remained an NARD goal throughout the decade. In addition to continuing efforts to work more closely with the American Pharmaceutical Association (APhA), the National Wholesale Druggists' Association (NWDA), the Pharmaceutical Manufacturers Association (PMA), and other traditional groups, Executive Vice President Woods and the executive committee also began informal meetings with the major pharmaceutical companies. Beginning in August 1979 as an informal meeting with sixteen of the industry's executives, NARD leaders began an

CHAPTER TEN — THE NINTH DECADE: 1979 – 1988

ongoing joint meeting with the manufacturers. Another important liaison was with the state associations. The regional meetings begun in the 1970s were popular with pharmacy leaders at the state and district levels. From these occasional get-togethers, Executive Vice President Woods began scheduling a regular meeting between NARD leaders and leaders of the state associations as part of the regular agenda at the annual convention. These meetings were especially important in planning strategy for legislation, membership campaigns, third-party payment initiatives, and other matters of mutual concern.

Of all NARD's concerns, legislation and governmental relations continued to dominate. Many of the issues were ongoing from the previous decade. These included making robberies of pharmacies a federal offense, providing

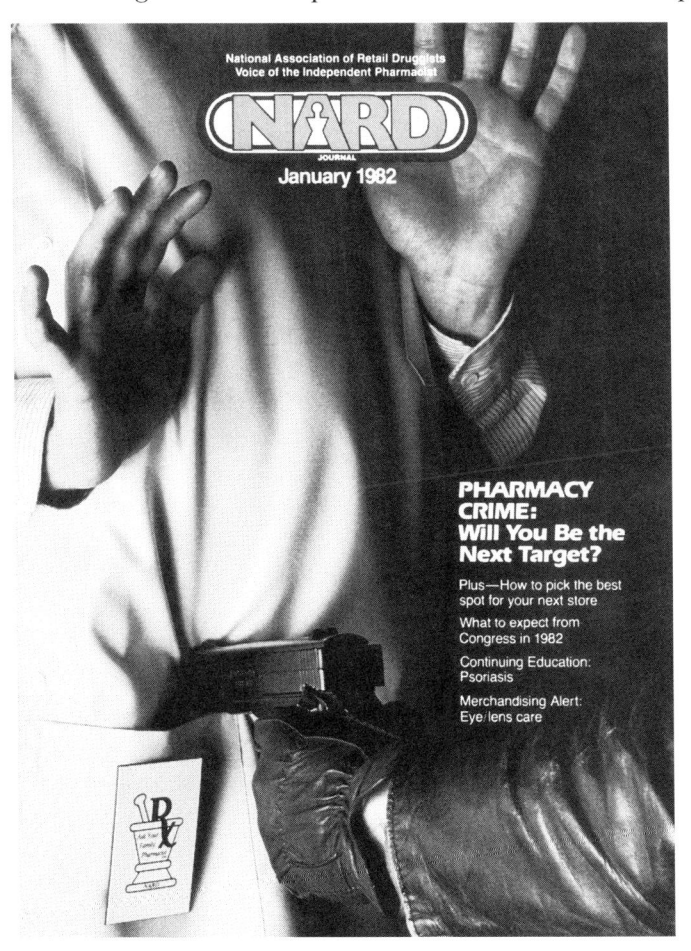

A decades' long struggle making pharmacy robbery a federal offense became a persistent Journal feature in the 1980s.

patients in third-party programs "freedom of choice" when choosing a pharmacy, allowing veterans covered by Veterans Administration programs to obtain pharmacy services from their local community pharmacists, amending antitrust laws to permit pharmacists to negotiate collectively with private and governmental health care program administrators, and establishing a two-tier regulatory system for small business.

New issues added in the eighth decade included legislation to cover medicines for home use as a benefit under Medicare, making prescribed drugs a mandatory benefit in state Medicaid programs, making prescribed drugs a mandatory benefit of any federally funded health program, amending the Drug Regulation Reform Act to eliminate mandatory price posting, reducing taxes for small businesses, and legislation to encourage adding mandatory prescribed drug coverage to private health insurance programs.

To implement this ambitious legislative agenda, NARD leaders established a "pharmacy alert program." This plan operated along the principle of a "telephone tree" whereby NARD leaders called state leaders, who then called key community pharmacists, and they in turn called their U.S. senators and representatives on specific legislative issues. The association did not abandon its traditional letter and telegram campaigns when needing lawmakers to support or oppose a bill, but the telephone alert system became the most effective lobbying method of choice.

NARD also began the new decade with a major reorganization of its committee structure. With executive committee approval, President Kenneth G. Mehrle decreased each committee's size, but increased the number of committees in operation. Members of the Executive Committee and association officers, including past presidents, were assigned to each committee. As President Mehrle noted, "I intend to place an accent on 'youth' in the committee appointments. We are looking for new ideas, new programs, and new energy. We also welcome the participation of more women pharmacists taking an active role in the committee system."

None of the key legislative issues NARD promoted made it out of committee in 1979. The association did win one indirect victory through the court system. The case in question, Royal Drug Co. Inc. vs. Group Life & Health Insurance Co., developed in Texas in the 1970s when the insurance company claimed exemption from antitrust laws in establishing a "fixed fee provider contract." A group of San Antonio pharmacists, led by the Royal Drug Company, challenged Group Life's position, charging that the fixed fee only added to the insurance company's profits. In a five-to-four decision, the U.S. Supreme Court upheld the pharmacists' position. NARD joined the Texas group with a "friend of the court" brief and celebrated the victory believing that the "fixed fee provider contract" was effectively set aside.

Other successes included NARD's hosting its first "Annual NARD Student Conference." This two-day meeting at NARD headquarters in February included selected student leaders from pharmacy colleges around the nation. Among the issues they discussed with NARD leaders and staff members included services the association offered its members, the student's specific needs, and the Doctor of Pharmacy (Pharm.D.) program. This program, having been established in the 1970s, had been developed with some reluctance by most pharmacy schools. NARD supported the program and degree, but wanted more course content on store merchandising and management rather than an increased emphasis on clinical pharmacy.

But as one student who was enrolled in the program told the conferees, she planned to "go back into the community to practice pharmacy...and she had been looked upon as 'an enemy' by her colleagues" for taking a job with an independent pharmacy." As another student said, "No one pushes community pharmacy.... It seems that when a student gets out of school, he perceives his only option as either employment in the chains or in hospitals." While Woods and the other NARD leaders did not necessarily like to hear such comments, it provided them with an understanding of the work they needed to do with students and the various pharmacy school programs.

When delegates gathered in Las Vegas for the eighty-first convention in October 1979, they heard reports of significant internal growth but little progress on the legislative front. The third-party payment issue dominated political discussions on Capitol Hill, but the association was unable to get favorable action on either its proposal to eliminate the fixed fee on prescriptions or to make drug coverage mandatory under Medicare.

President Mehrle strongly defended NARD's position on the third-party issue, saying, "When NARD goes to bat for the independent, it is talking of dollars and cents. It is talking about return on investment and a reasonable profit. Yes, profit is not a dirty word in NARD's vocabulary. Federal and state bureaucracies and the third-party czars don't like that kind of talk. They want to stroke our professional egos as an opiate (to) blind us to economic realities."

Executive Committee Chairman Neil Pruitt emphasized the association's membership growth, noting that the change in the bylaws in 1976 to "switch from store to individual membership" had greatly stimulated interest in NARD activities. Since making that change, some 5,000 "employee pharmacists" had joined the organization. He was also hopeful that APhA's ending its "compulsory affiliation" requirements would allow NARD to pick up some additional members. Executive Vice President Woods also emphasized the affiliation issue. APhA had affiliation agreements with nineteen state associations prior to 1979. As affiliates, states had access to workshops, seminars, and other benefits not available to non-affiliated states. States cooperating with APhA also actively recruited pharmacists for membership in the organization. By offering individual memberships, NARD could now offer an attractive alternative for the independent retail pharmacist. Woods was confident that NARD would pick up a significant number of individual memberships. "It is time," he said, "for many younger employee pharmacists to realize the need for them to support NARD and its new initiatives."

Before leaving Las Vegas, delegates elected Paul J. Dumouchel of Boston, Massachusetts president. John A. Johnson of Bellevue, Nebraska, was elected chairman of the executive committee. Delegates also voted to change the name of the John A. Dargavel Foundation to the NARD Foundation in an effort to attract a broader base of support. NARD Past President Frank Lobraico continued to serve as president of the foundation. The original mission of providing scholarships to students and emergency loans to pharmacists faced with catastrophic circumstances did not change.

The new year had hardly begun before NARD leaders learned that officials at the Department of Health and Human Services (HHS), the new name of the former Department of Health and Welfare, planned to require "patient package inserts" (PPI) on ten drug classes. The program was to be administered by the Food and Drug Administration (FDA).

The PPI concept was first introduced in the 1970s and reflected the growing sophistication and potency of modern drugs. The ten categories mandated by HHS officials included over 300 shelf items. For each drug in the PPI program, the manufacturer prepared a detailed explanation of the intended benefits of the drugs, possible side effects, and other factual data to allow the consumer to be better informed.

NARD had long favored providing information to consumers, but as Executive Vice President Woods explained, "we don't think government-mandated PPIs are the way to go." He explained that PPIs were expensive to produce, were ineffective in that there was no way to ensure that consumers read or followed the insert's directions, and placed an unfair administrative burden on the retail pharmacists.

However, HHS officials were adamant on trying the plan as a pilot program for three years. Ironically, the plan became entangled in bureaucratic "red tape" and presidential politics and was not implemented prior to President Jimmy Carter's leaving office. Newly elected President Ronald Reagan placed a moratorium on the PPI plan, and it was finally set aside.

To prepare community pharmacists for the PPI program and in recognition of the growing complexity of running an independent pharmacy, NARD leaders also began an energetic continuing education (CE) program. Contracting with the Massachusetts College of Pharmacy's Allied Health Services program, the association launched a year-long series of CE units. A major part of the costs for running the program was underwritten by Pfizer Laboratories. While the emphasis was on variety, each CE program had a common characteristic of having "practical, relevant and useful information to make (pharmacists) better able to counsel their patients." Pharmacists who completed twelve individual programs within twelve months received a "certificate" from NARD acknowledging their participation. The Pfizer CE program remains a regular monthly feature in the association's magazine to this day.

Another new membership service recognized the growing number of women in pharmacy. Following World War II, the number of women graduates from colleges of pharmacy steadily increased. By 1980 women represented over thirty percent of the profession and the percentage was increasing rapidly. This was a major development in the history of the association.

In recognition of the new circumstances, President Dumouchel appointed a special task force on "women in pharmacy" and charged the group with investigating the special concerns of women pharmacists. Helen Gouin was appointed to chair the group, which held its first meeting in June 1980. Par-

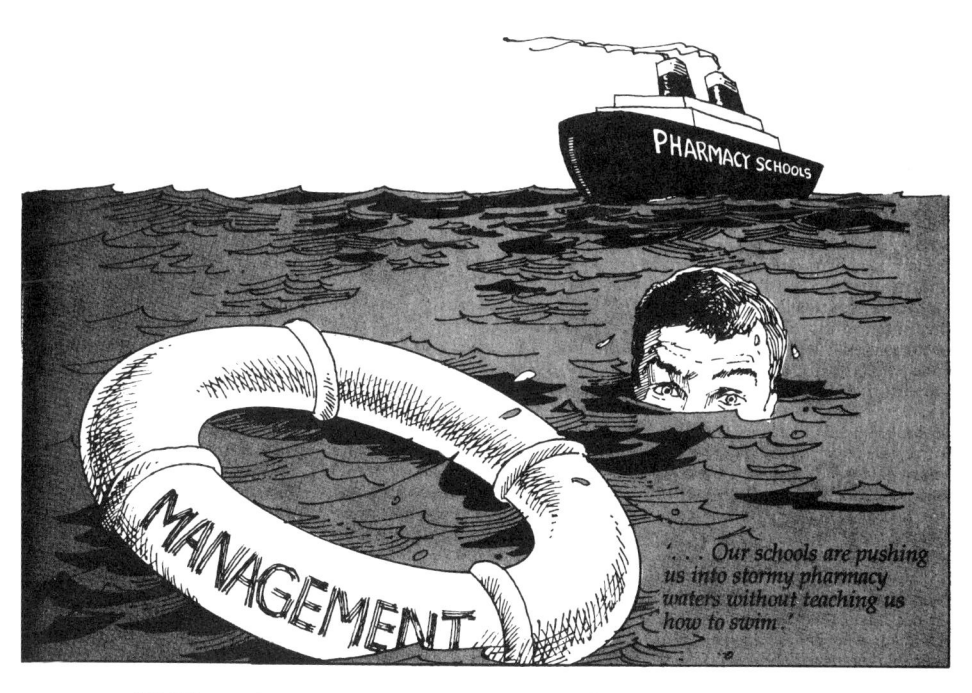

NARD sought more management courses in pharmacy school curricula, a historic concern of community pharmacy.

ticular attention was focused on the problems women pharmacists had in obtaining financing to purchase a pharmacy. Other matters related to issues of discrimination and working conditions relating to women. The task force also authorized the preparation of a brochure highlighting the role of women in pharmacy.

NARD also adopted a service mark for the profession of community pharmacy — "Ask Your Family Pharmacist." The service mark was inspired by two Ohio pharmacists who, while working for an NARD member, authored a popular newspaper column, "Ask Your Pharmacist," to make the public more aware of the pharmacist's crucial role in health care.

In the legislative field, NARD secured introduction of a "Prepaid Prescription Program Negotiations bill" in the second session of the ninety-sixth Congress. The proposal allowed independent pharmacists to be exempt from antitrust laws so that they could collectively negotiate with insurance companies or plan sponsors on reimbursement for third-party programs. Although not seen as a panacea, NARD leaders nevertheless believed the bill was an important step toward providing community pharmacists with some leverage to recover some of their costs in prescription pricing.

One bill NARD assisted in getting through Congress in 1980, the Omnibus Small Business Act, proved a major asset to young pharmacists. Although NARD was only one of some thirty sponsors, it was gratifying to the leadership to see the bill become law. Its major asset for pharmacy was a federal loan guarantee to employees who bought businesses from retiring owners when the owners financed the sale.

The eighty-second convention met in Atlanta, Georgia, in September 1980. President Dumouchel chose the theme "The New Independent" in his address to the House of Delegates. Noting that the population of community pharmacists had declined almost twenty-five percent since 1960, he said those that remained were "a new breed" who knew how to compete. This new breed of independent pharmacists had persevered "at great personal and financial sacrifice," but the struggle had been worth the effort. "We still swear by personalized service," he said, "we still deliver even though gas prices are now prohibitive. We still offer charge accounts, even though the cost of money these days is sky high...and we are still available twenty-four hours a day, seven days a week handling emergencies." It was this commitment to service that had given community pharmacy its identity, and Dumouchel was convinced the new pharmacists could not only compete, but even thrive in the decade of the eighties.

Executive Committee Chairman John Johnson noted the progress the association continued to make since moving its headquarters to Washington, D.C. He noted that the NARD leadership was particularly concerned with providing management training for its members. Since that topic was so seriously neglected in pharmacy school course offerings, NARD had offered a number of management workshops in the past year and would continue to do so. He admitted the association had not been able to move the pharmacy crime bill along in Congress, but pledged "to do everything in our power to bring about a reduction in the exposure of pharmacists to armed robbery."

Executive Vice President Woods emphasized the problems of "government encroachment." He told the delegates "the biggest danger to our survival that has developed in the 1970s and stares us in the face in the 1980s is not the competition from chains or from supermarkets and general merchandisers. Our greatest enemy is the monstrous government encroachment in health care. The government dictates to us how much we should pay for products, what we charge for professional services, and what we can or cannot dispense."

Before leaving Atlanta, the delegates elected Jesse M. Pike, Sr. of Concord, North Carolina as president. John Johnson was re-elected chairman of the executive committee. Delegates also voted to increase the association's annual membership dues from $60 to $80.

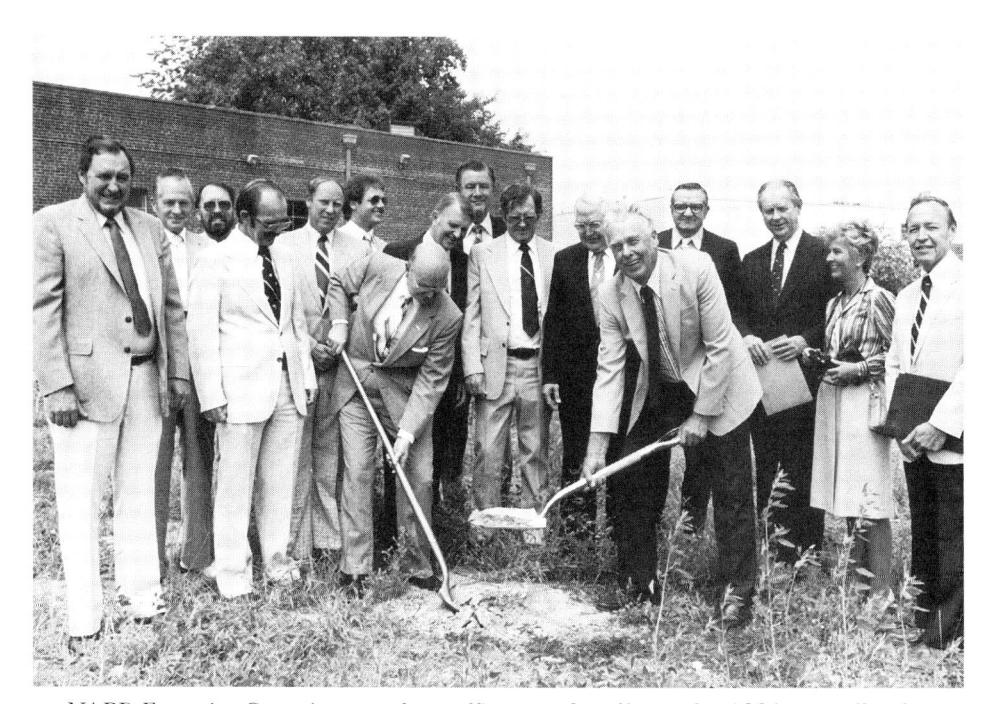

NARD Executive Committee members, officers, and staff attend a 1981 groundbreaking ceremony for the new NARD building in Alexandria, Virginia.

NARD began its eighty-third year preparing to look for a new home. Since moving to Washington, D.C. in 1977, the association had leased office space at 1750 K Street in the District of Columbia. However, the office staff had grown to some thirty members by 1981 and was in need of more space.

For a time the executive committee considered continuing the lease on the K Street space. Then property in Alexandria, Virginia became available, and the committee decided to buy rather than lease its new space. The lots at the intersection of Duke Street and Daingerfield Road in Alexandria had no building, and it would obviously take time to construct a new facility. But, executive committee members believed the long-term advantages outweighed the momentary inconveniences and approved the purchase (ultimately a very wise decision, given the soaring property values and build-up that occurred in that area during the next 20 years).

New staff in this year included John Rector who joined the association as Director of Government Affairs. Rector brought to the association an extensive background in drug issues as a former official of the Department of Justice as well as a long-time staffer and drug issues expert for Sen. Birch Bayh of Indiana. This background served the association well in the subsequent decades as NARD sought to overcome historic roadblocks in discriminatory pricing, physician dispensing, and mail order, among other issues. (Rector currently serves as general counsel to the association.)

Delegates for the eighty-third convention met in San Antonio in 1981. President Pike told the delegates about his efforts "to build better interprofessional bridges between doctors and ourselves." While he had some success, he acknowledged the task was more difficult than he had imagined and would need to be worked on over time. Part of the problem, he noted, was due to pharmacists not being in agreement on national goals. "It is difficult," he said, "to reach out to talk with doctors and dentists and others when there is so much divisiveness within pharmacy itself."

Pike also touted using a computer to the delegates. Although personal computing was still in its infancy, he said that he had "found the computer can not only increase your volume capability, (but also) can free up your time to allow you to render more, not less, personal service." Before leaving San Antonio, delegates elected Neil Pruitt of Toccoa, Georgia president and James Vincent as chairman of the executive committee.

In its eighty-third year the association's leadership continued to focus on the concept of "new." President Pruitt chose as his theme, "the New NARD." Whether "New Independent," the previous year's theme, or "New NARD," each represented efforts by Executive Vice President Woods and the executive committee to restructure NARD to attract and retain members.

New legislative initiatives were limited in 1982. Rep. John Paul Hammerschmidt of Arkansas introduced a bill (H.R. 3536) to permit veterans freedom of choice in selecting a pharmacy for their prescription drugs, and Rep. Hamilton Fish of New York sponsored H.R. 1571 to exempt pharmacists from antitrust laws when negotiating directly with third-party plan administrators. Neither of these proposals got beyond the "hearings" stage in Congress. For the most part, it was a year for watchful waiting on the legislative front and refining the association's internal structure.

Delegates to the eighty-fourth convention met in Boston in 1982. President Neil Pruitt told delegates that "giant chains are sweeping through this industry like a vacuum cleaner, sucking up hundreds of stores while the government stands idly by looking the other way." To combat this return to "merger mania," Pruitt urged community pharmacists to continue their emphasis on personal services and to monitor their merchandise selection. "Chains recognize," he said, that they "cannot compete with independents" in those areas. He reminded his listeners that the NARD leadership was working to remove governmental regulations wherever possible and to gain "estate tax exemptions and accelerated depreciation" so independent pharmacists would be in an even better position to compete.

Woods explained the association's efforts to effect legislation, particularly the "pharmacy crime bill," and to fend off efforts by HHS officials to modify various federal programs at pharmacy's expense. He also told delegates about his work as chairman of the Small Business Legislative Council

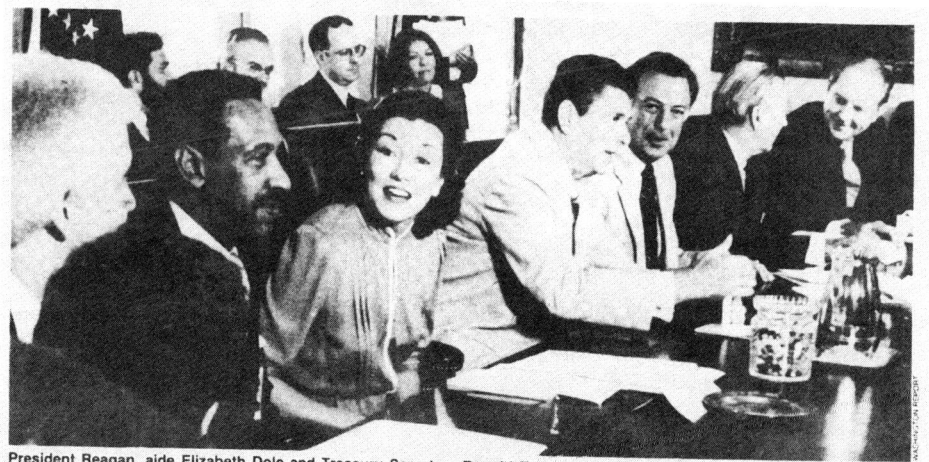

President Reagan, aide Elizabeth Dole and Treasury Secretary Donald Regan (second from right) met with small-business representatives who included, from far left, P.D. Hermann, Eugene Baker, William C. Burckhart and William E. Woods.

As chairman of the Small Business Legislative Council, NARD's Woods (far right) was invited to a briefing at the Reagan White House.

(SBLC) and the Joint Commission of Pharmacy Practitioners (JCPP). In both instances, he pushed for "tax reform for family-owned business" and less regulation "in third-party payment programs." He noted that the sharp downturn in the economy, which had lasted almost twenty-four months, had taken a heavy toll on community pharmacists.

Woods was also able to report that the headquarters staff moved into the new building in 1982. Located at 205 Daingerfield Road in Alexandria, the two-story brick building was the first permanent home for the association in its eighty-two year history. The concept of a permanent home for the association, first articulated more than 70 years previously, had finally been realized. And much of it was due to NARD officer and member contributions who helped swell the building fund established for this purpose.

Before leaving Boston, delegates elected John A. Johnson to be president; H. Joseph Schutte of Louisville, Kentucky was elected chairman of the executive committee. Delegates also created a new category of active membership to include "any registered pharmacist who managed an independent community pharmacy."

A few weeks before the Boston convention, the American public had become alarmed when the first product tampering of an over-the-counter (OTC)

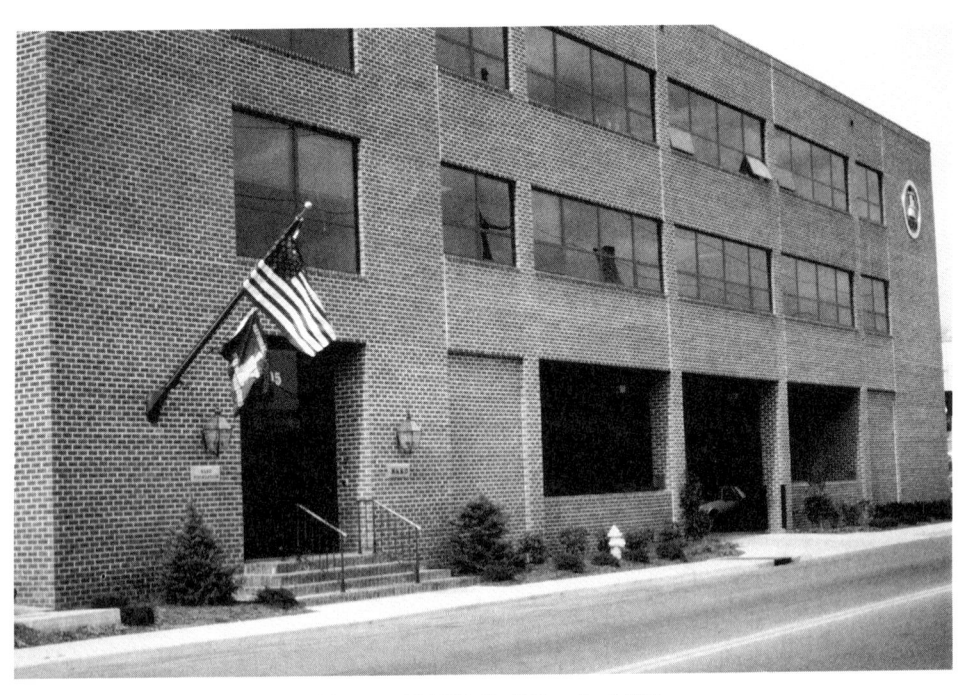

The new NARD Building in 1982

pain product was discovered in midwest supermarkets. Johnson & Johnson officials used the NARD convention to announce publicly for the first time that they were taking steps to produce tamper-resistant packaging. This one incident led to a widespread effort by all manufacturers to ensure product safety.

Public concern about product tampering continued for many months thereafter, and the NARD leadership played an active role in developing procedures to ensure product safety. The incident also gave them an opportunity to raise the point about OTCs being sold in "retail outlets far removed from pharmacy practice and the expert advice of a pharmacist." Chairman

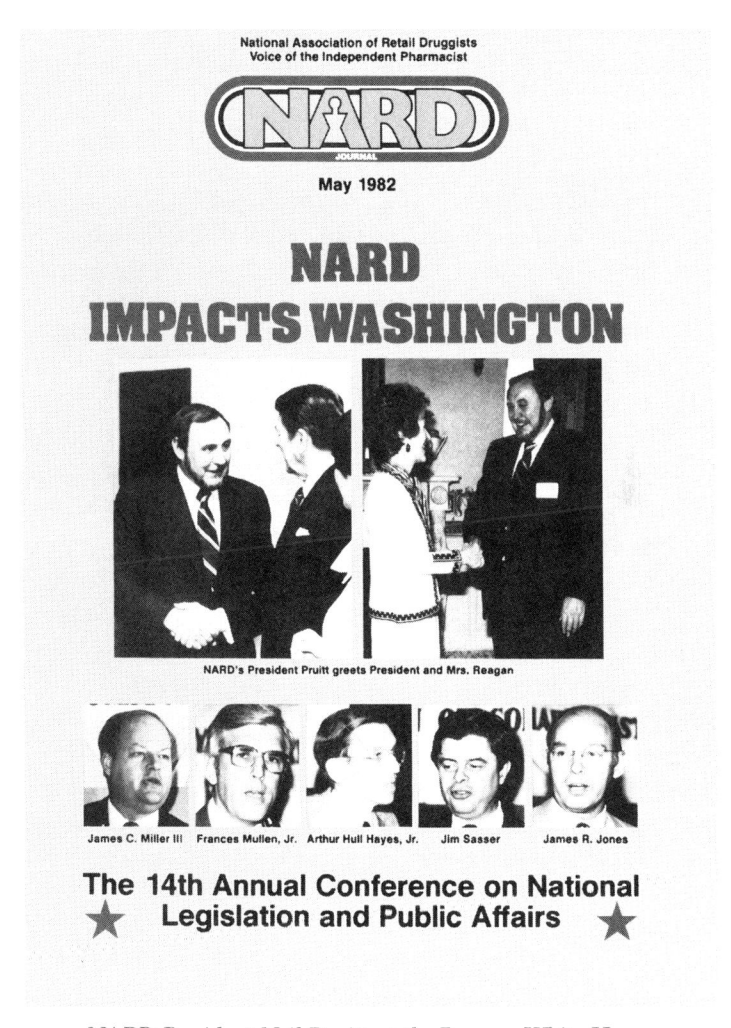

NARD President Neil Pruitt at the Reagan White House

Schutte pointed out that this problem had become more serious in recent years because of "the variety of former prescription medications now on the market as OTC products (and) all the safe packaging in the world won't protect the consumer as well as sound advice about how the drug should be used."

Moving into the new headquarters building provided more space and an opportunity for the association to offer new services. For example, the executive committee authorized Woods to create a new department to assist members wanting to enter or expand their activities in home health care business. This Home Health Care and Nursing Home Services Department was another indication of the changing nature of community pharmacy. Largely unknown just a decade ago, the industry had grown to a multibillion dollar business by the 1980s and was projected to double by the turn of the century.

Delegates to the eighty-fifth convention met in Las Vegas, Nevada in 1983. President Johnson emphasized the professional side of pharmacy in his address to convention attendees. It was commitment to honesty, integrity, and customer service that made it possible for community pharmacists to compete with the corporate chains and supermarkets. He said these qualities "were the cornerstones of independent retail pharmacy. Mass merchandisers and deep discounters in this business may not care or believe in quality service. Independents, however, do care because we deal with our customers on a day-to-day basis."

Johnson also suggested that the time was ripe for a "fair and equitable" reimbursement plan for third-party programs, including vouchers to expedite payments to pharmacists participating in the Medicaid program. "It is time to do away with conventional wisdom of the programs," he said. "You can drop them and go out of business quickly...or keep them and go out of business slowly. NARD's direct payment or voucher plan must become the law of the land."

Woods emphasized the association's involvement in the legislative process. He noted that in the past Congress — eight bills in the House and five in the Senate — were introduced with support from NARD. Each was still alive, said Woods, and he was confident they would become law. But to ensure that eventuality, he called upon the delegates to continue their "advocacy for the just causes of the independent. It is important to us that you support the various stances we take on your behalf."

Woods also talked about the new building and noted that it was "part of a broader agenda" to expand the association's services. One of those new areas was home health care. "We are the only pharmacy association," he said, "to have a home health care department, and we have been singled out by the national media for leadership in this area." Before leaving Las Vegas, delegates elected James Vincent of Yuma, Colorado president; H. Joseph Schutte was re-elected chairman of the executive committee. Health affairs writer and editor Todd Dankmyer was also named editor of the *NARD Journal* — a position he holds to this day.

NARD's eighty-sixth year proved to be a time of great success. The economy began to recover from its two-year recession at the beginning of the decade. Independent pharmacy sales increased eight percent on average, according to the *Lilly Digest,* and the leadership introduced new programs that were highly popular. Perhaps the one most talked about was Patient Information Leaflets (PILS), an NARD-sponsored alternative to the PPI program attempted by HHS officials. Unlike PPI, the PIL program was voluntary, and the information was prepared by experts of NARD's choosing. The leaflets proved highly popular with the membership, with more than 3 million having been distributed in the first year and another 5 million in print.

Success of a sort also came from a confrontation with the FDA. When the FDA proposed to switch to OTC status certain drugs formerly sold by prescription only, NARD objected to the lack of safeguards to protect the public. The agency at first ignored the association, but then NARD circulated two "citizen petitions" calling upon FDA to authorize OTC use for these drugs in a "pharmacist legend" category that would restrict the sale of these recently switched products to pharmacies only. The association urged the agency to include a label telling consumers to "consult your pharmacist" to ensure safe and proper use. The FDA did not embrace the NARD policy, but the petitions received widespread publicity and gave a boost to NARD's image of being on the side of the public when it came to ensuring safe medicine use.

Another reason for optimism was the major legislative victory NARD earned when Congress passed the "Pharmacy Crime Bill" (Controlled Substance Registrant or Pharmacist Protection Act). NARD leadership began lobbying for the bill in the early 1970s. However, opposition from the Drug Enforcement Administration (DEA) killed NARD-sponsored bills in 1970 and again in 1973. Association officials persisted. In a decade-long campaign, using the pages of the *Journal* to call attention to the growing number of drugstore robberies, subtly briefing lawmakers at the annual Legislative Conference, and enlisting store owners from throughout the nation to testify about the experience of being robbed or burglarized, NARD began to gain the upper hand.

When pharmacy crimes reached 11,786 in 1979, the *Journal* began printing a "pharmacy crime clock." From figures supplied by the Justice Department, the *Journal* showed that one in five robberies resulted in death or injury to victims, statistics that strongly disputed testimony of Justice officials.

By 1982 the weight of cumulative evidence began to have its effect. Iowa Senator Charles E. Grassley, after attending the association's Legislative Conference that year, introduced the NARD bill in the ninety-first Congress. Several House members, including Henry Waxman of California, Tom Luken of Ohio, and Tom Bliley of Virginia, supported the bill, and it began a tortuous path through the legislative process — a journey that took two years. Opposition from Justice's Drug Enforcement Administration (DEA) continued, but this time NARD's careful cultivation of key legislative officials paid off and the bill passed with ease. President Ronald Reagan signed P.L. 98-305 May 31, 1984.

According to NARD Legal Counsel John Rector, persistence on the "crime bill" re-established NARD as a political force in Washington. It convinced many legislators that the association would not give up, even in face of opposition. But to achieve such a victory, he said, community pharmacists "had to stay focused and take a building-block approach toward the legislative process."

NARD's eighty-sixth convention met in Miami Beach, Florida in 1984. President Vincent called the meeting to order and told the delegates it had been "a banner year for independent pharmacists." He used the convention's theme "Success — Go For It" to review the legislative success on the crime bill and noted the economic growth community pharmacists had experienced in the past year.

Vincent also called attention to other issues that still needed resolution, particularly mail order prescriptions and physician dispensing. With respect to mail order, he said, "I was on a panel...with a labor union representative who was telling his audience that mail order prescriptions were the greatest thing since sliced bread." Before that session was over, Vincent was able to convince that union leader the mail order system may not best serve his clients, but the NARD leader noted that there was a great deal of work to do to convince others.

With respect to physician dispensing, Vincent called attention to a drug distributor who did a national mailing "to all family physicians" promising them "$15,000 to $30,000 with no additional work" if they would dispense medications from their offices. He urged the delegates to make contact with their wholesalers and manufacturers to let them know of NARD's strong opposition to such a practice.

Executive Vice President Woods continued the upbeat tempo of the convention by recounting the legislative victory on the crime bill and the introduction of new services for the membership. He also informed the delegates about the association's special efforts to enlist state leaders to lobby for legislation endorsed by NARD.

In response to member requests, the association was formally adopting the title Doctor of Pharmacy (PD) for all practicing pharmacists, said Woods. He noted that academic leaders had been slow to respond to NARD on this issue, but twenty-two state associations had already accepted the association's recommendation on the title. Before adjourning their eighty-sixth convention, delegates elected John W. White of Tallahassee, Florida as president; Charles M. West, of Little Rock, Arkansas was elected chairman of the executive committee.

The association's eighty-seventh year got off to a rocky start. Two weeks after the Miami convention, a majority of the executive committee met in Kansas City to discuss Executive Vice President William Woods's job performance. NARD had made significant gains under his leadership, particularly in services to members and support for new opportunities in pharmacy, such as home health care. The headquarters staff had been greatly expanded, and the budget had increased four-fold to $4 million. However, Woods's volatile, confrontational management style had become a disruptive force both in the central office and among the executive committee members. NARD's relationship with other pharmacy organizations had also deteriorated due in part to the executive vice president's poor relationship with the other association executives.

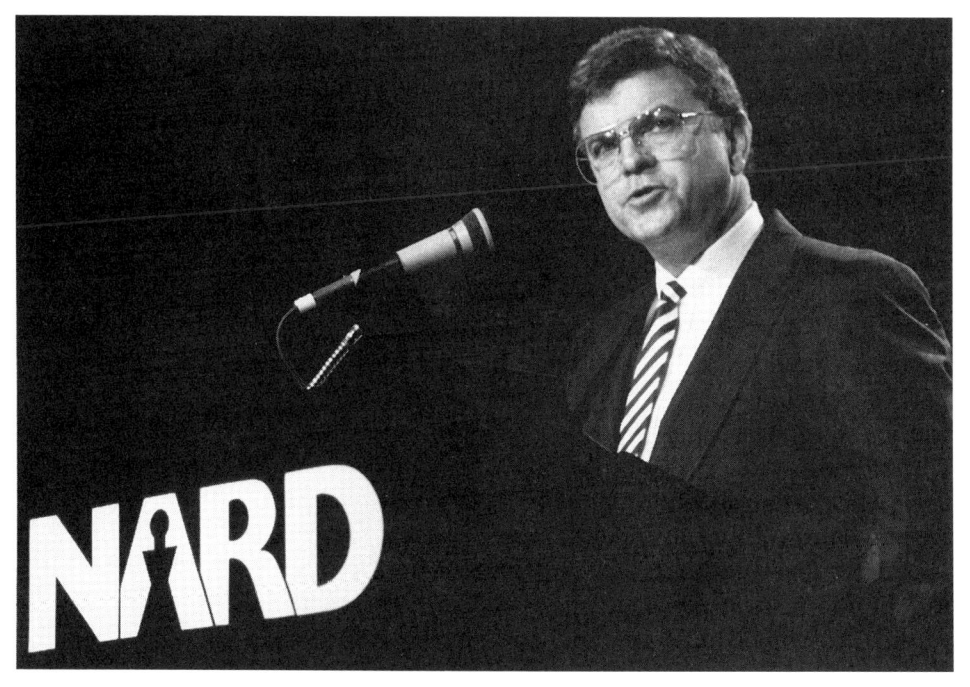

NARD Executive Vice President Charles M. West, 1984 – 1996

After much discussion, executive committee members reached a decision that Woods should be replaced. Chairman Charles West then called a special meeting of the full executive committee. Members came together at the Alexandria office on October 23, 1984, and voted unanimously to make the change. West, in fulfilling his duties as chairman of the executive committee, became interim executive vice president. Six weeks later, the executive committee made the appointment permanent. Committee members also chose Lonnie Hollingsworth of Lubbock, Texas to replace West as chairman.

A graduate of the University of Arkansas College of Pharmacy, West owned a pharmacy in Little Rock and was serving his ninth year as executive vice president of the Arkansas Pharmaceutical Association. He was the first NARD executive officer to have state association experience. Secretaries Thomas Wooten and Thomas Potts had both managed "city drug associations," but did not have statewide responsibilities. West brought what one pharmaceutical executive called "a sense of practicality and common sense to NARD that is somehow lacking...in virtually all who reside inside the beltway."

West had hardly settled into the executive vice president's office before an economic crisis erupted. Officials at HHS proposed to reduce Medicaid payments to pharmacists. Their decision was based on a price survey conducted by the Office of the Inspector General (OIG) in 1983. The survey identified what OIG officials interpreted as a "discrepancy" between pharmacists' Actual Acquisition Costs (AAC), and the Average Wholesale Price (AWP) as identified in the collected data.

West and NARD leaders argued that the difference between the AAC and AWP was an "earned discount." Pharmacists only received it if, by prior agreement, the wholesaler was willing to grant special incentives for such practices as buying in volume and/or paying invoices in a timely manner. This was simply good business, and the pharmacist should not be penalized for his or her initiative. Prior to the survey, Medicaid reimbursement to pharmacists had been based on the AWP plus a professional dispensing fee. NARD leaders wanted to preserve AWP.

OIG representatives saw the issue differently. They suggested that the cost after discount was in reality the Average Wholesale Price and recommended that Medicaid payments be based on that figure. Officials at HHS referred the recommendation to the Health Care Financing Administration (HCFA). After debating the issues much of 1984, HCFA officials in HHS's Region VI (the Southwest) decided to establish Actual Acquisition Cost (AAC) as the basis for Medicaid reimbursement and to implement the new policy July 1, 1985.

West charged that HCFA was attempting to "confiscate" pharmacists' earned discounts. "The OIG report ignores the fact that discounts are part of the profit structure and that such discounts are based on both private patient business and Medicaid business," he said. "Through its focus on only one component of the Medicaid program, the OIG and proponents of its recommendations can only yield uneven and unfair results." Accompanied by John Rector, he traveled to Dallas in December to meet with state pharmacy leaders in Region VI (Arkansas, Louisiana, Texas, Oklahoma, and New Mexico). In short order, that group developed a strategy to oppose the HCFA policy and implemented the "telephone alert" system to mobilize pharmacists' support.

Returning to Washington, West, Rector, and members of the executive committee enlisted support from the chain drugstores, the wholesale association, and APhA to assist in lobbying Congress. West also placed the issue prominently on the annual Legislative Conference agenda for May. Publicity generated from the conference, part of which was broadcast on C-SPAN cable network, led HCFA officials to delay and finally abandon the proposed policy. Pharmacists were able to keep the Average Wholesale Price (AWP) plus a professional fee as the reimbursement formula under Medicaid and thus keep their "earned discount."

In April 1985, West traveled to Boca Raton, Florida, for the annual meeting of the Pharmaceutical Manufacturers Association. In a speech that would resonate for more than a decade, he urged the manufacturers to abandon their discriminatory pricing practices and adopt single price policies for all competitors in the retail pharmacy marketplace. "We'll all be winners," said West, "manufacturers, pharmacists, and consumers." The manufacturers failed to heed that common sense advice, and the battle over pricing was again joined.

Delegates to the eighty-seventh convention met in New York City, New York in 1985. President White used the meeting's theme, "Accepting the Challenge," to tell delegates "the corner drugstore has grown up — because it had to given the intense competition that has grown up around it." To support that statement he called attention to a report released within the year by a leading trade magazine. That survey revealed that "the typical independent continues to be ahead of the chains" in all the major categories: number of prescriptions, new prescriptions, dollar volume per prescription, prescriptions per store, and in third-party prescriptions. That report also showed that community pharmacists dispensed over 80 percent of all Medicaid prescriptions.

As White noted, community pharmacy had been able to accept the challenge through efficient business practices that changed with the times. He highlighted the emergence of "Pharmacy Services Administrative Organizations (PSAOs)" — a term coined by NARD to describe the growing number of state and local networks of neighborhood pharmacists who were aligning to compete for third-party contracts in the still nascent managed care marketplace. White also noted the continued gains being made by pharmacists in the home health care market. "The service component is what makes independent retail pharmacy truly unique," he said, and he urged his colleagues to use the services provided by the association to better serve their customers.

Executive Vice President West reviewed the association's confrontation with HFCA over AWP in the Medicaid program. He estimated that NARD's victory on that issue would save pharmacists $128 million annually in Region VI alone. West also alerted delegates to new attempts to plug loopholes in the Robinson-Patman Act. He was particularly bothered by the problem of "drug diversion," whereby nonprofit hospitals increased their drug orders "under special hospital prices," then sold the surplus drugs to a broker. West said this was "unfair competition," and the NARD leadership planned to put a stop to it if they could. Before adjourning the convention, delegates elected H. Joseph Schutte president; Darwyn J. Williams of Webster City, Iowa was elected to chair the executive committee.

For much of its eighty-seventh year the NARD leadership planted the "seeds of legislation" and waited for them to produce. The typical issues of price discrimination, mail order, physician dispensing, and Medicaid/Medicare reimbursement continued to dominate the association's legislative agenda.

NARD's leadership in the PSAO movement accelerated. NARD hosted a PSAO conference in Kansas City, Missouri, attended by more than two hundred pharmacy leaders. The meeting targeted antitrust concerns and how best to legally organize and market pharmacy services to the growing array of employers, insurers, and other third parties now beginning to contract with PSAOs and other pharmacy entities.

A new computer software package, "The NARD Scriptwriter," was introduced for members. This program enabled small independent pharmacies to computerize without significant expense.

Delegates to the eighty-eighth convention met at Louisville in 1986. President Schutte reviewed the status of the agenda items on discriminatory pricing, mail order, and physician dispensing. On mail order, Schutte had a tragic anecdote to relate. An elderly patient was given the wrong medication on a mail order refill from the largest mail order company in the nation. As a result of that mix-up, the patient died.

An investigation of the incident revealed that the patient was taking four times the maximum recommended dosage. Schutte said, "Mail order dispensing, in which little or no drug therapy monitoring can be effected, represents a public health concern that must be addressed in legislative and regulatory forums." Before leaving the convention, delegates elected Lonnie Hollingsworth of Lubbock president; Donald W. Arthur of Tonawanda, New York was elected chairman of the executive committee.

The association leadership set "marketplace pricing" as its primary goal for the new year. In practice this meant continuing an aggressive relationship with HCFA over Medicaid pricing and renewing efforts to plug the loopholes in the Robinson-Patman Act.

To assist in the membership services area, West received approval from the executive committee to organize the Department of State Relations in

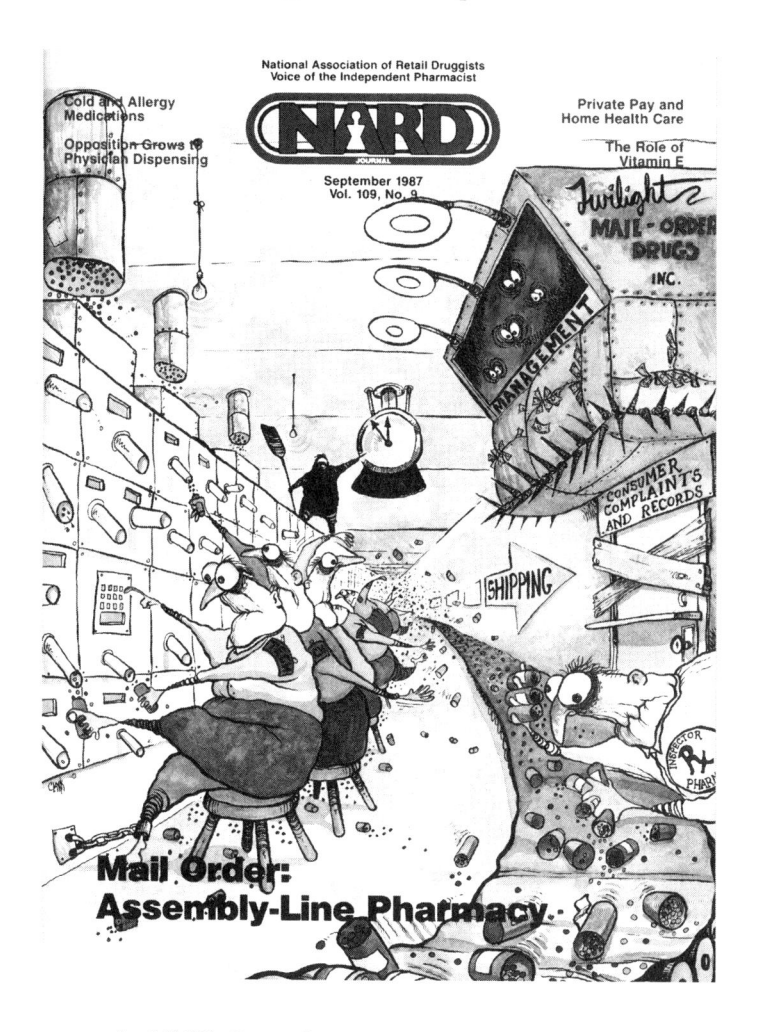

An NARD Journal view of mail order in the 1980s

the headquarters office. The initial focus of this new office was to promote an "affiliation program" between NARD and the respective state associations. This program was immediately successful. Nearly all of the state associations affiliated with NARD within months.

West also reorganized the headquarters staff to "departmentalize" the various services. Under Woods's administration all employees reported to the executive vice president. The new structure established department heads with line responsibilities for staff in their respective areas. Only the department heads reported to the executive vice president.

West also launched a new initiative to organize NARD student chapters at the various colleges of pharmacy. The focus of this program was to provide career guidance to pharmacy students and to encourage them to enter the world of independent pharmacy upon graduation. Too often, West said, "students have been steered toward 'safer,' low-risk positions on the payrolls of organizations. We want to instill student pharmacists with NARD's positive 'can do' attitude."

Delegates to the eighty-ninth convention met in Las Vegas in 1987. President Hollingsworth told the delegates about a series of new services developed in the preceding year to help community pharmacists remain competitive. These included Business Information Central, which was designed to help members with store management, customer relations, and expanding their product line. He also highlighted the work of the National Center for Independent Retail Pharmacy, which was issuing a new "Keys to Success" learning module, and the continued popularity of the PILS program.

Hollingsworth reminded his listeners that "twenty years ago, Dr. James Goddard, then the FDA commissioner, had the chutzpah to stand at a lectern like this one and predict the demise of independent retail pharmacy." Not only had that not happened, he said, but independent pharmacy was in an even stronger position than it was in the 1960s.

The association was also prepared to launch the Independent Pharmacy Matching Service, "designed to match graduating students with employers in independent pharmacies across the nation," said Hollingsworth. To further assist students, he announced that beginning in May 1988 graduating pharmacy students would be given six months of free membership in NARD.

The House of Delegates also voted to change the association's name. Younger members were bothered by "druggist" in the title and felt a need for change. After lengthy discussion, delegates agreed to drop the full name, National Association for Retail Druggists, in favor of the shorter acronym, NARD. As incoming President Darwyn Williams noted, the change "is the best kind of compromise. It enables us both to maintain that which is synony-

CHAPTER TEN — THE NINTH DECADE: 1979 – 1988   217

mous with our eighty-nine year tradition of service...and be responsive as well to the growing numbers in our profession for whom the word pharmacist most accurately reflects their role and stature."

Before leaving Las Vegas delegates elected Darwyn J. Williams of Webster City, Iowa as president; Joseph Mosso of Latrobe, Pennsylvania was elected chairman of the executive committee.

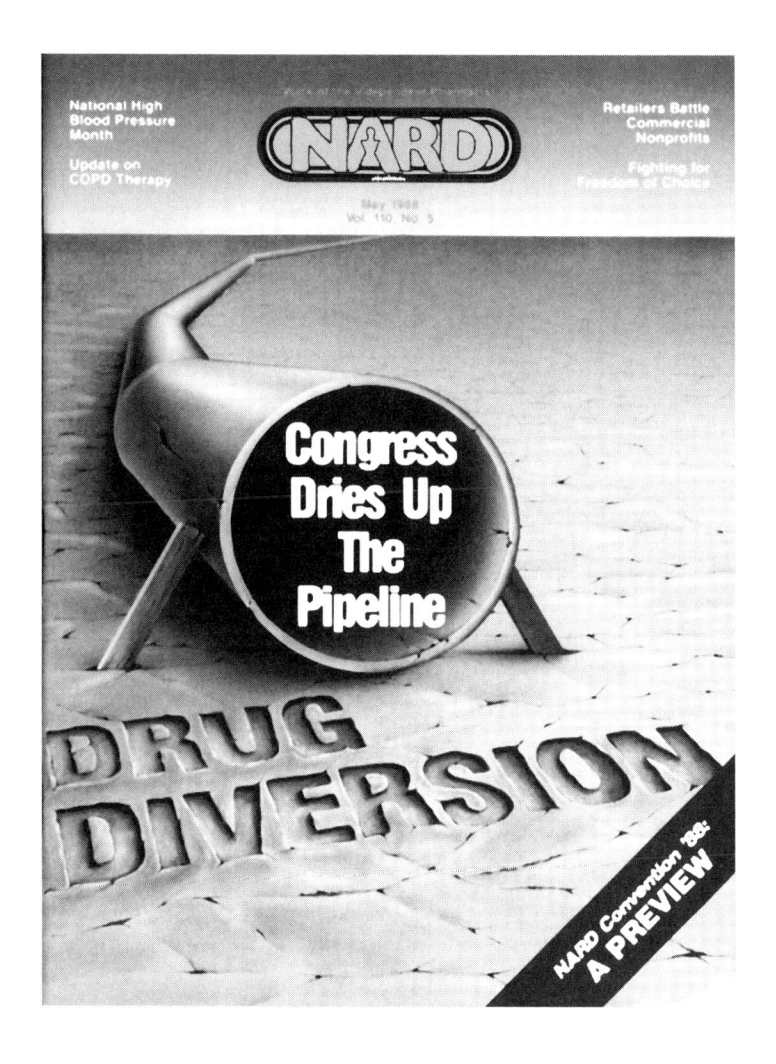

The last year of NARD's ninth decade saw major legislative successes reminiscent of the 1930s. A few short months before NARD's ninety anniversary in October 1988, a major victory was achieved in the association's war on drug diversion. Congress passed the Prescription Drug Marketing Act, introduced in the Senate by Spark Matsunaga of Hawaii as companion legislation to Michigan Representative John Dingell's bill (H.R. 1207), which had passed the House in spring 1987.

The bill was designed to stop "illegal prescription drug diversion," a practice that had grown progressively worse since 1938. In that year, Congress passed the Nonprofit Institutions Act, which permitted charitable nonprofit organizations to purchase drugs and other products at discount prices. The law was intended to benefit "pauper's hospitals" and similar charitable institutions.

However, over the years, numerous nonprofit hospitals began buying charity-priced prescription drugs in excess of their needs. The surplus was then sold, diverted, to individuals or groups for resale at inflated prices. To NARD leaders this practice violated the spirit of the original legislation, and in early 1984, they called the matter to the attention of several in Congress. Rep. Dingell, chairman of the House Energy and Commerce Oversight and Investigations Subcommittee, began hearings on the matter at NARD's urging. In short order he discovered an "extensive underground network of racketeering and conspiracy of counterfeit drugs" using the nonprofit loophole.

With information developed from the hearings, Dingell introduced legislation to prohibit "the resale of drugs and other products purchased by nonprofit institutions at discriminatory prices," the "re-importation of U.S. drugs shipped overseas," and the "resale of drug samples." The bill also would "require drug wholesalers to provide detailed records of the source of all drugs they purchased or sold."

Despite overwhelming evidence of how "drug diversion" hurt fair trade and abused the retail market, Dingell had trouble getting his bill out of committee and scheduled for a vote. It was only when Sen. Matsunaga introduced identical legislation in the Senate that the bill moved forward. After almost four years of hearings and debate, the Dingell-Matsunaga bill finally became law.

Following close on the heels of the drug diversion bill, Congress also passed the Medicare Catastrophic Coverage law in May. This legislation, too, was the product of an extended and intensive lobbying effort on the part of West, Rector, and their NARD colleagues. While broad in its coverage, the bill in its final form called for Medicare to cover "outpatient prescription drugs for catastrophic illness." It also "established a formula for reimbursing pharmacists" in the text of the bill, including indexing the pharmacist's dispensing fee to the Consumer Price Index. For the first time since Medicare was established, the program received funding to cover the costs of outpatient drugs.

NARD won still another "victory" with a Freedom of Information suit against the Federal Trade Commission (FTC). The issue involved the executive committee's attempt to find information about physicians who were selling drugs to patients for profit. In the late 1970s, NARD leaders worked with the FTC to develop information on "physician dispensing" of prescription medication. However, in the 1980s, FTC officials not only ceased to investigate in this area, they intervened in a number of states to block attempts by local legislators to regulate physician dispensing.

West and members of the executive committee wanted to know why the FTC had changed its policy and why these officials were not using data already compiled to limit physician dispensing practices. FTC refused all requests for its files on physician dispensing, and NARD filed suit forcing the agency to release the records.

Association leaders then used that information to develop a new bill, introduced by Rep. Ron Wyden of Oregon, to prohibit physicians from dis-

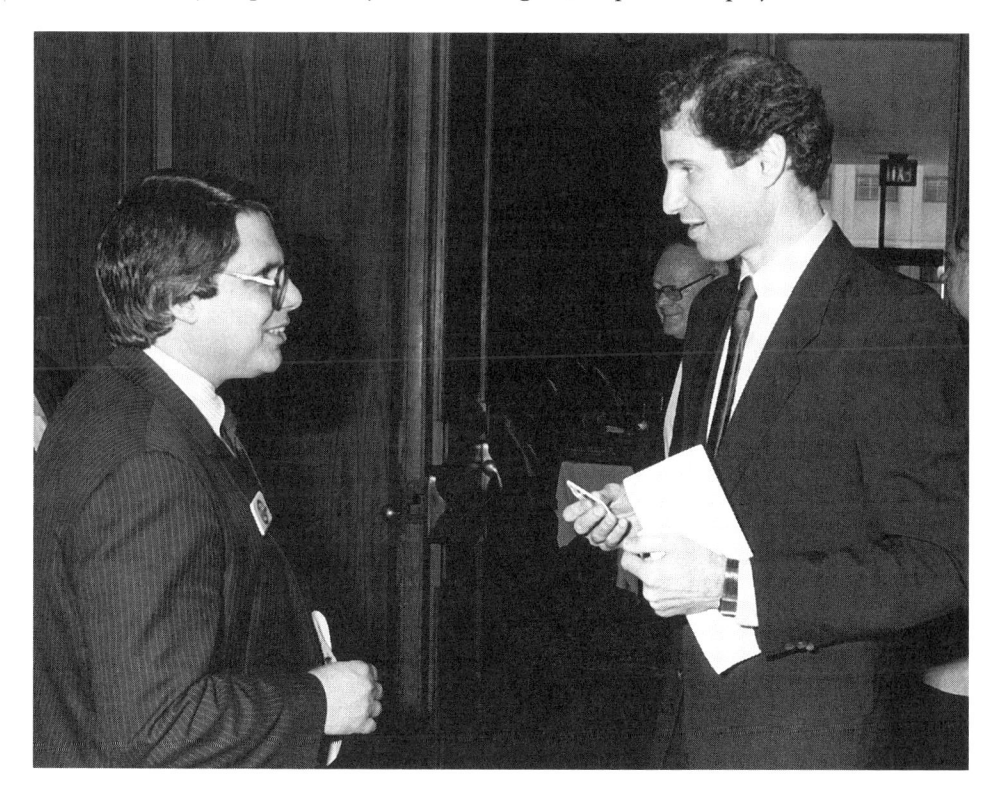

NARD's General Counsel John Rector (left) discusses physician dispensing bill with its sponsor, Oregon Rep. Ron Wyden.

pensing prescriptions for profit. The association also launched a two-year public relations campaign exposing physician dispensing as both anticompetitive and as jeopardizing the essential checks and balances that are preserved when physicians prescribe and pharmacists dispense medicines. The bill ultimately did not pass, but the growth of physician dispensing was effectively stopped in its tracks.

Given these high profile successes, delegates to the ninetieth convention in Atlanta in 1988 were in a enthusiastic mood. President Williams said, "my presidential year witnessed the ultimate ascendance of the nation's pharmacists." He was referring not only to the legislative accomplishments, but also to a recent Gallup Poll that identified pharmacy as "the most respected and ethical among all professions." It had been a long climb from the late 1950s when Senator Kefauver's investigation into drug pricing cast a great shadow of disrepute over pharmacy.

Williams also reminded delegates that the public's expression of confidence was due in large part to the independent's commitment to patient counseling, and he encouraged his colleagues to keep up the good work. "If you are now counseling thirty percent of your customers," he said, "step up that number to forty. If it's already forty, make it fifty percent. I don't think it is possible to counsel your patients too much. Consumers everywhere are starving for good service."

Executive Vice President West reviewed the successful legislative year and also noted that NARD had made important gains in other areas. Among these was the launch of The Prescription Network (RxNET), a for-profit subsidiary established to help PSAOs compete for national and regional contracts for pharmacy services. The NARD Management Institute was another service for which the membership could be proud. After the Institute was approved, West hired Dr. D.C. Huffman, a pharmacy administration expert at the University of Tennessee, to head the program. A new newsletter for the association's student chapters was also introduced. But the key to continued success, West said, was to remember the convention theme "Independents '88: Winning Together. That's how we ultimately will prevail over those who would take away our patients."

NARD finished its ninth decade in a strong position. The legislative victories paid dividends for years to come. The vote of confidence in public opinion polls gave the association's strong lobbying efforts even more ammunition for its regular bouts with Congress. The executive committee also used this time to do strategic planning and prepared a ten-year plan outlining priorities and strategies for achieving those objectives. Thus, the association entered its centennial decade with a well-designed plan for meeting the needs of its members and the American public.

Chapter Eleven

The Centennial Decade: 1989 – 1998

Community Pharmacists Tackle the New Marketplace

NARD entered its tenth decade with a strong feeling of optimism. Membership had increased for the third year in a row. The ninetieth convention had sold a record amount of exhibit space; contributions to the organization's political action committee, National Association of Pharmacists Political Action Committee (NAPPAC), reached an all-time high; advertising in the *NARD Journal* exceeded $1 million for the first time; and the association's budget exceeded $5 million. Moreover, the political successes of the previous year provided a solid basis on which to build in the coming decade.

The NARD leadership had also adopted a long-range strategic plan for the organization. Among other things, the plan called for increased attention to discriminatory pricing, the growing number of prescriptions being sold through mail order, the emergence of "managed care" programs, and the "exceptional number of mergers" that were affecting the entire pharmaceutical industry, including community pharmacy. Rather than take on all of these issues at one time, the executive committee studied each issue carefully with respect to how and when the issue in question should be made a priority.

Cost containment was the common denominator for each issue in the association's strategic plan. Since the inception of Medicaid/Medicare in the 1960s, the federal government and private insurers had been seeking ways to limit costs. By the 1980s new third parties had joined in the search for profits from the government-subsidized health programs. Health care providers, secured by federal underwriting and pressed by a decade-long cycle of inflation, raised prices for their products and services at a rapid rate. This revolution in medical costs forced Corporate America and others to look for new ways to control how much they paid for health care coverage for their clients and employees.

The cost of prescription drugs quickly became a central issue in the search for cost containment in the health arena. After remaining fairly stable for almost two decades, drugs in several categories began to rise rapidly in the 1980s. It was at this juncture that the NARD leadership chose to begin its new legislative assault on discriminatory pricing.

The discriminatory pricing issue reached a crescendo in 1989 when it was given top billing at NARD's twenty-first Annual Conference on National Legislation and Public Affairs. As Executive Vice President West declared to loud applause from meeting attendees, "this year's target issues are discriminatory pricing, discriminatory pricing, and discriminatory pricing." President Donald Arthur said that "discriminatory pricing represents the most serious and far-reaching problem, both in terms of fair competition and public health and welfare, facing the pharmacy profession today.... NARD's awareness of the problem is acute, as is its resolve to solve it.... What we want is equal access to prices."

This rallying cry found receptive ears in Congress. At NARD's urging, Senator David Pryor of Arkansas, chairman of the Senate Special Committee on Aging, announced at the Legislative Conference that he would hold hearings that summer "to examine prescription drug prices and discriminatory pricing." Sen. Pryor acknowledged that NARD would be a star witness at the hearings because, in speaking to the pharmacy leaders, "we feel that you are out there on a daily basis in the trenches; you're the ones who have to be on the front line trying to explain these cost increases to these people. They do not understand them, I don't understand them, and the Congress does not understand them. But it's you who bear the brunt of this discriminatory process."

The glare of the public spotlight was turned on the issue on July 18, 1989. In large measure, NARD served as the stage manager, whetting the interests of national radio-TV-newspaper media whose cameras and reporters documented the Senate Special Committee on Aging's first hearing examining prescription drug prices. (For the better part of a decade, NARD officers and staff had skillfully developed mass media interest in the pricing disparities and other marketplace challenges facing the independent. Time and again, it proved to be commonplace to read about these challenges in such prestigious newspapers as the *New York Times* and *Wall Street Journal* or to see them dramatized on network TV newscasts.)

More than 200 people crowded into Room 628 of the Dirksen Senate Office Building for the Pryor hearing, while another 500 politicos waited in the nearby Russell Senate Office Building for a chance to get into the hearing. Although many of the observers had to sit on windowsills, stand in the aisles, or crane to hear from the doorway of the hearing room, few left during the five-and-a-half-hour session. The attendees heard a riveting story about the insidious effects of price discrimination on America's health care system.

CHAPTER ELEVEN — THE CENTENNIAL DECADE: 1989 – 1998   223

For his part, Sen. Pryor dispelled any of the remnants of the odious Kefauver-type debate of the 1960s. At every opportunity he made it clear that the community pharmacist was not to blame for rising drug prices. Pryor had invited nineteen of the leading pharmaceutical manufacturers to testify. Only one, Amgen Inc., accepted the invitation. Lacking industry input, the senator turned to NARD's West and General Counsel John Rector for expert testimony. Pryor's inquiry revealed from one New York investment firm that since the late 1970s, "but most noticeably in the last three years, pricing has become the major force in generating revenue growth" for the drug companies. Between 1986 and 1988, Pryor noted that eleven of the top drug manufacturers had an "average stock earnings record better than 78 percent" of other American manufacturers.

Drug companies frequently blamed their high product costs on the time and expense involved in researching and developing new drugs. However, Pryor noted that over two-thirds of the new drugs brought on the market in the 1980s represented copies or enhancements of existing formulas, so-called "me too" drugs, and made little or no contribution to "new therapies." At the same time these companies were receiving "tax breaks well in excess of $1

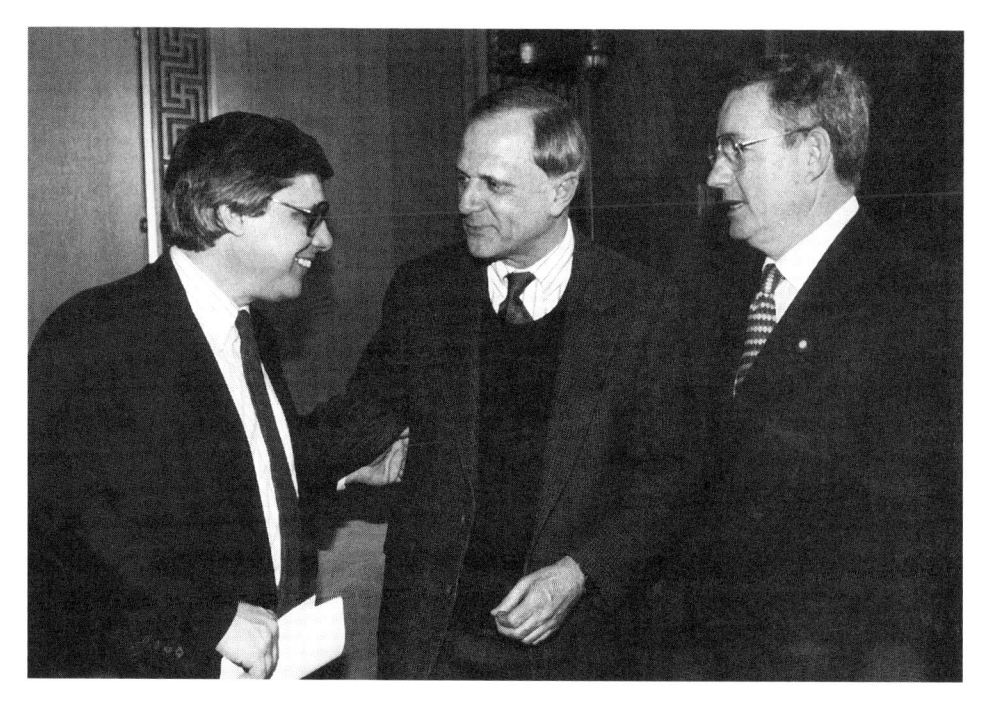

NARD's John Rector, Sen. David Pryor, and NARD's Calvin Anthony confer during a break in the discriminatory pricing hearings.

billion." Finally, the senator noted that another factor in high prescription prices may be due to "who you are and what deal you can strike with the manufacturer." He stated that "hospitals and the Department of Veterans Affairs get the best price," sometimes as little as one/one hundredth of what the community pharmacists paid. "The public buying at community pharmacies" he said, "gets the worst prices, because the pharmacies have to pay high prices, too." The Pryor hearings led to congressional legislation the following year.

Third-party programs were another issue NARD challenged in 1989. With almost forty percent of all prescriptions being paid for by third parties, the matter had enormous implications for pharmacy. To assist community pharmacists in evaluating third parties and other store operations issues, the NARD leadership, through its Management Institute, developed a "cost to dispense analysis" for prescription drugs, which provided a basic formula for pharmacists to use in evaluating the pros and cons of various third-party programs.

A potentially huge third-party program, outpatient prescription drug coverage for seniors under Medicare, went by the boards in 1989 — only one year after congressional passage. Seniors railed against perceived discrimination in the financing of the new benefit, and Congress was forced to repeal

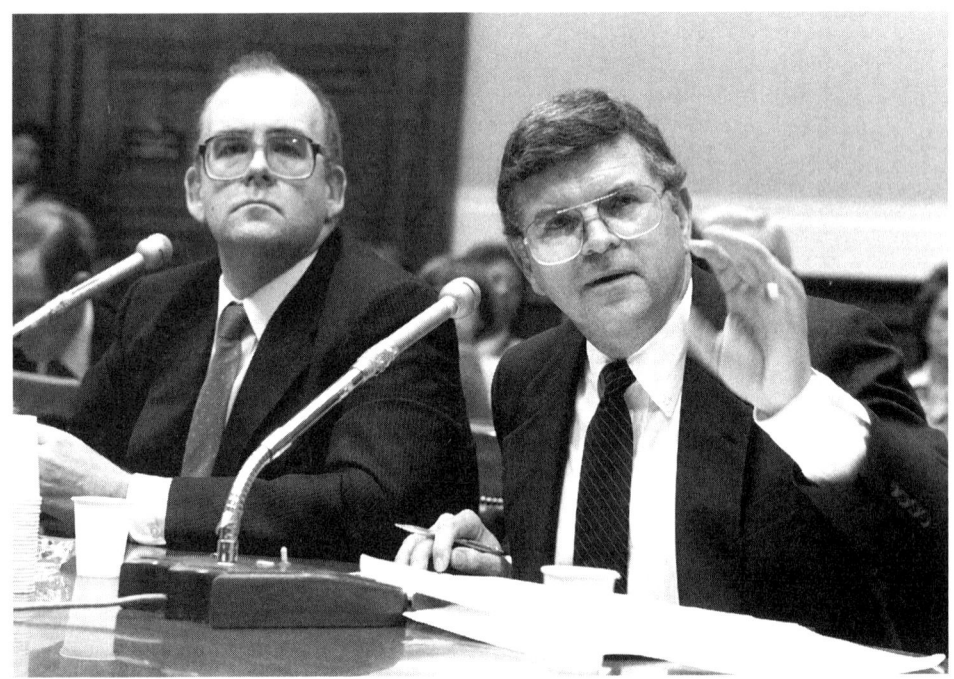

NARD's Charles M. West testified frequently in congressional hearings on key association issues during the 1990s.

the law before it went into effect. The ninety-first convention was held in San Antonio, Texas in 1989. President Donald Arthur used the convention theme, "Independents '89: Shaping Pharmacy's Future," to encourage pharmacists to get involved in political and community affairs as well as the practice of pharmacy. Noting that current figures indicated about 70 licensed pharmacists per 100,000 population, he said that it was "impossible to tell how many were actually practicing." However, he estimated that many were not and that was "causing a reduction of hours and even closing of some pharmacies."

A community pharmacy forced to reduce its store hours obviously played into the hands of the chain and supermarket drug stores. Arthur said part of planning for the future involved knowing basic data such as the demographics of the pool of pharmacists. To better understand that phenomenon, he told the delegates that NARD had joined with other national pharmacy groups to do a "comprehensive study of pharmacist supply and demand." Data from that survey also allowed the NARD leadership to study the "impact of women in pharmacy." With women making up sixty percent of pharmacy school enrollments, Arthur said the association "must make plans now that will enable us to adapt successfully to the changing demographics of our profession." Delegates elected Joseph Mosso, of Latrobe, Pennsylvania president; Calvin J. Anthony of Stillwater, Oklahoma was chosen chairman of the executive committee.

In the new year, the NARD leadership continued to focus the association's legislative initiatives on discriminatory pricing and third-party programs. With respect to membership services, the Management Institute maintained a strong presence with lead articles in the *Journal* and workshops that provided continuing education training on a variety of issues.

The executive committee also prosecuted the issue of "freedom of choice" — preserving the right of patients to continue to have their prescriptions filled at the pharmacy of their choice. NARD announced a nationwide campaign to enact consumer choice statutes in state legislatures throughout the country. To that end, the NARD staff compiled a NARD "Consumer Freedom of Choice Legislation Manual." The manual was distributed to every state association and was highly popular with state leaders. By convention time, six new states had used the manual to help get state freedom of choice laws passed.

President Mosso identified "pharmacy education" as the major theme for his presidential year. He devoted a great deal of time to visiting with students in pharmacy colleges throughout the nation, discussing curriculum with pharmacy deans and faculty, and trying to educate the educators about independent pharmacy.

As a follow-up to a staff report of his committee, Sen. Pryor at the twenty-second NARD Legislative Conference outlined legislation designed to address drug prices in state Medicaid programs. Three days later on May 10, 1990, he introduced S.2605, the "Pharmaceuticals Access and Prudent Purchasing Act of 1990" (PAPPA). NARD, the National Association of Chain Drug Stores (NACDS), and the American Pharmaceutical Association (APhA) issued a joint statement expressing their support for the legislation, noting that the initiative "is fair, wise, and workable." They were joined by nine other organizations representing the elderly. NARD said to its members, "Simply put, this is the most important piece of legislation affecting pharmacy to be introduced in decades."

With the strong support of the association membership and the Bush administration, a similar bill — the Medicaid Anti-Discriminatory Drug Price and Patient Benefit Restoration Act — passed Congress in near record time and became law in October. In its essence this bill required drug manufacturers, beginning February 1, 1991, to provide state Medicaid programs a 12.5 percent rebate or the manufacturer's best price, whichever was lower, on each of their products dispensed to Medicaid recipients. After two years, manufacturers were required to offer state Medicaid programs the lower of a 15 percent rebate or the manufacturer's best price. Existing agreements negotiated by state Medicaid programs and manufacturers were automatically included in the new program.

NARD leaders were nearly euphoric with their victory. Executive Vice President West said that "pharmacists will now stop bearing the burden of cost containment alone. This is a tremendous victory for NARD and the independent retail pharmacists it serves, and represents a giant step in the association's efforts to eliminate discriminatory pricing in the pharmaceutical marketplace."

The ninety-second NARD convention convened in Nashville, Tennessee in 1990 during National Pharmacy Week. The meeting coincided with Pryor's bill becoming law, further fueling the enthusiasm and good will among the delegates. President Mosso talked with them about the importance of professionalism and shared the results of several public opinion polls. Each poll compared the community pharmacist with those practicing in a chain pharmacy.

By every index — e.g., number of prescriptions, refills, sales volume, Medicaid prescription volume — community pharmacists outperformed their chain counterparts. Mosso noted that this public acclaim was no accident. He said that the improvement in the retail pharmacists' image coincided with NARD encouraging all pharmacists to become more involved in patient counseling. He urged the delegates, "talk to (your) customers, counsel (your) patients, each and every one of them — face to face. Nothing less is acceptable.... You can never be too busy to counsel."

Executive Vice President West reviewed the association's legislative accomplishments and discussed third-party issues with the delegates. He noted that a particular problem with third party was the disagreement over the professional fee that pharmacists charged for dispensing a prescription. He reminded his listeners that when that issue had been discussed in the distant past, the prevailing opinion was that a fixed dispensing fee would "make the pharmacist more professional."

However, with the advent of Medicaid, the fee had become the center of attention in every effort to negotiate cost containment for prescriptions. West suggested that pharmacists should have learned their lesson on that issue. "We must never again attempt," he said, "to enhance our professionalism at the expense of our economic stability." Before leaving Nashville, delegates elected William S. Katz of Newington, Connecticut president; Calvin Anthony was re-elected chairman of the executive committee.

The ninety-third year in NARD's history saw a lull in legislative action, but a significant growth in member services. Soon after giving his inaugural address, President Katz appointed two task forces to address specific needs among the membership. The first of these produced a publication, "Protecting Your Family's and Your Pharmacy's Future," which was intended as a guide to assist families in times of family tragedy. Making decisions on whether to sell or keep operating a pharmacy after the owner's death or incapacitation and how to do estate planning in advance of tragedy were some of the topics covered.

Katz charged the second task force with finding ways to retain more retired pharmacists as NARD members and to better utilize the expertise of those pharmacists. Among the ideas that came from this group was a "NARD Peace Corps" that would match retired pharmacists with business expertise with members having difficulty in some aspect of their business.

In November 1990, administrative and legislative officials reached agreement on the federal budget for the coming year. The changes in Medicaid created by Sen. Pryor's bill proved to be a major sticking point in the discussions. Bush Administration officials wanted to reduce pharmacy fees, while congressional leaders held to the language in the bill. The issue was finally resolved when budget officials reached agreement for a four-year moratorium on prescription fees paid to pharmacists. This compromise was included in the 1991 Omnibus Budget Reconciliation Act (OBRA).

The new year also saw a new association formed under NARD's affiliation. The National Home Infusion Association (HHIA) was a reflection of NARD's continuing efforts to develop specialized programs for members seeking to serve niche markets. In some ways this organization was an extension of the home health care services movement, which NARD recognized as a member need in the early 1980s.

NARD's ninety-third convention met in Baltimore, Maryland in 1991. President Katz reviewed his initiatives from the two task forces he formed during the year. Among other key programs he discussed was the formation of a nationwide Diabetes Care Club to provide independents with the marketing and merchandising they needed to build a specialty in diabetes products and services. Katz said that under his leadership NARD's goal had been to "keep our members in business (and) doing our level best to prepare the next generation of pharmacists for independent pharmacy ownership."

Executive Vice President West told the delegates about the leadership's efforts to work out a payment plan on Medicaid with the Health Care Financing Administration (HCFA) and to develop legislation to protect independent pharmacy's interests in third-party programs. But he reserved some of his choice words for mail order prescriptions.

Earlier in the year representatives from the industry had asked the Federal Trade Commission to investigate NARD for possible antitrust violations. West assured his membership that the association would not be intimidated, and said "we are not going to go away on this vital consumer issue." West also deplored a decision by the Hallmark Company to provide its employees a "prescriptions by mail service." He noted that the company had for decades turned to community pharmacists to move its products. He noted that "unregulated, substandard pharmaceutical care" could hardly be considered a benefit for employees.

In the final analysis, he asked, "how can anyone advocate clinical pharmacy and not question mail order in the same breath?" Hallmark was installed as the first member of NARD's "Hall of Shame," later renamed the Mail Order Dishonor Roll.

However, as deplorable as the mail order and price discrimination issues were, West told the delegates that legislation alone would not solve the problems. In addition to legislation, he urged pharmacists to become more concerned and involved in their profession. He reminded delegates about the "passion of the people of the Soviet Union, who rejected communism for democracy...even laying down their lives to assure freedom for their children."

While he was not asking community pharmacists to lay down their lives, nevertheless, he said, "some measure of real passion is required for us to succeed. Commitment — resolve — determination — passion. We must make those four attributes part of our professional behavior each and every day." Before leaving Baltimore, delegates elected William L. Scharringhausen of

Park Ridge, Illinois president; Calvin Anthony was re-elected chairman of the executive committee.

Third-party issues continued to dominate NARD activities in its ninety-fourth year. Three major attempts were made to implement major drug benefit programs, while largely bypassing community pharmacy. The first was a plan by Arizona Senator John McCain to mandate mail order pharmacy for all active and retired military personnel. Tipped off that the bill was forthcoming, West activated the "pharmacy alert" hotline and generated enough protest from community pharmacists to block the proposed measure. Sen. McCain then tried to attach a similar measure as an amendment to the Department of Defense appropriations bill. While not able to defeat this proposal outright, NARD was able to get it modified to require a study comparing the benefits of "retail pharmacy networks" with mail order pharmacy.

Freedom of choice had also continued to be a bellwether issue for the association, and particularly in the managed care environment in which health plans sought to proscribe where patients could obtain their health care, including pharmacy services. Even the federal government got into the act in 1992 when the Office of Personnel Management (OPM), through Blue Cross/Blue Shield, administering the Federal Employees Health Benefits Program, announced its intention to restrict the pharmacies federal employees could use in filling prescriptions.

NARD leaders challenged that plan for denying consumers "freedom of choice" in selecting a pharmacy. By activating once again the pharmacy alert hotline, West called upon NARD members to flood OPM, the President, and their representatives in Congress with phone calls, telegrams, and letters protesting the action. The call to action worked, and OPM backed away from the discriminatory plan.

NARD delegates met at the association's ninety-fourth convention in Seattle, Washington in 1992 amid a national debate on health care reform and national health insurance. NARD President Scharringhausen used an ophthalmologic metaphor to warn the membership about the dangers of myopia, hyperopia, and astigmatism. He called upon his listeners to have 20/20 vision about the issues, problems, and opportunities facing community pharmacy.

The president also called attention to a member survey the association conducted in September. He noted the importance of "face-to-face patient counseling, patient profiling, home delivery service, and 24-hour emergency service," which a majority of NARD members reported they were providing.

To reinforce the importance of the valuable services community pharmacists provide — both to consumers and payers — Scharringhausen said the association was launching a multiyear educational campaign bearing the slogan "The Family Pharmacist: Your Best Benefit." As part of the campaign, said Scharringhausen, NARD's Management Institute had targeted corporate "benefits managers" with printed materials detailing the valuable services that community pharmacists provide. Scharringhausen noted that "it is these kinds of professional services that have long separated the nation's independents from the pack. And now would be absolutely the worse time to turn our backs on that tradition. Because...that tradition is coming full circle. Patient-centered, hands-on pharmacy care, not robots and automation, is what the world wants and needs now."

Executive Vice President West in his address to the House of Delegates reminded them "we have a serious problem with third-party reimbursement." Part of the solution to that problem, he noted, was to be political in "action, vigilance, and perseverance." He reported on the "action" association leaders had taken on the McCain bills, the OPM action, and continued efforts to assist state associations with consumer freedom of choice laws in their respective states.

But, he said, members must continue to maintain "vigilance" on attempts by various interests to undermine the "best price" provisions in the Medicaid law and steps by federal agencies to unilaterally issue regulations that adversely affect community pharmacy. Certain issues, such as requiring insurance companies to be subject to antitrust laws and mail order, simply require "perseverance," said West. At Seattle, delegates elected Donald Moore of Kokomo, Indiana president; Gene Graves of Little Rock, Arkansas was elected chairman of the executive committee.

A significant milestone in the association's history occurred during the next several years when the organization's stature and visibility was measured at the highest level of government — the Executive Branch. The genesis of this was the 1992 presidential campaign. As the campaign heated up, more and more discussion was devoted to health care reform in general and national health insurance in particular. NARD, long an opponent to federally mandated programs, took the position that any such program must include an outpatient prescription drug program, address discriminatory pricing, protect the consumers' right to choose a pharmacy, and include adequate compensation for pharmacists for their services.

Two weeks after the NARD convention in Seattle, Washington, Bill Clinton was elected president and Al Gore, vice president. NARD sought to bring to the health care reform debate historic core issues it believed needed to be carved into any reform plan. In an August 1996 *NARD Journal* interview with West, the former executive vice president recalled how other pharmacy leaders reacted to NARD's position. "In 1992 when health care reform became a primary issue in the months leading up to the presidential election, the Joint

Commission of Pharmacy Practitioners (JCPP) created a work group to develop a position paper on health reform. The hope was that JCPP could issue a joint health reform statement that everyone could support."

West continued, "The work group eventually presented a paper for consideration in the fall of 1992. When we reviewed the JCPP document here at NARD, we saw two glaring omissions — discriminatory pricing and consumer freedom of choice. We developed a revised document that added those two bedrock issues for the nation's independents. I chaired the next meeting of JCPP at which health reform was debated. I presented NARD's revised position paper and went around the table asking if any of the groups would support it. Not one group did."

"I told JCPP that we could not support a statement on health reform that did not include the two core issues of putting an end to discriminatory pricing and preserving consumer choice. After that, the die was cast. NACDS was not at that JCPP meeting. I called Ron Ziegler, my counterpart at the chain

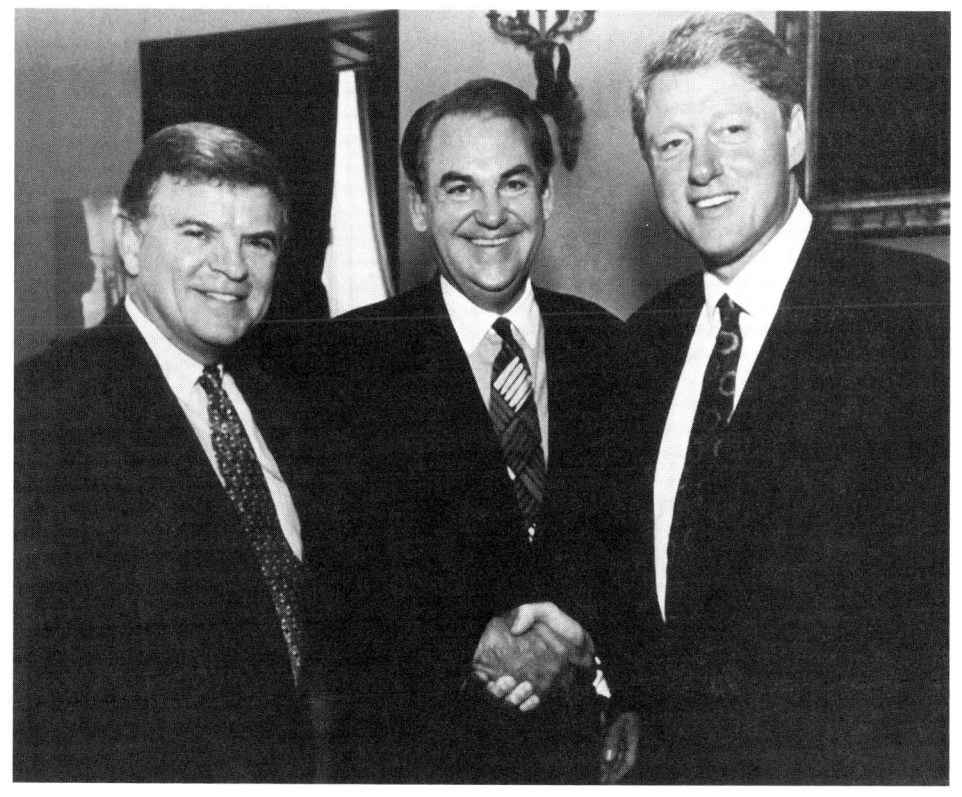

NARD's Charles M. West, NACDS's Ron Ziegler, and President Bill Clinton at a White House briefing during the health care reform initiative.

drug store group, and asked him if he wanted to join us in a coalition on health care reform (that addressed these two core issues). The answer was yes, but it took a little while, because the chains were with us in opposing discriminatory pricing, but divided on freedom of choice. Finally, in February 1993, the NACDS board agreed to support our position on choice, and the NARD-NACDS Coalition was born (the Community Retail Pharmacy Coalition)."

This new entity provided most, if not all, the pharmacy data being assembled by a White House task force that was developing plans for the Clinton administration's new health care reform proposal that year. Much of 1993 was devoted to consultation with the Clinton task force. NARD President Donald Moore, West, Rector, and key members of the executive committee were in frequent contact with members of the health reform team. Community pharmacy's position on health care reform was the primary topic for the association's twenty-fifth Legislative Conference in May, which had the largest attendance in its history.

By summer, NARD's focused persistence had paid off again. Almost every political issue the association had dealt with since 1984 was addressed in the first draft of the bill the administration would present to Congress. West and Rector were invited to the White House to review the document.

For pharmacy the proposed legislation allowed outpatient pharmacy benefits for all prescription drugs, equal access to price discounts for all purchasers involved in the Medicare/Medicaid drug programs, reimbursement at the lower of the ninetieth percentile of actual charges or estimated acquisition cost plus a $5 dispensing fee indexed to the Consumer Price Index, and a manufacturer rebate program modeled on the 1990 Medicaid best price law. Physician self-referrals and ownership of pharmacies was prohibited. Insurance companies were brought under antitrust regulation. A new home infusion benefit was added, and health care providers would be permitted "safe harbors" to collectively negotiate terms for participation in the program. Later, consumer freedom of choice was also added to the package.

There were a few negatives to the comprehensive health care package. For example, community pharmacists, as all small business with fifty or fewer employees, would be required to phase-in health coverage for their employees. There was also a great deal of flexibility at the state level in structuring health care benefits. But, to the NARD leadership's way of thinking, these were details that could be resolved and were minor when compared to the overwhelming number of cherished NARD principles that had been included.

The optimism that NARD leaders felt with respect to the president's health reform initiative was reinforced by news of a lower court ruling in Arkansas against the huge deep discount chain, Wal-Mart. The court found that Wal-

Mart had used predatory pricing methods against three local independent pharmacists. While it was only the first step in what promised to be an extended court fight, it was obviously a landmark decision for community pharmacists.

Ironically, just as community pharmacists seemed to have everything going their way, news came of a proposed merger between Merck & Company and Medco Containment Services Inc. This union of the nation's largest pharmaceutical manufacturer and the largest mail order prescription company revived the specter of anticompetitive practices. The merger, which NARD denounced as an "unholy alliance," made passing the president's health reform bill all the more crucial for community pharmacists.

Delegates convened the ninety-fifth convention in Indianapolis, Indiana in 1993. President Moore reviewed some of the political successes of the past year and noted that each success was the product of planning. "We have a clear set of long-range goals," he said, "that we keep sharply in focus when deciding how to allocate our limited resources.

He also reminded the delegates that "it is possession of nuts and bolts management skills that is contributing to the success of independents and placing in jeopardy those who lack them." In view of that strength, he urged them to take advantage of the training opportunities offered by the NARD Management Institute. "I am committed," he said, "to training our pharmacists to be the best in the country. Patient counseling...is our opportunity to shine. And further diversifying our professional services, finding the niche that works best for you, is where more and more independents are headed. Whether it is home health care, long-term care, home infusion, ostomy, diabetes or elder care, the future bodes well for you in niche marketing."

Executive Vice President West told the delegates that "we are on the threshold of regaining control of our future and eliminating the greatest threat to it — discriminatory pricing." He elaborated on the provisions in the Clinton health reform proposal and said "most of our priorities have been incorporated into the president's health care reform legislation. Never have we had such a great opportunity to solve so many of our problems with one piece of legislation."

West urged the delegates to remain politically active to see the landmark legislation successfully through Congress. He cautioned them to "be very careful not to be taken in by the steady flow of disinformation that has already begun. It's designed to divide us and to undermine our very real chances for success."

Before leaving Indianapolis, delegates elected Calvin J. Anthony of Stillwater, Oklahoma president; Kenneth Epley, of Salem, Oregon was elected chairman of the executive committee.

In the fall of 1993, as the health reform debate was heating up, a group of community pharmacists, 1,346 in fifteen states, filed class-action lawsuits against a number of drug manufacturers and wholesalers. These suits were ultimately joined with a consolidated group of seventy cases scheduled for trial in February 1996 in Chicago. The pharmacists charged the drug manufacturers with discriminatory pricing and antitrust violations of the Sherman Act by "using patents to block normal market forces in a lockstep manner." While the suit did not directly involve NARD, it cut to the heart of the problems inherent in the discriminatory pricing system that NARD had made its highest priority for years.

For NARD 1994 reversed the gains made in 1993. The high excitement of being on the inside track and all but custom-making legislation to benefit community pharmacy in 1993 met with increasing obstacles and frustrations in 1994. The Clinton health reform initiative had been introduced in Congress as H.R. 3600, the Health Security Act (HSA), and routinely referred to Michigan Representative John Dingell's House Energy and Commerce Committee, among others. The bill began to be challenged from a variety of sources. A well-financed lobby led by physicians, insurance providers, and

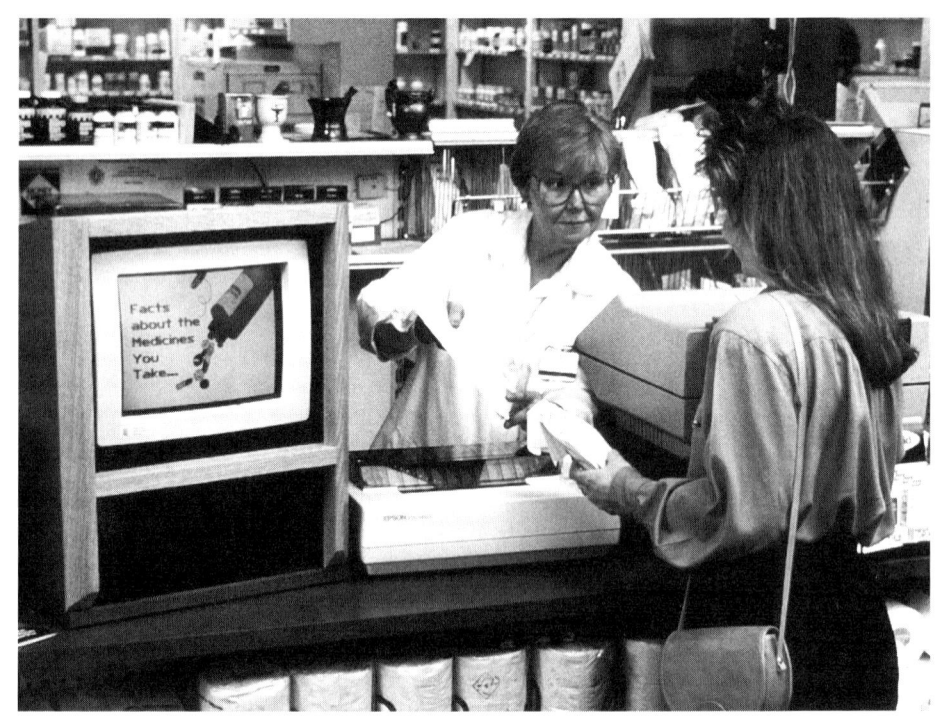

The pharmacy counter of the 1990s with in-store televised patient information as well as face-to-face counseling

major pharmaceutical companies began to attack individual segments of the comprehensive bill.

One of the earliest attacks came from Merck-Medco. With merger agreements now finalized, the company moved to amend the HSA to radically restrict the outpatient Medicare prescription drug benefit to a small network of pharmacies that emphasized mail order pharmacy. That action was the "last straw" for West and the executive committee. In a strongly worded letter to the company president P. Roy Vagelos, West wrote, "It has become clear to us that Merck has changed its philosophy regarding the role of America's independent pharmacists.... Your company is committed to anti-consumer, anti-community pharmacy...that makes a mockery of any serious commitment to high-quality service."

But the hearings continued to go badly for White House interests. President Clinton used his office to rally support wherever he could — including inviting NARD's West to join the presidential party during a visit to a community pharmacy in Connecticut. NARD President Calvin Anthony and Executive Committee Chairman Ken Epley also traveled extensively and spoke to numerous pharmacy groups promoting health care reform.

But the comprehensive nature of the HSA, the dramatic changes it proposed for some aspects of health care, particularly the insurance industry, and the approaching congressional elections proved too much for the bill. By mid-August leaders in Congress were ready to table the issue and reopen discussions after the November elections. The reform initiative as legislation ultimately slipped into oblivion. But the legislative stirrings prompted the health insurance industry to initiate numerous managed care "reforms" that proved inimical to independent pharmacy's interests.

The ninety-sixth convention met in Boston, Massachusetts in 1994. President Anthony reviewed the year's intense political and marketplace challenges. He told the delegates that "we must regain control of our professional destiny. Others are brokering our assets...drug makers, insurance companies, academics, and bureaucrats. We should control our profession."

To regain that control, he emphasized that we must "gain equal access to prices, intervene in the care of our patients, document that care and work to get paid for it, train our staff to the highest possible levels, gather and disseminate more and better information about the market power of the nation's independents, find our market niche and make the most of it, install the entrepreneurial spirit in the independent pharmacists of tomorrow, and work to ensure that our patients continue to have the right to patronize the pharmacy of their choice."

Anthony reminded his listeners, "we will always be able to succeed (because) we are smart and extremely effective politically, we have positive attitudes, we are cost-efficient, and we genuinely care about the patient. When you hear buzzwords like 'pharmaceutical care,' you know what it means. It means what you and I have been doing for ten or twenty or thirty years. It is a way of life for us. We will succeed because we care."

Executive Vice President West remained undaunted in the face of the failure of the Health Security Act. The long campaign, said West, "established community retail pharmacy as a force to be reckoned with. We now know that we can solve problems in one manner or another. It doesn't have to be health care reform at the federal level. (Our) force is being felt at the local and state levels as well and can be dealt with effectively in the state legislatures."

West also praised the delegates for their response to his numerous calls for help and noted "during one critical seven-day period, you responded to our call with more than 25,000 calls to the offices of 100 U.S. senators. We have no doubt that we are a force to be reckoned with, because our message was right, our concern for the consumer was genuine, and our work was good." NARD had activated its newly created Fax Alert Network of thousands of independent pharmacies to mobilize members to action.

Finally, the executive vice president recommended that the association organize a "Home Town Pharmacy Service" patterned after the floral delivery system. This would be a safe, cost-effective alternative to mail order pharmacy. If employers insist on a mail order option, let's give them one. However, rather than have the prescription being delivered by the mail man, the home town pharmacists would have the responsibility for getting the order to the patient and thus the patient-pharmacist relationship remains intact." Before leaving Boston, delegates elected Gene Graves of Little Rock, Arkansas, president; Kenneth Epley was re-elected chairman of the executive committee.

Few could have anticipated the political upheaval that came with the November 1994 congressional elections. Republicans gained control of both houses of Congress and, along with that control, the chairmanship of all committees. The political ideology of many of the new leaders was significantly different from their predecessors, but NARD was well positioned to work with them. Many in the Republican leadership had been cultivated as part of bipartisan efforts in the past and had been featured speakers at Legislative Conferences.

NARD shifted the legislative fight on discriminatory pricing from Washington to the states. Joining with NACDS, Rector and other association leaders drafted a "model bill" to prohibit discriminatory pricing practices by pharmaceutical companies. Before the year was out, the model bill had been introduced in thirty state legislatures.

Another major development in the professional services arena was the formation of the National Institute for Pharmacist Care Outcomes (NIPCO). NIPCO was created in May 1995 to optimize patient health through pharmacist-directed disease management and wellness programs, as well as to ensure that pharmacists would receive compensation for nondispensing services. The Institute quickly became a leader in the burgeoning pharmacist care movement, launching disease state management certificate programs for pharmacists in diabetes care, cardiovascular care, respiratory care, and pharmacist care skills training.

In announcing the formation of the Institute, NARD President Gene Graves said that "the Institute will play a leadership role in developing patient outcome and disease management programs for independent community pharmacists. The Institute will also enable us to more rationally organize the services we now have to assist our members in providing pharmacist care and to dramatically expand the pharmacist care services we offer." NARD Vice President for Professional Affairs Kathryn Kuhn, R.Ph., was named NIPCO's executive director.

As part of the Institute's effort to help pharmacists get paid for providing these professional services, NARD created the NARD Pharmacist Care Claim Form for pharmacists to submit to third parties for payment. The claim form includes codes to identify the type and level of services provided, and enjoys widespread use today.

Also during 1995 (and again in 1996) NARD launched a massive multimedia campaign nationwide to bring greater public awareness to the unfair, anticonsumer practices of many health insurance carriers and health plans. The managed care environment had become so oppressive for many pharmacists that a groundswell of member support for a public display of their concerns evolved over a year's time into public demonstrations throughout the country. On September 20, 1995, some 200 community pharmacists converged on Times Square in New York City to kick off NARD's high profile "High Noon for Your Local Pharmacy" campaign. (The scene was reminiscent of a march on Washington by the nation's independents to lobby for fair trade legislation nearly 60 years previously.)

Just prior to the Times Square rally, NARD leaders held a press conference at a hotel in midtown Manhattan at which many of community pharmacy's complaints about managed care or "mangled care," as NARD President Gene Graves noted, were explained to members of the national press corps. "Our main criticism of managed care, or third-party pharmacy, West said, "is that it has insinuated itself between the practitioner and the patient. Arbitrary — and exclusionary — contractual arrangements have denied patients access to the pharmacy provider of their choice."

Thousands of community pharmacists in every state in the country participated in High Noon. The *NARD Journal* in November 1995 arrayed dozens of pages and photographs quoting newspaper accounts in over 25 major cities of similar protests, rallies, and press conferences. As the *NARD Journal* noted, "pharmacist participation and consumer response to the High Noon protest were astounding. Participation was phenomenal. Some independents drew hundreds of people to their pharmacies. Many draped their pharmacy in black, donned black High Noon armbands, and dimmed their lights at noon." The campaign was the product of year-long planning by the NARD staff. High Noon Pharmacist Action Kits were developed, which included ad slicks, bag stuffers, a guide to media outreach, and a "top 25" list of unfair

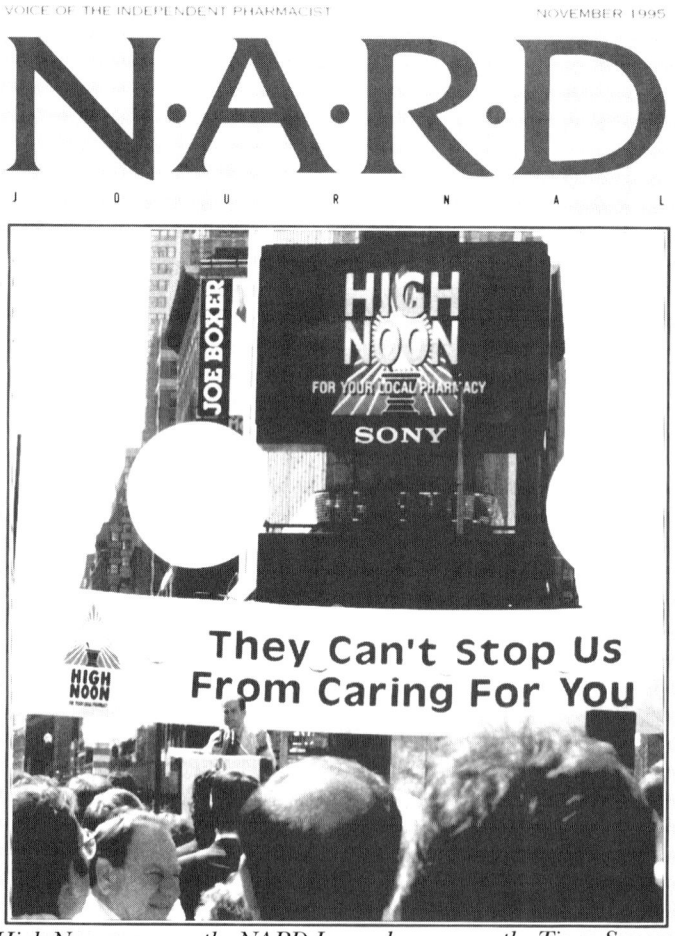

The High Noon scene on the NARD Journal cover was the Times Square rally September 20, 1995.

practices by health insurance companies, among other items. A High Noon for Pharmacy Fund was also established for member contributions to be used "to battle third-party injustices in the marketplace."

Also in 1995, the debate over a single Pharm.D. entry-level degree for pharmacists prompted controversy. For NARD's leaders and members, it was a matter of equity. In the 1970s, a number of colleges of pharmacy began offering an additional year of training, from five to six years, and certifying a terminal degree for that program — the Pharm.D. By the 1990s the Pharm.D. degree was almost universal in the profession. NARD, while always supporting additional training, had reservations about the "two-class" system the new degree created. Before seeing its membership divided into two factions — one with the new Pharm.D. degree and one with the traditional B.S. degree — association officials suggested that colleges "grandfather" all the baccalaureate degree holders. Some institutions did just that, but the matter became a state-by-state issue.

Delegates returned to Las Vegas in 1995 for their ninety-seventh convention. President Gene Graves described the past year as one of change. He told the delegates they were in the midst of a "Health Care Revolution" that had been "initiated for one reason — money. This revolution," he said, "is being waged simply as a financial issue, but it has vast ramifications for the fundamental rights of the people to choose their health care providers and to continue to have access to quality health care."

Graves urged his listeners not to be discouraged by "the crisis," because "over the long haul" community pharmacy would emerge the winner. It would do so because "the crisis will eliminate the apathy of our professional colleagues, or it will eliminate them." Also, "the revolution generates tremendous business and professional opportunities...because of the pharmacists' accessibility to the patient," Graves said.

"The American Health Care Revolution is a war about money and people. But who is championing the cause of the people? Pharmacists are the most accessible health care professionals to the people. We are the most trusted professionals by the people. We can significantly reduce the cost of health care for the people.... Therefore, we as community pharmacists must accept our role as the champions of the people."

Executive Vice President West continued the theme of revolution, but in a different vein. "Community pharmacists have been exploited by third parties," he said, "Faceless intermediaries are negotiating with, and profiting from, our hard-earned professional assets every day. They don't own a pharmacy; they hold no pharmacy license. But they are growing richer and richer while we struggle to survive. We can't continue to believe...that all people are dealing in good faith. We have been exploited enough."

West's stirring words proved to be anti-climatic. As he neared the end of his speech, he said, "I would like to close by making an announcement. There is a certain and profound truth in the biblical verse, 'To everything there is a season and a time for every purpose under the heavens.' I find the season has come for me to announce my retirement from NARD." The decision would become effective July 1996.

This unexpected statement stunned the audience. While West had been contemplating retirement for several months, few knew about his decision and it caught the delegates by surprise. He announced that Calvin Anthony would be his successor. Before the delegates left Las Vegas they chose Louis Mitchell of Swedesboro, New Jersey as president; Kenneth Epley continued to serve as chairman of the executive committee. The House of Delegates also approved a recommendation from the executive committee to create the Charles M. West Distinguished American Award. Sen. David Pryor was chosen as the first recipient.

The anticipated change in NARD leadership did little to the association's high profile initiatives, including its unrelenting campaign against discriminatory pricing. In March 1996 NARD received some good news on that issue from an unexpected source. The Federal Trade Commission announced its intention to investigate the pricing policies of the nation's pharmaceutical companies. Over the past decade association leaders had asked more than thirty times for such a review to be undertaken. Responding to the news, Executive Vice President West said, "We hope that the outcome of this long-awaited FTC investigation will be a cease-and-desist order...to the manufacturers."

There was more good news on the discriminatory pricing front. In February 1996, thirteen of the defendant pharmaceutical companies in the largest antitrust litigation ever involving any one industry in history offered $600 million to settle the case. As the association noted in its *NARD Newsletter,* "the $600 million settlement offer is a clear validation of NARD's long-time stand against the ill-conceived pricing policies that have plagued our members and their patients for years."

But the proposed settlement would not provide injunctive relief from future discriminatory prices, an essential component NARD argued, of the final resolution of these legal actions. Moreover, the agreement imposed "extraordinary confidentiality restrictions on the millions of documents of evidence...and would have a harmful effect on other pricing lawsuits now pending...as well as future litigation."

In view of these issues, NARD leaders advised the plaintiffs not to settle. NARD's Rector voiced the association's opposition to the proposed settlement in the *Wall Street Journal* and on CNBC's "The Money Wheel" program.

The plaintiff pharmacists agreed and, with NARD's assistance, mounted a major letter writing campaign urging Judge Charles Kocoras not to accept the offer.

Judge Kocoras agreed with the plaintiffs, saying that he had found "the record replete with instances of collusive behavior, parallel conduct, uniformity of reposes, mutual awareness of each other's policies and practices, and various incriminating quotes on the part of the defendants." He also cited company memoranda and other records showing that industry officials made statements indicating a collective belief that retail pharmacies should not get discounts.

In June 1996, Judge Kocoras approved a $351 million settlement offered by eleven drug manufacturers to settle the litigation. Other defendants later settled out of court, leaving four in litigation as of this writing. The offer guaranteed community pharmacists "equal access to discounts" from those companies — a historic concession — and it allowed pharmacists to take the companies to court again should they violate the terms of the settlement.

West called the ruling "an important first step toward eliminating the discriminatory pricing that has for so long disadvantaged our members in the marketplace." General Counsel Rector, who had been at the forefront of the price issue for more than a decade, said "the settlement means that these...companies must now provide community pharmacists equal access to prices (and that will ultimately) "result in a decline in drug prices" for the consumer.

The "transfer of power" in the Executive Vice President's office occurred smoothly and quietly in late July. NARD President Louis Mitchell described the change as a winning relay team. "We have the perfect baton passing duo," he said. "We know what we have and we know what we're getting, and they're in lockstep."

Tributes to West's tenure were captured in the respected *Dickinson's Pharmacy* newsletter: "Pharmacy history will record that Charles M. West did more for the cause of community pharmacy than any national figure before him." His years of experience as a state association executive made him an effective political lobbyist. He took NARD's strong political presence in Washington and made it even stronger. His national legislative legacy is comparable to that of John Dargavel.

"But, with his unique background in state association affairs, he also led NARD to assist state pharmaceutical associations in aligning their constituencies with key NARD issues — freedom of choice, nondispensing reimbursements, antidiscriminatory pricing, among other legislation developed and pursued at NARD's urging. He brought all fifty state pharmacy associations into affiliation with NARD, and the Student Outreach Program he launched in 1987 had resulted in 30 NARD student chapters being organized at the nation's pharmacy colleges by the time he left office."

New Executive Vice President Calvin Anthony was thoroughly familiar with the interworkings of the association. Anthony was a store owner in Stillwater, Oklahoma, and an NARD officer and executive committee member for ten years before assuming the high post. Over the years he developed, then sold a number of pharmacies to young pharmacists beginning their careers in community pharmacy. He served on the board of directors of the National Home Infusion Association, as well as on the advisory council of the Oklahoma University College of Pharmacy. A leader in his community,

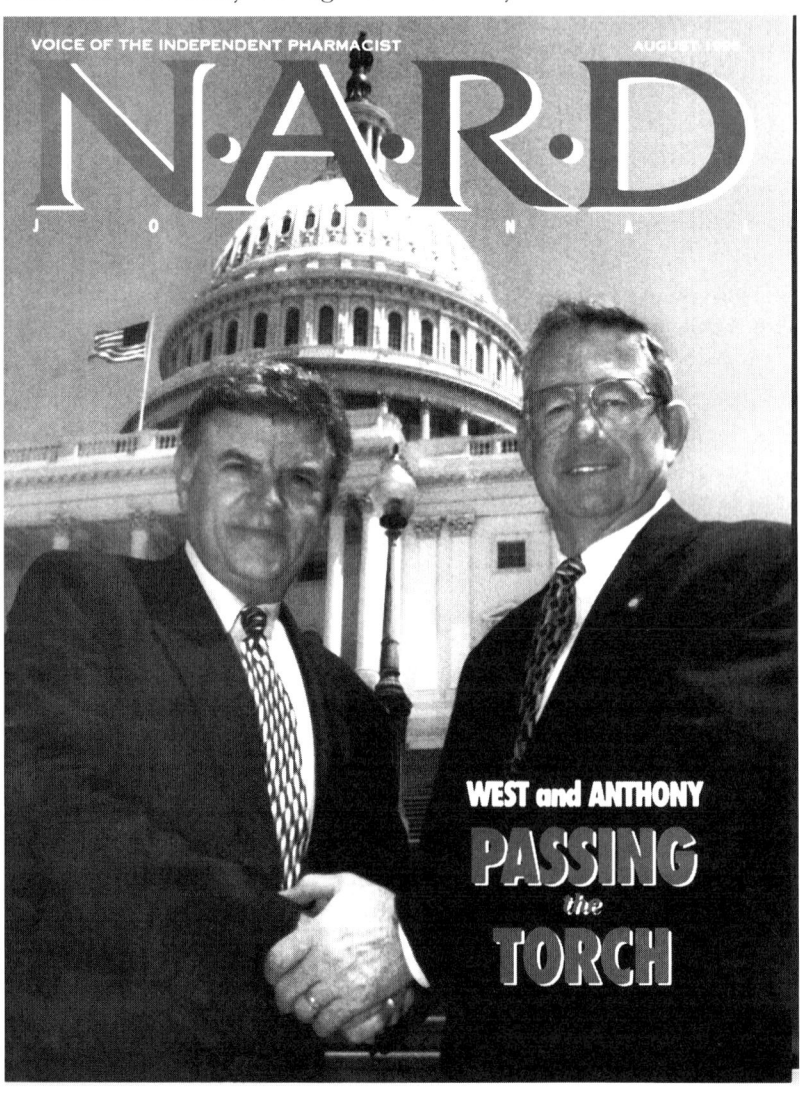

Anthony served as president of the Oklahoma Pharmaceutical Association, past vice president of the Stillwater Chamber of Commerce, and former chairman of the Stillwater Federal Savings Bank. As a legislative leader, he served as mayor of Stillwater and two terms in the Oklahoma state legislature, where he chaired the state's health reform task force.

As the association's eighth executive officer, Anthony held firm to the association's longstanding fight for pricing equity. But he also immediately sought to mend fences with a variety of interests that had borne the brunt of NARD's advocacy in the long battles over drug diversion and discriminatory pricing, among other issues.

At the time of his appointment, Anthony outlined four objectives for the near future. First, he wanted to "keep our members in business"; second, he sought to "keep NARD and independent pharmacy in the forefront of political activism"; third, he planned "to advance pharmacist care and compensation for pharmacist care services"; and fourth, he hoped "to improve the financial health of the nation's independent pharmacies."

In September 1996 High Noon II was launched with the slogan, "Pharmacist Care: There Ought to Be a Law." Dozens of white-coated independent pharmacists — many wearing gags — rallied in the nation's capital to warn that many insurers and managed care companies were putting their patients' lives at risk. NARD President Louis Mitchell announced at the rally that NARD was launching a 50-state campaign to enact pharmacist care legislation across the country. Mitchell noted that four states had recently enacted pharmacist care laws and that twenty more had plans to introduce such legislation.

In the fall of 1996, the leadership also had to prepare for a momentous occasion in the association's history — changing the name of the organization. For ninety-eight years the acronym NARD had been synonymous with the tenacious heritage of both the association and of its independent retail pharmacist members. Delegates who gathered in New Orleans, Louisiana, for the ninety-eighth meeting of the association felt a high sense of purpose. Seldom had the House of Delegates seen so much symbolic change in the organization.

The new name, the "National Community Pharmacists Association," had in fact been decades in the making. From time to time throughout the association's history, members had recommended a change in the organization's name to better reflect current directions of the profession. After nearly ninety years, delegates at the annual meeting in 1987 voted to cease the use of the name, National Association of Retail Druggists, in favor of the acronym NARD, which was synonymous with independent retail pharmacy. That was a transitional step, however. The longer-term objective was to fashion a name that better captured the vital role pharmacists play in the community as health care professionals. Previously recommended by the Committee on Form of Organization and finally ratified by the 1996 House of Delegates, the name, National Community Pharmacists Association (NCPA), has been well received by the members, the general pharmacy community, and by the public.

When the new name of the association was overwhelmingly ratified by the delegates at the 1996 convention, Executive Vice President Anthony announced that "this is the culmination of a transition in our organizational identity that began nearly a decade ago. That transition is now complete, and we are prepared to move forward aggressively into the next century as the organization representing the professional and proprietary interests of the nation's independent community pharmacists."

The 1996 convention also marked a quantum leap for NCPA as it launched itself into the electronic age. The first step was a state-of-the-art satellite telecommunications network called NPTV: Your Neighborhood Pharmacy Network. In announcing plans for the venture, Executive Vice President Anthony, who was the major proponent of the new service, said, "this new digital satellite technology will allow NCPA to bring all kinds of educational programming directly to our members, right in their pharmacies.

"One of our greatest challenges as an association representing thousands of small businesses and pharmacists across America is the task of providing timely information and education. Only a small number of our members can attend our meetings for education and information. With this new, exclusive 24-hour satellite channel, we will bring that information right to them, including legislative updates, pharmacy news, consumer information, continuing education, and other programs. All our members will have to do is turn on the television. This technological leap will help us accomplish our pharmacist care goals."

Another form of electronic communication with its members was launched at the 1996 convention. The association officially plugged into the world wide web at www.ncpanet.org. "With more than 95 percent of our members fully computerized, it is a natural step to offer the website as a valuable new communications vehicle (for our members)," said Anthony. "As the site grows, the nation's consumers will also be able to turn to our website for valuable information on their medicines and how their community pharmacist can help them better manage their health."

The association's new name also precipitated a change for the monthly *NARD Journal*. After researching several options, the magazine was renamed *America's Pharmacist*. The first monthly issue with the new name appeared in March 1997.

Before adjourning the ninety-eighth convention in 1996, delegates elected Dennis Ludwig of Boulder, Colorado president; W. Whitaker Moose of Mount Pleasant, North Carolina was chosen chairman of the executive committee.

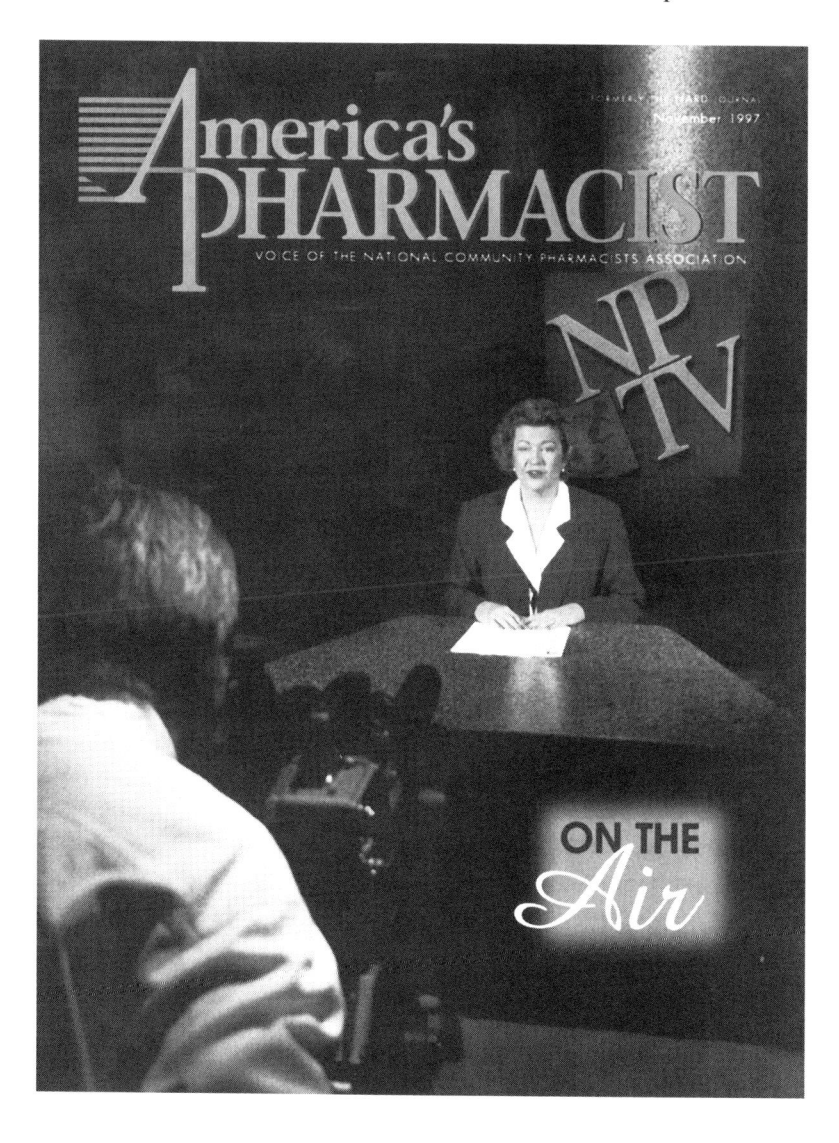

Executive Vice President Anthony used much of the new year meeting with his counterparts in health care and pharmacy associations and establishing his style within the organization. He also spent time working on the development of the satellite television network announced at the prior convention. After holding focus groups with pharmacists to learn what kinds of programming would best serve their needs, NCPA developed a six-week pilot program that was broadcast over the summer. Follow-up surveys were encouraging, and the NCPA leadership decided to proceed with the nationwide launch of NPTV in December 1997.

In other activities, the association again confronted a federal attempt to mandate the amount and kind of written prescription drug information pharmacists provided to their patients when dispensing prescriptions. After vigorous lobbying and the establishment of a task force, including NCPA, to review options to the proposed mandatory "Medguide" plan, the Department of Health and Human Services backed off and agreed instead to a voluntary action plan to increase the levels of drug information being provided to patients.

NCPA was a key participant in the development of the action plan. One of the plan's recommendations, included at Anthony's urging, was a provision that "strongly encouraged third-party payers, including government, to provide payment for oral and written prescription communication."

To help implement the voluntary plan, NCPA convened at association headquarters in 1997 a landmark meeting of all of the nation's pharmacy organizations to plan a National Symposium on Oral Counseling. The meeting and the subsequent symposium proved to be a rare, but noteworthy example of how on certain issues the diverse interests in pharmacy could in fact achieve a high level of consensus.

Third-party issues continued to be a source of contention for the association. For example, without explanation or warning, PCS began charging a $35 "research fee" to pharmacists for providing information. Given that pharmacists were doing much of PCS's work, the fee seemed most inappropriate and NCPA members appealed for help. The association leadership met with PCS officials and not only succeeded in persuading them to drop the fee, but also to refund more than $100,000 previously charged.

Face-to-face meetings played a key role in addressing several other important issues facing independents. Merck & Co. had instituted a restrictive distribution plan for its new AIDS product Crixivan utilizing mail order and circumventing the nation's community pharmacies. Officials at Serono Labs later made a similar decision about their AIDS product. Anthony met with executives from both Merck and Serono and stressed that it was NCPA's position that all FDA-approved products should be available to all licensed pharmacies. Eventually, they agreed to revise their plans and provide community pharmacists access to the products.

Delegates returned to Denver for the ninety-ninth convention in 1997. President Dennis Ludwig welcomed association members to his adopted state and told them "there is life beyond the dispensing fee. At this meeting we are introducing several tools to help you mold your pharmacist care practice."

One of those new tools was a new electronic "claims transmission service." NCPA President Dennis Ludwig noted to convention-goers that the costs to transmit third-party claims had reached an average of $3,000 per year for many pharmacies. To assist members in reducing these costs, the association had developed a new electronic switch called "Valu-Switch," which reduced costs from an average of 12 cents to 8 cents per claim. Valu-Switch would also allow pharmacists "to regain control of pharmacy data," he said.

Ludwig stressed that the association was committed to helping its members receive payment for their professional services. "You are the leaders of the pharmacist care movement in America. You know better than anyone what professional care and quality is all about. Your pharmacist care must be just innovative enough that patients expect to pay something for the value they receive.... You'll get paid for pharmacist care the day you charge for it."

Executive Vice President Anthony assumed the role of a talk show guest on the association's new NPTV satellite network to address the delegates. In addition to explaining how the network had been developed and some of the benefits he expected the network to provide, Anthony also reviewed some of the highlights from his first full year as executive vice president.

Among those achievements was passage of two important pieces of legislation: pharmacist compounding provisions in the new law reforming the federal Food and Drug Administration — language that preserved the pharmacist's traditional right to compound — and enactment of a new law that would compensate pharmacists for diabetes education and other professional services under Medicare.

Anthony told the attendees that NCPA was committed — legislatively and in the marketplace — to doing all it could to help independent pharmacists be paid for not only dispensing products, but also for providing vital pharmacist care services. He also announced plans to create a Third-Party Contract Negotiations Task Force — signaling yet another attempt to find a way to empower pharmacists to collectively negotiate the terms of the services they provide without running afoul of the antitrust laws.

For all the excitement about the new member services, the ninety-ninth convention may well be remembered as the time of the "great blizzard." Twenty-four inches of snow fell on Denver, closing the airport for a time and paralyzing the city for several hours. The inconvenience of getting to and from the convention hotels made the meeting a memorable event. Before leaving Denver, delegates elected Ken Epley president; C. Robert Blake of West Union, Ohio was chosen chairman of the executive committee.

In preparing for the centennial year, NCPA President Ken Epley said in his address to the Denver convention audience that he would focus on three main goals during his term. One of these would be "to pass measures allowing pharmacies to negotiate insrance contracts. A second goal would be "to make sure NPTV is up and running in every pharmacy we can get it in." As a third goal the new president wanted to continue to advance pharmacist care and see to it that as many pharmacists are trained to provide and are getting paid for providing pharmacist care."

NCPA was leading the charge on behalf of the profession to achieve that last goal. Since its inception in 1995, NCPA's NIPCO has accredited nearly 7,000 pharmacists who have participated in disease management in certification programs.

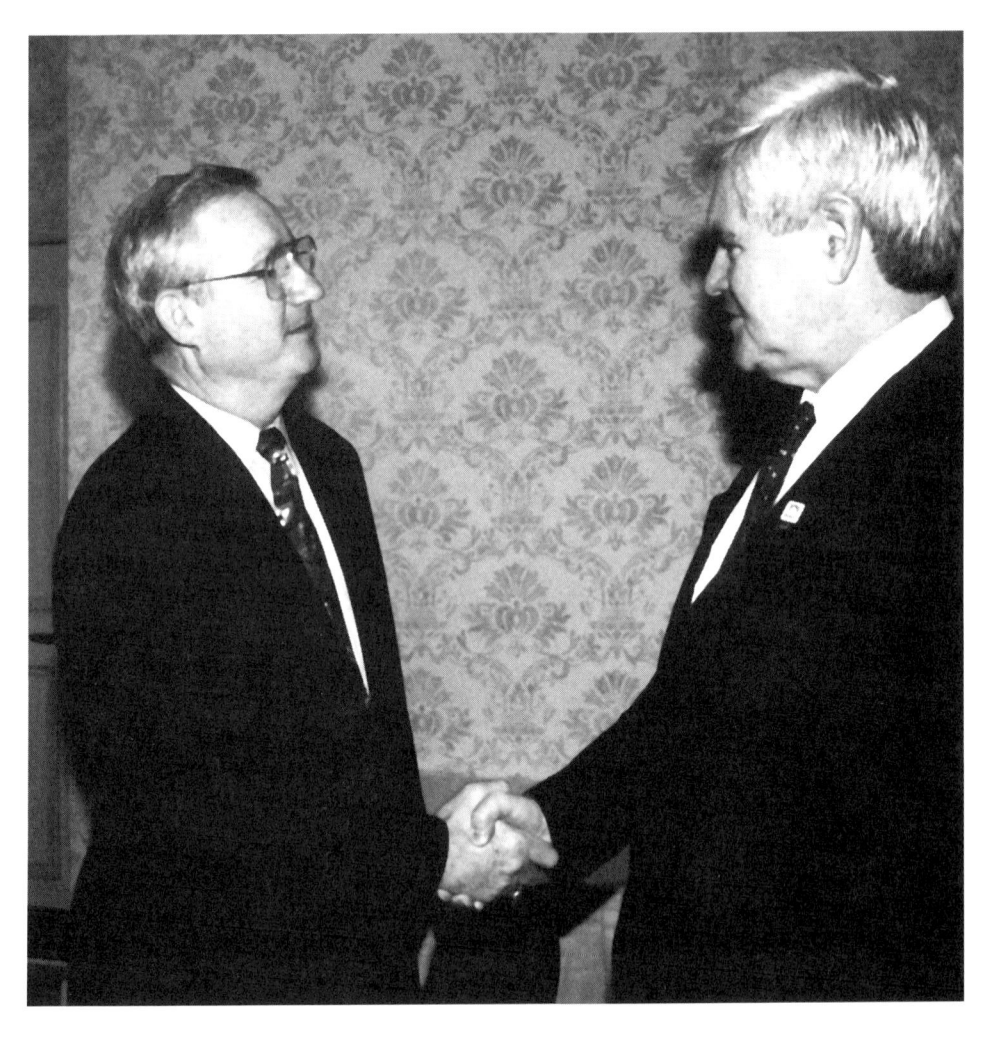

NARD's Calvin Anthony greets House Speaker Newt Gingrich.

The association pulled off a coup of sorts at its 1998 Legislative Conference, getting Speaker of the House Newt Gingrich of Georgia to address the attendees. Gingrich sounded themes that were reassuring to independents challenged by an increasingly integrated, depersonalized managed care marketplace. Gingrich said that he envisioned a coming "paradigm shift" that would transform the health care system into a model of "personal health and personal health care." Large, impersonal health delivery systems, including "direct mail order pharmacies are, I think, the wave of the past," said Gingrich.

Potential help on the third-party negotiations front arrived in July 1998 with the introduction of California Representative Tom Campbell's Health Care Coalition Act. NCPA's Third-Party Task Force had recommended congressional legislation as one of the remedies to the antitrust obstacles facing pharmacists, and the bill was given further impetus when the American Medical Association joined NCPA in supporting it.

In Mississippi a state-based pharmacist care model for the entire nation was under way by summer 1998 after the state received a mid-spring approval from the Health Care Financing Administration to pay pharmacists under Medicaid for disease management on a "per-encounter" basis. Mississippi became the first state to include pharmacist payments under what was called the "Other Licensed Practitioner" law. The rule stated that financial participation is provided for "medical care or any other type of remedial care recognized under state law furnished by licensed practitioners within the scope of their practice as defined by state law. The bill specified payments for pharmacists "specially credentialed" in such services as diabetes care and asthma, lipids, and coagulation management.

NCPA, NACDS, and the National Association of Boards of Pharmacy worked with Mississippi pharmacy leaders to develop an approved credentialing system. The three groups also formed the National Institute for Standards in Pharmacist Credentialing to develop a national model and process for credentialing pharmacists in disease statement management. It is hoped that this model will ultimately be adopted by public and private payers nationwide. As NCPA President Kenneth Epley noted, "this is a model for what pharmacist care payment should be. It recognizes the valuable role that pharmacists play in patient care while compensating us for our services."

Looking to the future, President Epley said, "I think people will be surprised both by how much we have changed over the years and also by how little we have changed.... We've changed so little because we are still are providing personalized care to people on a one-on-one basis. Yet we've changed a lot because of all the vast technological advances and the dramatic evolution in the pharmacy marketplace."

President Epley's words were also true in a historical sense. The 100-year history of NARD/NCPA had been a long-running chess match. The issues have remained extraordinarily consistent. But the strategies for playing the game have been exceptionally creative and never-ending. Of all the players, NARD has emerged as a master. Outnumbered in almost every fight, outspent in all, it still has won most of the time.

Calvin Anthony perhaps said it best in noting that "sooner or later all roads lead to price." But it was an exceedingly difficult road with unexpected curves, steep hills, long valleys, potholes, and not a few dead ends. The spirit of survival and sheer resilience of America's independent pharmacists, combined with the relentless tenacity of its organization, have made an incredible team. From the members who made up the critical mass to the leaders who gave it direction, the association never lost its focus — to be the voice of independent community pharmacy: nothing more, nothing less, nothing else.

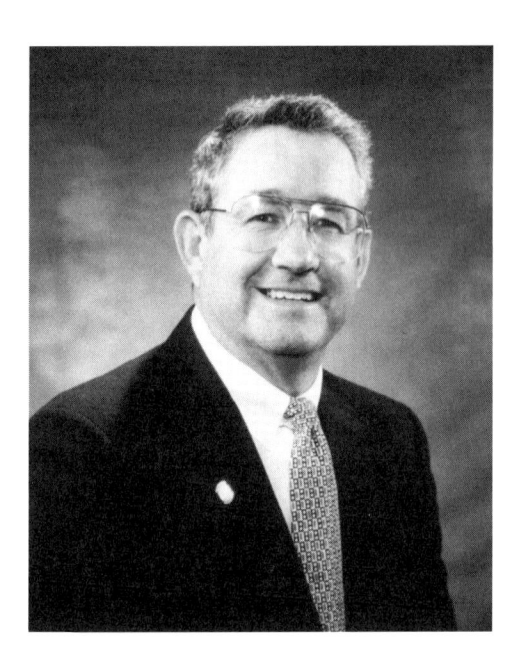

Calvin J. Anthony, NARD Executive Vice President, 1996 – to present

Epilogue

And now for the next 100 years. Epilogues usually conclude a well-rounded story with a convenient beginning, middle, and end. Epilogues often are a retrospective, looking back rather than looking forward. But NCPA's story today is the future, some of which is being written today. NCPA has a vision for its future and its members. What lies ahead?

The future of the community pharmacist will be exciting — full of new and old challenges and abundant opportunities. More prescriptions are being written and more innovative new medicines introduced than ever before in American history. An aging population is requiring more and better medicines and more personalized pharmacy services. These trends present real opportunities for community pharmacy. For, while the vicissitudes of the marketplace have reduced the number of independent pharmacies, there is more business than ever before waiting to be captured by today's independents. The latest data from the *1998 NCPA-Searle Digest* confirm this. Sales in the average independent pharmacy topped $1.65 million last year — a dramatic 14.3 percent increase from the previous year. Net profits remain tight — particularly in the private insurance marketplace — but new marketplace opportunities are emerging to compensate for those narrow margins.

The best opportunities lie in pharmacist care and specialized professional services — in an ever-expanding array of market niches ideally suited to the hands-on, professional expertise of today's independent. NCPA has positioned community pharmacy to capitalize on these opportunities now and in the future.

NCPA has, through its National Institute for Pharmacist Care Outcomes, accredited the training of more than 7,000 pharmacists in disease state management services. NCPA has embarked on a bold new credentialing initiative intended to not only ensure the quality of those disease management services, but also, importantly, fair payment for those services. NCPA has advanced federal and state legislation to enable community pharmacists to be compensated for providing professional services. NCPA has worked closely with private payers and regulators to demonstrate the value to the health care system of compensating pharmacists for compliance monitoring and a wide range of professional services — to prove that these services not only enhance the lives of patients, but save the system literally billions of dollars.

The challenge for community pharmacy will be to deliver on the enormous promise of pharmacist care. It will be up to today's and tomorrow's independent pharmacists to demonstrate, once and for all, that pharmacy is indeed the best bargain in all of health care.

The future will also be about new alliances. To remain independent, independents need to be prepared to give up some of their independence. Provider networks, payor and wholesaler affiliations, franchises, buying groups — all of these alliances will prove critical to success in a managed care-dominated marketplace.

The new millennium will have its own sets of challenges and, hopefully, some of them won't be discriminatory pricing or physician dispensing. These are old battles, well fought and won. New challenges lie in surviving in a managed care environment, fine-tuning pharmaceutical delivery services to ensure fair compensation, enhancing professional knowledge through credentialing to deliver the highest levels of personalized pharmacist care, and continuing to refine the mission of the profession.

That mission is more likely to be fulfilled in a marketplace where independents have regained control of their professional destiny. NCPA is committed to finding a legal way to help accomplish that by gaining pharmacists the power to negotiate with insurers on the terms of the pharmacy services they provide. Thankfully, the pendulum is swinging away from a health system dominated by insurers and fiscal intermediaries and back toward providers and consumers, who want to have some say over the health care they receive. That is good news for independents — the most trusted professionals in the eyes of the American public for a decade.

Speaking at the 1998 NCPA Legislative Conference, Speaker of the House of Representatives Newt Gingrich forecast a coming "paradigm shift" that would transform the health care system into a model of "personal health and personal health care." Driven in part by advancing technology, Gingrich envisioned a system where the power in health care would indeed return significantly to the people.

That is a future that NCPA and the independent pharmacists of America will welcome — and do all it can to realize. Who better to provide individualized, cost-effective, professional care in the new millennium than independent pharmacists?

Critics have been writing about the demise of the independent for decades. Perhaps it's time for a new story line. There are another 100 years ahead for the independent — more strong and relevant to pharmacy and health care than ever before — and many more stories are yet to be written.

— Calvin J. Anthony, NCPA Executive Vice President

Highlights From The 100-Year History Of NARD/NCPA

NARD Meets Its Destiny in St. Louis –1898

Federal government implements a "stamp tax" on proprietary medications to help finance the Spanish-American War. Incensed pharmacists who would bear the tax burden seek to organize to oppose the tax.

Leonard Tillotson, Thomas Wooten, and other pharmacists call for organizational convention October 17 in St. Louis, Missouri.

On October 19, delegates from 21 states agree on common goals, adopt a constitution, elect officers, and write resolutions. The National Association of Retail Druggists is created.

The First Decade: 1899 – 1908

1898

Chicago pharmacist Thomas V. Wooten is named NARD's first Executive Secretary. Dues are 25 cents.

1901

"Organization Department" is created to develop membership through the use of field representatives.

A Tripartite Plan of retailers, wholesalers, and manufacturers — aimed at preventing price cutting at both the wholesale and retail levels — is reintroduced by NARD. Executive Committee Chairman Simon Jones augments the plan to include a "direct contract" with each party and a "serial numbering system" allowing products subject to price cutting to be tracked.

1902

Delegates approve a "Publicity Department." *N.A.R.D. Notes,* with Editor Charles M. Carr, makes its first appearance on October 18, 1902. Price is 50 cents (or included with membership). Wooten uses *N.A.R.D. Notes* to launch a major campaign against price cutters.

1903

Dr. Miles Medical Company of Elkhart, Indiana, agrees to the Tripartite Plan with its direct contract, serial numbering component. More than half of the wholesale houses sign agreements with Miles.

Dues increases to 50 cents, then $2.00.

NARD leads petition drive to reduce tax on alcohol, saving its members $1 to $2 million a year in excess revenue taxes as "licensed liquor dealers."

NARD opposes American pharmaceutical companies obtaining patents and trademarks on drugs manufactured in foreign countries when said formulas or chemicals were in the public domain in the U.S. NARD wants U.S. to join other countries that refuse to grant these patents.

NARD membership swells to 25,000 independents in its first five years.

NARD's work on behalf of West Coast pharmacists in the struggle to keep Owl Drug from price cutting brings national attention. President Theodore Roosevelt meets with NARD officials during the association's Washington, D.C. convention.

1904

NARD delegates vote unanimously to raise dues to $4.00.

The NARD Constitution is amended to give Executive Committee "full authority to act in the interim between annual meetings" — a reflection of the membership's confidence in the national leadership.

Secretary Wooten raises concerns about mail order drugs and physician dispensing.

St. Louis World's Fair organizers declare October 14, 1904 "Druggist Day."

1906

Food and Drugs Act is enacted by Congress.

"Earthquake Fund" set up by NARD to help earthquake victims in San Francisco. Special "California Relief Edition" of *N.A.R.D Notes* appeals for help.

Women's Organization of the National Association of Retail Druggists (WONARD) organizes to "unite more closely the families of the druggists." Founding President is Emma Gray Wallace.

1907

U.S. Court of Appeals in the Sixth Circuit rules that the direct contract plan violates the Sherman Antitrust Act.

First Pharmaceutical Exhibition at a NARD convention features 30 exhibiting drug manufacturers.

1908

Secretary Wooten and Chairman Simon Jones announce their retirements. Philadelphian Thomas Potts replaces Wooten as Executive Secretary.

N.A.R.D. Notes begins to accept advertising.

The Second Decade: 1909 – 1918

1910

NARD opposes pharmaceutical mail order industry, which aligns with agricultural groups to get favorable postal privileges through parcel post legislation.

With Tripartite Plan declared unconstitutional, pharmacists become interested in "cooperative buying" through local buying clubs, which NARD encourages.

A "Telephone Committee" is formed to help members understand the value of purchasing new "pay" telephones for their customers' use in their stores.

1911

Price protection is still an issue. A modified Miles-Boehm Plan based on a coupon system is proposed in Congress, but fails.

1913

NARD finds an ally in the price protection war in the new American Fair Trade League.

N.A.R.D. Notes changes its name to *The Journal of the N.A.R.D.*

1914

Journal Editor Charles Carr resigns and is replaced by Hugh Craig.

Harrison Narcotics Act is signed into law by President Woodrow Wilson, requiring pharmacists to keep detailed records on narcotics prescriptions.

1916

World War I causes disruptions of shipments of supplies and drugs to pharmacists and their customers.

1917

The U.S. is at war. Attempt to pass a Pharmaceutical Corps bill fails, but NARD earns for independents an "essential industries" qualification to ensure priority for receiving materials and finished products for the war's duration.

Executive Secretary Thomas Potts resigns and is replaced by Pennsylvanian Samuel Henry.

The Third Decade: 1919 – 1928

1919

With WWI's end, Executive Secretary Samuel Henry urges early discharge from military service for druggists. "Spanish Influenza" epidemic allows many to return home.

1920

On January 16, 1920, the sale of beverage alcohol is prohibited. National prohibition enforcement provisions are known as the Volstead Act. Community pharmacists become the gatekeepers of enforcement and are required to pay a special franchise tax for a liquor license.

So-called "talcum shops" emerge as retail competitors.

NARD successfully eliminates "war tax on medicinal products."

NARD is accepted for membership in the tenth U.S. Pharmacopeial Convention.

Volume discounts by manufacturers become a concern.

Chains and department stores with health products and sundries begin to grow.

1921

NARD's "Live and Let Live" slogan is amended to "Live and Help to Live" in recognition of the growing health enhancing role of the profession.

1922

Johnson & Johnson launches a national advertising campaign that supports retail pharmacists with a "Try the Drug Store First" slogan. The campaign becomes an annual promotion called "First Aid Week."

1923

Independents account for 50,000 of the nation's 52,000 drug stores.

The average independent pharmacy records $25,000 in annual sales.

1924

NARD launches another annual promotion called "Pharmacy Week" to enhance the public's perceptions of the professional side of retail pharmacy.

1925

NARD's President acknowledges and welcomes at the convention the increasing number of women pharmacists in the profession.

The Fourth Decade: 1929 – 1938

1929

The Great Depression begins to cause sales decreases that ultimately reach 25 percent annually in some drug stores. Chains are hit much harder than independents.

1930

At NARD's urging, Representative Kelly of Pennsylvania introduces a bill to allow manufacturers to set the retail price for their trademarked products before they leave the factory. Senator Capper of Kansas adds his support. Bill does not pass, but is a model for state legislation.

"Pine board store" emerges, in which a well-financed "silent partner" enters an economically depressed area, opens a pharmacy, uses "cheap labor," and buys in large volume. As these practices begin to affect big business, Congress becomes interested in stopping such "predatory price cutting."

California passes a "junior" Capper-Kelly Bill with hope that a similar victory for the nation is possible.

Secretary Wooten dies.

1931

Leonard Tillotson, the "Father of NARD," dies.

John Dargavel, a young activist in the Minneapolis Association of Retail Druggists, becomes President of NARD and seeks a more activist approach toward issues.

NARD takes on its first full-time legal counsel in Washington.

NARD targets "unfair trade practices."

1932

The Journal of the N.A.R.D. gets a "new look" and becomes a biweekly publication.

President Dargavel lambastes "secret allowances and rebates," calls on manufacturers to extend "equal privileges to all with special privileges to none."

1933

President Franklin D. Roosevelt signs the "Fair Trade Code" into law, which is a disappointment for NARD. However, it does for the first time prohibit "selling below the manufacturer's list price."

Roosevelt's New Deal overshadows hope for the Capper-Kelly Bill.

John Dargavel is elected NARD's fourth Executive Secretary, succeeding Samuel Henry. George Bender is named the new editor of the *Journal*.

1934

NARD sets theme of "35 in 34," targeting a goal of 35,000 members.

1935

American Retail Federation (ARF) tries to silence all efforts to standardize prices and labor codes. NARD calls ARF a monopoly and encourages a congressional investigation, spearheaded by Representative John Cochran of Missouri and then Representative Wright Patman of Texas. Hearings uncover a grocery chain that received over $8 million in secret rebates.

NARD President establishes an advisory board to his office, made up of the presidents from each state association, to lobby political leaders in various jurisdictions for specific legislation.

1936

NARD galvanizes the nation's independents to action on price discrimination. "Independents' Day" rally in Washington, D.C. attracts 1,700 from 36 states in support of the Robinson-Patman Anti-Discrimination bill. Senator Joseph Robinson of Arkansas joins NARD ally Wright Patman in sponsoring the bill. The Robinson-Patman Anti-Discrimination Act, signed on June 19, 1936, by President Roosevelt, requires a seller to extend to all customers the same price for the same kind and quantity of goods.

1937

Maryland Senator Joseph Tydings's National Fair Trade Enabling Bill incorporates key provisions favored by NARD. Arkansas Representative John Miller introduces a similar measure in the House. Initial reservations of President Roosevelt dissolve in the face of NARD lobbying and Rep. Patman intervention. Roosevelt signs the Tydings-Miller Fair Trade Law on August 17, 1937.

Business Week magazine extols NARD's formidable clout on Capitol Hill, labeling NARD "the most powerful trade association today."

1938

The Federal Food, Drug, and Cosmetic Act becomes law.

The Fifth Decade: 1939 – 1948

1939

The Journal is redesigned and enlarged — 40 pages to 100 pages. New departments debut featuring both the professional and merchandising aspects of store ownership.

NARD supports Rep. Patman's Federal Chain Store Tax.

Hospitals are receiving drugs and supplies for much less than retail.

1940

Efforts to repeal the Tydings-Miller law are underway.

Air conditioning and fluorescent lighting makes store design more appealing.

As World War II emerges, NARD, the Post Office, and other organizations participate in "Retailers for Defense" Week, September 15-20, 1940.

1940 (continued)

A Defense Savings Stamp is printed and sold to retail outlets. Stamps are then exchanged for Defense Savings Bonds. Pharmacists throughout the nation participate in the program.

1941

Executive Secretary Dargavel declares manufacturer-hospital deals on prices an "unholy alliance."

U.S. and Japanese relations deteriorate as World War II threatens to engulf the U.S.

Physician dispensing surfaces again as a growing concern.

1942

Executive Committee outlines four plans for cooperating with the National Defense Effort: calls on pharmacists to make their stores "civilian defense centers," forms committee to develop surveys and supply information to the Office of Price Administration for drug procurement and allocation, establishes a consumer information bureau on drugs and health supplies to inform consumers on price trends and market conditions affecting supplies, and extends annual First Aid Week to a full year program.

1943-46

No NARD conventions are held because of difficulties with travel, shortages of staff in pharmacies owing to the large number of pharmacists serving in the military. The *Journal* holds an "in print" convention during these years.

1947

Dargavel calls for a "grand strategy" in the war to preserve independent business.

1948

Dargavel assails "capitalistic collectivism" as forces of monopoly and corporatization threaten small business.

NARD celebrates its 50th anniversary with a large turnout at the New York City convention.

The Sixth Decade: 1949 – 1958

1949

President Truman announces his "Fair Deal" legislative package, including a national public health program. NARD opposes "socialized medicine."

Supermarkets begin to expand into pharmacy. Drug stores begin to lose health and other products to other outlets.

Dargavel denounces manufacturer discounts. He says that "the issue of discounts must be pushed to a satisfactory conclusion before it is too late to overcome the downswing of business."

NARD focuses on the need to educate the public about the problems facing community pharmacists. "One of the dangerous situations we face is the ignorance of the public relative to the necessity of business," says Dargavel. The leadership is concerned that if consumers don't understand these principles, they could be easily influenced to support legislation that would open the doors to cut-throat competition.

1950

NARD learns that a Senate bill will be introduced in the new Congress that will undermine the Robinson-Patman Act. Dargavel urges the nation's independent pharmacists to send "an avalanche of letters to President Truman." It works. President Truman tells reporters he was deluged with "piles of telegrams and letters" urging him to veto the measure. He vetoes the bill, and Rep. Wright Patman calls it "one of the greatest victories of NARD."

1951

The U.S. Supreme Court rules a section of the National Fair Trade Law (Tydings-Miller Act) unconstitutional. This is a blow to NARD and other small business allies. The unconstitutional section prohibits "willingly and knowingly advertising, offering for sale or selling any commodity at less than the price stipulated in any contract entered into pursuant to the provision of Section I of this act, whether the person so advertising, offering for sale or selling is or is not a party to such contract, is unfair competition and is actionable at the suit of any person damaged thereby."

Dargavel announces to convention attendees that "too many druggists still depend on others to fight for the things that involve the welfare of every independent drug store and the profession of pharmacy in general." He announces that the NARD leadership has a new bill that will be introduced in the next session of Congress to restore fair trade protections.

NARD Executive Committee members are accused of being "pinks" because of strong support for North Carolina Representative Carl Durham's and Minnesota Senator Hubert Humphrey's bill that would legalize refills except for restricted drugs, allow orally authorized (telephoned) prescriptions, establish a uniform legend, and require manufacturers to affix that legend to all controlled medicines. Many other pharmaceutical organizations oppose the bill.

Durham-Humphrey Amendments are signed into law October 26, 1951 — a big victory for NARD.

1952

Connecticut Representative John McGuire, at NARD's behest, introduces and ultimately gains passage of the McGuire Act. The law restores some of the fair trade protections lost with the repeal of the Tydings-Miller Act.

John A. Dargavel Memorial Foundation (now NCPA Foundation) is founded to support loans to pharmacy students.

NARD's leadership recommends creating a specialty department for the "baby boom."

1953

"The traditional position of pharmacy is in jeopardy," says NARD, as a result of physician dispensing, chain stores, and undercutting on price maintenance.

NARD implements a national public relations campaign, including an ad in the *Saturday Evening Post*. "There is no more essential merchant in your town than your modern independent pharmacist," says the ad.

The U.S. Supreme Court rejects a challenge to the McGuire Act by a huge supermarket chain, preserving the act's fair trade provisions. NARD is elated.

1955

Media reports begin to target pharmacists for "overpriced prescriptions."

The American Medical Association (AMA) supports physician ownership of pharmacies.

1956

Dargavel tells NARD convention "the independent druggist and small retailers in general will have to live with the changes that come with the postwar revolution in distribution."

U.S. Supreme Court decision facilitates some price discounting, undermining fair trade.

1958

John Dargavel celebrates his twenty-fifth year as NARD Executive Secretary. He tells the '58 convention, "I am confident that NARD will continue to march with progress and that it will grow in influence to be even more significant to the independent retail pharmacist than it is today. Of that I am certain."

The Seventh Decade: 1959 – 1968

1959

The American Association of Retired Persons begins to develop a mail order pharmacy program.

Hospitals begin opening their own pharmacies for outpatient care.

Labor unions begin contracting with specific pharmacies (usually a chain) for pharmacy needs.

Phil Jehle, chief counsel to the Senate Small Business Committee, is hired as NARD's Washington Representative.

Arkansas Representative Oren Harris introduces a new fair trade bill. It faces huge opposition and is ultimately tabled.

1960

Tennessee Senator Estes Kefauver announces an investigation into "the high costs of drugs." Although mostly aimed at manufacturers, the negative publicity spills over into the retail setting.

The Harris bill is reintroduced and again fails. Dargavel blames independents for providing only "meager support for the bill."

1961

The Federal Trade Commission files suit against 37 pharmaceutical manufacturers — requiring them to make their pricing policies available. Most respond that they have a "uniform, single-price system," but the fine print reveals the existence of discounting to select customers.

New fair trade legislation, the Fair Competitive Practices Bill, is introduced into both houses of Congress. The bill fails.

John Dargavel dies of a heart attack upon his return from the October 1961 NARD Convention. He is 67 and has served for 28 years as NARD's Executive Secretary. Tributes to Dargavel pour in to NARD from Congress and throughout the United States.

Former Executive Committee Chairman Willard Simmons of Texarkana, Texas is named Executive Secretary.

1962

Association steps up efforts to collaborate with AMA, but the talks break down over physician dispensing.

The Veterans Administration announces plans to discontinue its Hometown Pharmacy Program in spite of huge opposition from NARD and congressional ally Wright Patman.

Model state law on physician dispensing is developed.

1963

NARD develops a model state law on physician ownership of pharmacies. Executive Secretary Simmons announces plans to reach out to "women in pharmacy."

1965

Vice President Hubert Humphrey, a pharmacist, speaks at the NARD Convention.

President Johnson's "Great Society" Medicaid/Medicare initiatives become law. Medicare presents opportunities in the home health care and nuring home arenas, but fails to include prescription drugs as a mandatory benefit. The states are given considerable control over Medicaid outpatient drug benefits.

1967

NARD launches a national public relations campaign emphasizing community pharmacists' contribution to public health. The campaign includes the film, "Bartlett and Son," and a drug education program in the Chicago public school system.

The Eighth Decade: 1969 – 1978

1969

Medicaid accounts for about 15 percent of the average independent pharmacy's business.

NARD holds its first Legislative Conference in Washington, D.C. Senator Phil Hart of Michigan, the lead-off speaker, targets physician dispensing.

NARD expands its drug abuse education program nationally and is recognized for its efforts by the Nixon administration.

NARD Executive Committee Chairman Avellone calls third-party payment "the number one concern of pharmacy today." The association urges support for "usual and customary" reimbursement.

1970

NARD and the National Association of Chain Drug Stores (NACDS) develop a standard drug claim form to use in third-party payments.

NARD opposes efforts to abolish "anti-substitution" laws.

1971

Prescription drug sales reach a then historic high of 46.6 percent of sales. Net profits sink to a new low of 3.6 percent.

1973

All issues take a back seat to the overwhelming changes created by Medicare/Medicaid.

NARD seeks to have legislation introduced to allow pharmacists to supply medicine to patients at home under Medicare.

Efforts continue, without success, to gain passage of legislation that would enable retail pharmacists to meet with third-party administrators and negotiate the terms under which pharmacists would be paid for their services.

NARD celebrates its "Diamond Jubilee Anniversary" in Portland, Oregon. Vice President Gerald Ford, in the wake of Vice President Spiro Agnew's resignation, is the keynote speaker.

The Office of Veterans Affairs' new mail order pharmacy program prompts concerns.

U.S. Supreme Court upholds a North Dakota law requiring a pharmacist to own the pharmacy in order for it to be licensed.

1974

NARD forms the National Association of Pharmacists Political Action Committee (NAPPAC), the first PAC in pharmacy.

NARD-supported "Ask Your Pharmacist" labeling on over-the-counter medicines is derailed by the AMA. The physician-only reference is retained on the label.

NARD President Shinnick deplores growing price discrimination. "We ask no special favors, no special discounts for ourselves, just an opportunity to buy on equal terms and equal prices."

1976

A proposal to change the name of the organization to the National Association of Independent Pharmacists is offered, then tabled.

Maximum Allowable Cost (MAC) pricing goes into effect for Medicaid.

Willard Simmons resigns as Executive Secretary after 16 years of service. NARD Associate General Counsel William E. Woods, a pharmacist and lawyer from Texas, is named to replace him. In a by-laws change, the title is changed to Executive Vice President.

The Executive Committee votes to move the headquarters office from Chicago to Washington, D.C.

NARD creates the Health Supports and Appliances Program to certify pharmacist specializing in these areas — a forerunner to the pharmacist care certification movement.

1978

NARD is one of the founding members of the Joint Commission of Pharmacy Practitioners (JCPP), a group created to provide a forum for all of pharmacy's national organizations to discuss issues of common concern.

NARD's headquarters staff in Washington is expanded dramatically from five to thirty, and the budget exceeds $2 million for the first time.

The Ninth Decade: 1979 – 1988

1979

NARD expands its committee system to gain more member involvement in association affairs.

NARD introduces its "Ask Your Family Pharmacist" service mark to distinguish the professional services of independent pharmacies from the rest of the retail pharmacy marketplace.

1980

NARD begins regular meetings with state pharmacy associations at the convention.

"Pharmacy Alert" system is established — a "telephone tree" of pharmacy leaders and practitioners across the country who call their elected officials on specific legislative issues at NARD's urging.

Royal Drug Co. Inc. vs Group Life and Health Insurance Co. is a key lawsuit filed by a group of pharmacists in which they charge that a "fixed fee contract" only adds to the insurance company's profits. The insurance company claimed exemption from antitrust laws in establishing the contracts. In a 5-4 decision, the U.S. Supreme Court upholds the pharmacists' position. NARD is a "friend of the court" in the lawsuit.

NARD fights a proposed "patient package insert" mandate by the Food and Drug Administration (FDA).

NARD begins a monthly continuing education program in the *NARD Journal*.

NARD assists in getting the Omnibus Small Business Act passed by Congress. The law establishes a federal loan guarantee to employees who bought businesses from retiring owners when the owners financed the sale.

NARD supports congressional legislation to exempt pharmacist from the antitrust laws when negotiating collectively with insurers on third-party programs.

1981

Former U.S. Senate aide and Justice Department official John Rector joins NARD as General Counsel.

1982

NARD builds and moves into offices in Alexandria, Virginia, a suburb of Washington, D.C.

NARD creates the first Department of Home Health Care Pharmacy Services in a national pharmacy organization.

1983

NARD launches its own voluntary Patient Information Leaflets (PILs) as an alternative to the FDA's ill-fated mandatory proposal.

NARD-generated citizen petitions call upon the FDA to establish a pharmacist legend category for drugs newly switched from prescription to OTC status. This category, says NARD, would ensure safe and proper use of these drugs by consumers. The campaign receives widespread publicity.

NARD holds its first annual Home Health Care Conference.

1984

The "Pharmacy Crime Bill" (Pharmacist Protection Act) passes Congress, making the robbery or burglary of a pharmacy a federal crime. This is a major victory for NARD. It had been a top NARD priority since the early 1970s.

NARD launches the Legislative Defense Fund to build a war chest for legislative action.

NARD formally adopts the Doctor of Pharmacy (P.D.) designation for all practicing pharmacists.

1985

NARD Executive Committee Chairman Charles West of Little Rock, Arkansas, replaces William E. Woods as NARD's Executive Vice President.

NARD coins the term Pharmacy Services Administrative Organization (PSAO), to describe new state and local entities emerging to contract with employees for third-party contracts.

NARD holds a PSAO meeting in Chicago to analyze the antitrust concerns associated with the PSAO movement.

NARD's West spearheads opposition to a federal Health Care Financing Adminstration initiative to undermine Average Wholesale Price (AWP) reimbursement in the Medicaid program. NARD argues that the proposed reimbursement change would confiscate the "earned discounts" pharmacists receive for prudent business practices. The "earned discounts" effort succeeds in preserving millions of dollars for participating pharmacies in the Medicaid program.

West delivers "We'll All Be Winners" speech at the Pharmaceutical Manufacturers Association Annual Meeting — urging manufacturers to abandon discriminatory pricing voluntarily.

1986

NARD forms a Department of State Relations to coordinate relationships and common legislative goals with state associations.

NARD's Student Chapter Program is launched, reaching 38 student chapters at pharmacy schools by 1998.

Independent Pharmacy Matching Service is created to match buyers and sellers of independent pharmacies.

NARD hosts its First Annual PSAO Conference in Kansas City, Missouri.

1987

Representative Ron Wyden of Oregon introduces legislation to limit physician dispensing for profit. NARD works closely with Wyden on the bill and launches a two-year public relations campaign against the practice. The bill ultimately founders, but the growth of physician dispensing is effectively stopped — a huge NARD victory.

NARD introduces a spring mid-year educational meeting called Rx Expo. It incorporates the specialty programming of the previous Home Health Care Conference, plus many more market niches.

NARD changes its name from the National Association of Retail Druggists to NARD.

1988

The Prescription Drug Marketing Act passes the Congress, culminating a two-year legislative effort by NARD to expose abuses of the Nonprofit Institutes Act that fuel drug diversion. NARD points to discriminatory pricing as the root cause.

The Medicare Catastrophic Coverage Act is passed, extending outpatient coverage to seniors for the first time. NARD lobbies for and gets Average Wholesale Price reimbursement, plus a $4.50 dispensing fee indexed to the Consumer Price Index.

Pharmacists voted the nation's most trusted profession in the Gallup Poll for the first time — beginning a decade-long run at the top.

RxNet is launched to help local and state PSAOs compete for regional and national third-party contracts for pharmacy services.

The Centennial Decade: 1989-1998

1989

NARD focuses on the rising costs of prescription drugs. Executive Vice President West and key NARD staff testify before Arkansas Senator David Pryor's Senate Special Committee on Aging on the discriminatory pricing practices of drug manufacturers.

NARD launches the Management Institute. One of the Institute's first projects is to develop a "cost-to-dispense analysis" as a basic formula for pharmacists to use in pricing prescriptions and evaluating third-party contracts.

The Medicare Catastrophic Coverage Act is repealed by Congress after a backlash from seniors over the financing of the new coverage.

1990

NARD announces a consumer "freedom of choice" campaign to preserve the rights of patients to patronize the pharmacy of their choice. NARD compiles the NARD Consumer Freedom of Choice Legislation Manual and a model bill, which are distributed to every state association. Six new state laws are passed in the first year.

Senator Pryor introduces "best price" legislation to require drug manufacturers to offer their best prices to the Medicaid drug program. This landmark legislation, passed in October 1990, attacked discriminatory pricing at its core. Declared West, "This represents a giant step in the association's efforts to eliminate discriminatory pricing in the pharmaceutical marketplace." Senator Pryor's Medicaid law also includes a first-time-ever moratorium for four years on pharmacists' reimbursements cuts in the Medicaid program.

1991

NARD launched its Mail Order Dishonor Roll in the *NARD Journal*, highlighting companies that consign their patients to "substandard, unregulated pharmacy practice through mail order.

NARD launches the National Home Infusion Association to help independents capitalize on this growing market niche.

The NARD Diabetes Care Club (now the Diabetes Care Center Certification Program) is launched.

1992

As planks in the Democratic and Republican platforms for the presidential race, NARD urges that any health care reform program must include an outpatient prescription drug program, protect consumer freedom of choice, address discriminatory pricing, and pay pharmacists for their services.

The Family Pharmacist: Your Best Benefit education campaign is launched. It targets consumers and corporate benefit managers who are determining the kinds of pharmacy services their employees will receive.

NARD meets with top officials of the newly elected Clinton administration to present "A Pro Competitive Agenda for the Pharmaceutical Marketplace," outlining NARD's position for health care reform.

1993

NARD joins with NACDS to form the Community Retail Pharmacy Health Care Reform Coalition, which provides most of the pharmacy information being assembled by President Clinton's health care reform task force. NARD and the coalition work full time on health care reform. Almost every issue the association has dealt with since West's tenure began is addressed in the first draft of the bill. West and key staffers are invited to the White House to review the first draft.

Independent pharmacist Dwayne Goode successfully sues Wal-Mart for predatory pricing practices.

Merck & Company and the nation's largest mail order pharmacy, Medco Containment Services, announce plans to merge. NARD blasts the merger as an "unholy alliance" and objects to the Federal Trade Commission about the anticompetitive nature of the merger.

President Clinton's health care reform bill is introduced in Congress and includes virtually all of NARD's priorities, including providing community pharmacies equal access to drug manufacturers' prices. It marks the first time an American president has endorsed the elimination of discriminatory pricing.

Pharmacists in 15 states file class-action lawsuits against several drug manufacturers and wholesalers, charging price discrimination and price-fixing violations of the Sherman Act.

1994

The administration's health reform bill fails after multimillion-dollar lobbying efforts by drug manufacturers and the health insurance industry.

1995

NARD forms the National Institute for Pharmacist Care Outcomes. NIPCO begins certifying community pharmacists across the nation in disease state management, including diabetes, cardiovascular care, respiratory care, osteoporosis, pharmacist care skills, and immunizations.

NARD creates the Pharmacist Care Claim Form (PCCF) to help pharmacists document and bill for pharmacist care services.

NARD drafts a "model bill" prohibiting discriminatory pricing, and the bill is introduced in 30 state legislatures.

NARD implements an immense consumer public relations campaign, "High Noon for Your Local Pharmacy," a national day of protest. The campaign culminates on Sept. 20 with rallies across the nation, including one in Times Square.

Charles West announces his plans to retire in 1996. Former NARD Executive Committee Chairman and President Calvin Anthony of Stillwater, Oklahoma, is named his successor.

1996

Under heavy pressure from NARD, the FTC announces its intention to investigate the pricing policies of the nation's drug manufacturers.

Thirteen pharmaceutical manufacturers offer a $600 million settlement in the landmark discriminatory pricing class-action lawsuit brought by pharmacist groups. After a major letter writing campaign from independents opposing the settlement because it fails to provide injunctive relief that give pharmacists equal access to prices. Presiding Judge Charles Kocoras rejects the offer. He says, "the record was replete with instances of collusive behavior."

Later in the year, eleven manufacturers offer a $350 million settlement that does give independent pharmacists "equal access to discounts." It is a historic victory and vindication of NARD's decades-long battle against price discrimination.

Calvin Anthony assumes role as NARD Executive Vice President.

NARD House of Delegates votes to change the association's name to the National Community Pharmacists Association (NCPA).

1997

NCPA launches its website — www.ncpanet.org.

NCPA launches NPTV, a satellite television network broadcasting 12 hours daily in pharmacies across the country.

NCPA launches Valu-Switch, an electronic claims service to reduce transmission costs to independents.

NCPA forms the Task Force on Third-Party Contract Negotiation. The group is charged with finding a legal way to allow independent pharmacists to collectively negotiate professional services in third-party contracts.

NCPA is a key player in preserving the pharmacist's traditional right to compound medicines in legislation reforming the Food and Drug Administration.

NCPA works with Representative Nita Lowey of New York to build support for her Prescription Drug Benefit Equity Act, which would establish a level playing field for neighborhood pharmacy and mail order in third-party contracts.

Congress enacts legislation supported by NCPA to compensate pharmacists for providing diabetes education and consultation to Medicare beneficiaries.

Anthony underscores the association's commitment to carry community pharmacy into the new millennium by "getting pharmacists paid" for not only dispensing products, but also for providing vital pharmacist care services. These services are "the best bargain in health care," declares Anthony.

1998

Sparked by a Mississippi Medicaid initiative that will pay pharmacists for disease management services, NCPA forms a coalition with the National Association of Chain Drug Stores and the National Association of Boards of Pharmacy to create a national model and process for credentialing pharmacists in disease state management. The model is based on the Pharmacist Care Model developed by NCPA's NIPCO. The three groups announce the creation of a National Institute for Standards in Pharmacist Credentialing.

In part as a result of the ongoing work of NCPA's Third-Party Task Force, congressional legislation is introduced to allow pharmacy to collectively negotiate third-party contracts. The American Medical Association joins with NCPA in endorsing the bill.

NIPCO becomes a leader in the pharmacist care movement. In three years, more than 7,000 pharmacists complete NIPCO-accredited disease management programs.

The 1998 *NCPA-Searle Digest* records still narrow 3.1 percent net profits, but record average sales per pharmacy of $1.65 million — a healthy 14.3 percent increase over the following year.

Past Presidents Of NARD/NCPA

TERM	PRESIDENT	FROM	WHERE ELECTED
1898-99	Henry Hynson	Baltimore, MD	St. Louis, MO
1899-00	Simon Jones	Louisville, KY	Cincinnati, OH
1900-01	William Anderson	Brooklyn, NY	Detroit, MI
1901-02	James Seeley	Detroit, MI	Buffalo, NY
1903-04	B.E. Pritchard	Pittsburgh, PA	Washington, DC
1904-05	Thomas Voegeli	Minneapolis, MN	St. Louis, MO
1905-06	M.T. Breslin	New Orleans, LA	Boston, MA
1906-07	Charles Mann	Detroit, MI	Atlanta, GA
1907-08	Thomas Potts	Philadelphia, PA	Chicago, IL
1908-09	William Elkin Jr.	Atlanta, GA	Atlantic City, NJ
1909-10	Charles Huhn	Minneapolis, MN	Louisville, KY
1910-11	H.B. Guilford	Rochester, NY	Pittsburgh, PA
1911-12	H.C. Shuptrine	Savannah, GA	Niagara Falls, NY
1912-13	Henry Merritt	Plains, PA	Milwaukee, WI
1913-14	James Finneran	Boston, MA	Cincinnati, OH
1914-15	Samuel Henry	Philadelphia, PA	Philadelphia, PA
1915-16	M.A. Stout	Bluffton, IN	Minneapolis, MN
1916-17	Robert Frick	Louisville, KY	Indianapolis, IN
1917-18	Walter Cousins	Dallas, TX	Cleveland, OH
1918-19	Charles Harding	Cincinnati, OH	New Orleans, LA
1919-20	Theodore Hagenow	St. Louis, MO	Rochester, NY
1920-21	J.J. Possehl	Milwaukee, WI	St. Louis, MO
1921-22	Ambrose Hunsberger	Philadelphia, PA	Denver, CO
1922-23	Curtis Gladding	Hartford, CT	Detroit, MI
1923-24	J.H. Webster	Detroit, Mi	Boston, MA
1924-25	F.R. Peterson	Portland, OR	Washington, DC
1925-26	Frank Stone	Washington, DC	Memphis, TN
1926-27	Samuel Davis	Nashville, TN	Philadelphia, PA
1927-28	William Oren	Indianapolis, IN	Kansas City, MO
1928-29	Denny Brann	Des Moines, IA	San Francisco, CA
1929-30	Thomas Roach	Oklahoma City, OK	Minneapolis, MN
1930-31	J.H. Riemenschneider	Chicago, IL	Atlantic City, NJ
1931-32	John Dargavel	Minneapolis, MN	Detroit, MI
1932-33	John Goode	Asheville, NC	Boston, MA
1933-34	Monte Powell	Denver, CO	Chicago, IL
1934-35	Harvey Henry	Los Angeles, CA	New Orleans, LA
1935-36	Charles Ehlers	Cincinnati, OH	Cincinnati, OH
1936-37	George Secord	Chicago, IL	Pittsburgh, PA
1937-38	Thomas Smith	Wilmington, DE	St. Louis, MO
1938-39	John Witty	Portland, OR	Chicago, IL
1939-40	Albert Fritz	Indianapolis, IN	St. Paul, MN
1940-41	Samuel Watkins	Dora, AL	New York, NY

Year	Name	City	Convention
1941-42	Hugh Beirne	New Haven, CT	Cleveland, OH
1942-47	J. Otto Kohl	Cincinnati, OH	Chicago, IL
1947-48	John Tripeny	Casper, WY	Chicago, IL
1948-49	Edgar Bellis	New York, NY	Atlantic City, NJ
1949-50	Frank Moudry	St. Paul, MN	New York, NY
1950-51	Charles Gilson	Centredale, RI	Long Beach, CA
1951-52	Elbert Gibbs	Birmingham, AL	Minneapolis, MN
1952-53	A.C. Mayerson	Chicago, IL	St. Louis, MO
1953-54	M.V. Hardesty	Louisville, KY	Chicago, IL
1954-55	G.M. Eisele	Hot Springs, AR	Houston, TX
1955-56	John McKeighan	Flint, MI	Atlantic City, NJ
1956-57	Charles Seward	Pasadena, CA	Cincinnati, OH
1957-58	H.E. Henderson	Seattle, WA	Minneapolis, MN
1958-59	Angus Taylor	Minneapolis, MN	Philadelphia, PA
1959-60	Ralph Rooke	Richmond, VA	St. Louis, MO
1960-61	Tom Sharp	Nashville, TN	Denver, CO
1961-62	Bert Corgan	Denver, CO	Miami Beach, FL
1962-63	Frank Lobraico	Indianapolis, IN	New York, NY
1963-64	T. Donald Perkins	San Diego, CA	Chicago, IL
1964-65	Leonard Dueker	St. Louis, MO	San Francisco, CA
1965-66	J.C. Cobb	Tishomingo, OK	Washington, DC
1966-67	Charles Dunnington	Brockton, MS	St. Louis, MO
1967-68	George Wilharm	Minneapolis, MN	Houston, TX
1968-69	Michael Perhach	Binghamton, NY	Boston, MA
1969-70	Chris Haleston	Portland, OR	Las Vegas, NV
1970-71	Nick Avellone	Bay Village, OH	Atlantic City, NJ
1971-72	E. Crawford Meyer	Louisville, KY	New Orleans, LA
1972-73	George Benson	Seattle, WA	Chicago, IL
1973-74	Harold Shinnick	Chicago, IL	Portland, OR
1974-75	E. Boyd Garrett	Nashville, TN	Las Vegas, NV
1975-76	William Wickwire	Los Altos, CA	Miami Beach, FL
1976-77	Salvatore D'Angelo	New Orleans, LA	San Francisco, CA
1977-78	Sam McConnell Jr.	Scottsdale, AZ	Washington, DC
1978-79	Kenneth Mehrle	Cape Girardeau, MO	New Orleans, LA
1979-80	Paul Dumouchel	Waltham, MA	Las Vegas, NV
1980-81	Jesse Pike Sr.	Concord, NC	Atlanta, GA
1981-82	Neil Pruitt	Toccoa, GA	San Antonio, TX
1982-83	John Johnson	Bellevue, NE	Boston, MA
1983-84	James Vincent	Yuma, CO	Las Vegas, NV
1984-85	John White	Tallahassee, FL	Miami Beach, FL
1985-86	H. Joseph Schutte	Louisville, KY	New York, NY
1986-87	Lonnie Hollingsworth	Lubbock, TX	Louisville, KY
1987-88	Darwyn Williams	Webster City, IA	Las Vegas, NV
1988-89	Donald Arthur	Tonawanda, NY	Atlanta, GA
1989-90	Joseph Mosso	Latrobe, PA	San Antonio, TX
1990-91	William Katz	Newington, CT	Nashville, TN
1991-92	William Scharringhausen	Park Ridge, IL	Baltimore, MD
1992-93	Donald Moore	Kokomo, IN	Seattle, WA
1993-94	Calvin Anthony	Stillwater, OK	Indianapolis, IN
1994-95	Gene Graves	Little Rock, AR	Boston, MA
1995-96	Louis Mitchell	Swedesboro, NJ	Las Vegas, NV
1996-97	Dennis Ludwig	Boulder, CO	New Orleans, LA
1997-98	Kenneth Epley	Salem, OR	Denver, CO